for

Jenai, Xóchitl, Dagda, and Creo

Disclaimer

Practicing the poses depicted in this book may be harmful and hazardous to your health. If you choose to practice any of the poses in this book, you do so at your own risk. These instructions are not intended to take the place of personal instruction by a trained yoga teacher in a classroom or private session. Prior to practicing yoga, it is paramount that you consult with a qualified professional regarding any health issues, injuries, or physical limitations.

If you choose to practice hatha yoga, the guidance and support of a skilled teacher is essential. Additionally, not all exercise or physical practices are suitable for everyone. Consult your doctor before you practice yoga.

To reduce the risk of injury, never force or strain while practicing yoga. If you feel pain, stop and seek medical attention immediately.

The creators, producers, and performers of the *Yoga Resource Practice Manual* cannot guarantee that this product is suitable and safe for everyone. If you choose to practice yoga, you do so solely at your own risk.

Any liability, loss, or damage in connection with the use of the *Yoga Resource Practice Manual*, including, but not limited to, any liability, loss, or damage arising from the performance of the exercises demonstrated or described here, or any advice or information contained within this product, is expressly disclaimed.

• • •

Credits

Pose photographs feature Darren Rhodes
Written instructions by Darren Rhodes
Photography & design by MiLo (Michael Longstaff)
Editing by Ellen Huang and Gretel Hakanson
Published by Yo Productions/Tirtha Studios, LLC

www.shopatyo.com

table of contents

photo indexes   3

pose page number below each photo

practice instructions   35

360 poses arranged alphabetically by Sanskrit name

A-Z index   451

arranged alphabetically by Sanskrit name

introduction

If I am any kind of yogi, I am a hatha yogi. The reason I meditate, practice *pranayama*, study scripture, chant the "Hanuman Chalisa" daily, and found my teacher Lee Lozowick is because of hatha yoga. Even if I could no longer practice (which was the case from June 2009 to June 2010), I would continue to study and teach hatha yoga. My commitment to hatha yoga, for better or for worse, is lifelong.

My mom and dad were my first yoga teachers. They did not give me formal instruction, but rather led by example. I noticed without noticing that my mom practiced hatha yoga daily throughout my entire childhood. I observed my dad reading scripture, meditating, and devoting himself to what is called *The Work* in the Gurdjieff tradition.

When I graduated from Sarah Lawrence College, I sought out and studied with many master hatha yoga teachers from a variety of traditions. I studied with some of these teachers briefly and others for years. The style of hatha yoga I now teach is called *yogahour*, which is a synthesis of what I have learned from the teachers and traditions that have influenced me. Yogahour breaks down alignment instructions into three categories: shape, safety, and refinement, which is the same format used in this eBook. Yogahour is a flow-style practice, which means teachers must get students into and out of each pose safely and succinctly. To accomplish this, the teacher must teach only the essential shape, safety, and refinement instructions for each pose, which is exactly what I aim to offer in this eBook.

The 400 photos in the *Yoga Resource* library were originally taken in 2005 by Milo (Michael Longstaff). The purpose of these photos was to create a poster divided into three syllabi: *basics*, *expanding*, and *radical expansion*, which were the names of the YogaOasis (yo) studios classes (the Tucson, Arizona-based yoga studios I have directed since 1998). We wanted to give students a visual reference of the syllabi of poses from which these classes would draw from. As the project got underway, we realized this poster would be a useful resource for more than just yo students. We therefore turned the poster project into a product called *From Tadasana to Savasana*. Since that first photo-shoot back in 2005, Milo and I have continued to refine and replace many, if not most, of the original photographs. For example, we replaced seventy photos for this project.

I was raised in a spiritually-oriented community whose aim, as my granddad put it, was to "discover and develop one's unique talents for the sake of others." This book is my attempt at that: I hope it informs and inspires your practice; please practice.

– Darren Rhodes

foreword

Where does the body end and the mind begin? Where does the mind end and the spirit begin? They cannot be divided as they are interrelated and are but different aspects of the same all pervading divine consciousness.

– B. K. S. Iyengar

The literal translation of the Sanskrit word *hatha,* as in hatha yoga, is "to force or to strike." Hatha yoga, then, is the yoga that utilizes a force of effort to strike at the habitual patterns of thought and energetic constrictions interfering with the direct knowledge of who we most truly are. Practicing hatha yoga requires tremendous willpower, determination, and resolve because of its difficult postures, breathing techniques, mudras, and kriyas.

In the preface to this book, Darren Rhodes, my friend, calls himself a hatha yogi. I cannot disagree with him: The clear, concise instructions accompanying the over 400 beautiful and inspiring photos in this book demonstrate his mastery of the art of asana. And yet, much in the way that modern hatha yoga master B. K. S. Iyengar asks us to consider where the body ends and where the mind and spirit begin, I must ask where the yoga of posture ends and the yoga of devotion begins?

The way I see it, Darren Rhodes is first and foremost a bhakti yogi. Known as the yoga of devotion, bhakti yoga reminds us that any action can be performed as a prayer, an offering or a ritual of sacred remembrance. What you hold in your hands is not simply a compilation of pictures and alignment protocols but the outcome of a lifetime of study, practice, and personal devotion to an art using the body to fashion form, to express beauty, and to cultivate awareness while fostering virtues such as acceptance, commitment, honesty, and integrity. How could anyone achieve such symmetry in form, such beauty in expression, such depth of understanding without devotion? How could anyone write such detailed descriptions and helpful instructions for others without the desire to make an offering? Only a bhakti yogi would pour his personal time and resources into a project with such excellence, finesse, and artistry. Yes, Darren Rhodes is a bhakti yogi, and this book constitutes a devotional offering that will benefit generations of yoga practitioners to come.

I met Darren Rhodes in 2001 and have had the good fortune to enjoy an ever-deepening friendship and teaching partnership with him. We also share the same spiritual teacher, Lee Lozowick. As his friend and sister in sadhana, I have personally witnessed the fire of devotion living behind the asanas depicted in the pages of this book.

In 2003, Darren told me he wanted to be able to do all of the postures in B. K. S Iyengar's book, *Light on Yoga*. This goal fueled Darren's efforts for many years and created an enduring relationship with the book, *Light on Yoga*, by B. K. S Iyengar. The impressive syllabus poster, *From Tadasana to Savasana*, and the self-published book, *Yoga Resource*, grew from Darren's accomplishments. This ambitious goal also brought injury, doubt, and personal clarity to Darren, and became a rite-of-passage and trial-by-fire through which he became much more than a limber, capable asana practitioner: He developed and evolved into a man of impressive character, great conviction, and unshakable courage.

When Darren asked me to write the foreword for his book, I leapt at the opportunity to contribute to what I believe is an invaluable resource for practitioners at every level of proficiency. Both beginners and advanced practitioners can use this book because yoga only asks us to meet ourselves where we are and to honestly work from that point while never failing to reward our sincere efforts.

Where does your body end and your mind and spirit begin? Where will your practice of asana end and the practice of your devotion begin? Use this book as a guide for your practice. Find out.

– Christina Sell

Founder and Director, The San Marcos School of Yoga & Live the Light of Yoga Programs; Author, *Yoga From the Inside Out: Making Peace with Your Body Through Yoga* and *My Body is a Temple: Yoga as a Path to Wholeness*

key anatomical terms

front view · back view · side view

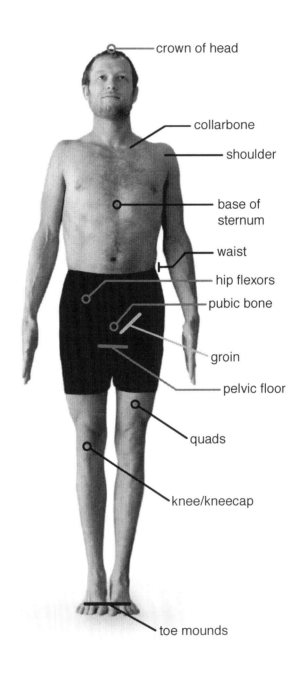

crown of head

collarbone

shoulder

base of
sternum

waist

hip flexors

pubic bone

groin

pelvic floor

quads

knee/kneecap

toe mounds

key anatomical terms

front view · **back view** · side view

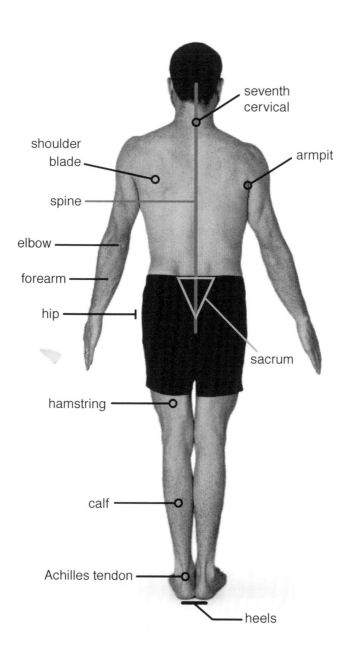

seventh
cervical

shoulder
blade

armpit

spine

elbow

forearm

hip

sacrum

hamstring

calf

Achilles tendon

heels

key anatomical terms

front view • back view • **side view**

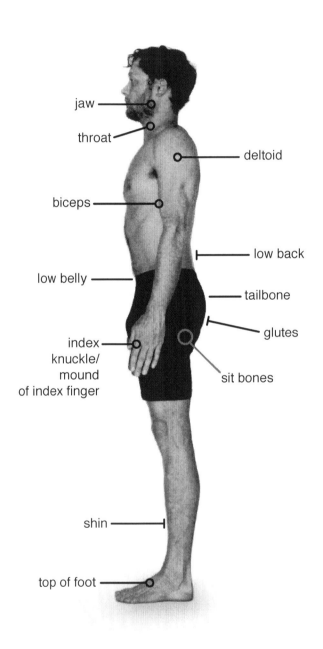

jaw

throat

deltoid

biceps

low back

low belly

tailbone

glutes

index
knuckle/
mound
of index finger

sit bones

shin

top of foot

how to use the Yoga Resource Practice Manual

The *Yoga Resource Practice Manual* features detailed practice instructions for 360 yoga poses. It is intended to serve as a comprehensive guide for yoga practitioners of all levels.

Poses are arranged alphabetically by sanskrit name and feature practice instructions in three sections: **shape** guides students on entering and exiting the basic form of each pose, the **safety** section lists key actions focused on helping students optimize the benefits of practice (including alternatives or modifications as needed for varying ability or special conditions), and the **refinement** section offers additional insights including advanced variations, philosophy, and/or inspirational stories.

Some poses feature additional photographs illustrating variations or modifications of the main pose.

how to locate a pose

you know what it looks like

Use the 10 visual indexes *(beginning on pg. 3)*
Peruse the visual indexes to locate a pose. Use the page number listed under the photograph to locate the instructions for that pose within the book. Variation photos will also appear in the photo indexes.

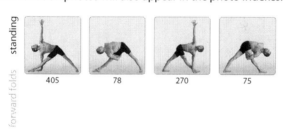

you know the name of the pose

Use the A-Z index *(beginning on pg. 451)*
All poses are listed in the A-Z index section alphabetically by Sanskrit pose name. Below each pose name is an english translation, variants, a list of categories in which the pose appears in the visual indexes, and the page number for the pose.

adho mukha svanasana
downward-facing dog pose
forward folds
36

photo indexes

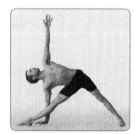

(page number)

standing

forward folds

backbends

twists

arm balances

inversions

seated

prone

supine

core

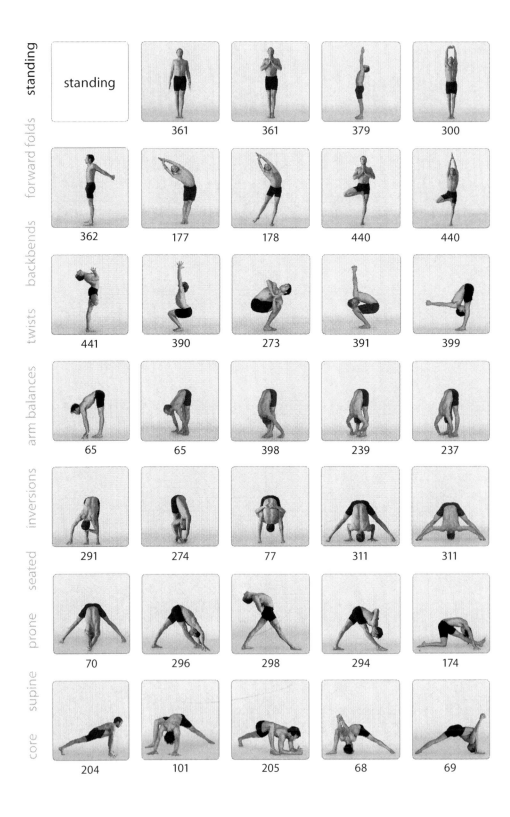

standing

361   361   379   300

362   177   178   440   440

441   390   273   391   399

65   65   398   239   237

291   274   77   311   311

70   296   298   294   174

204   101   205   68   69

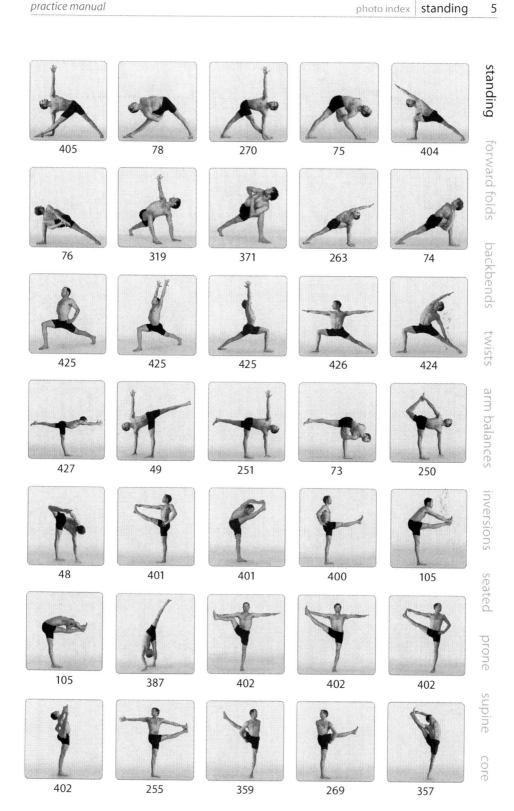

standing

forward folds

backbends

twists

arm balances

inversions

seated

prone

supine

core

405	78	270	75	404
76	319	371	263	74
425	425	425	426	424
427	49	251	73	250
48	401	401	400	105
105	387	402	402	402
402	255	359	269	357

standing

forward folds

backbends

twists

arm balances

inversions

seated

prone

supine

core

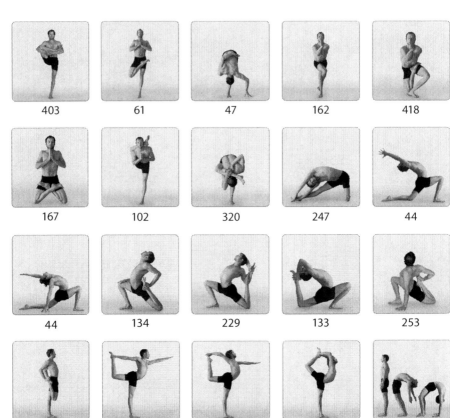

403   61   47   162   418

167   102   320   247   44

44   134   229   133   253

115   231   232   233   363

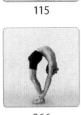

366

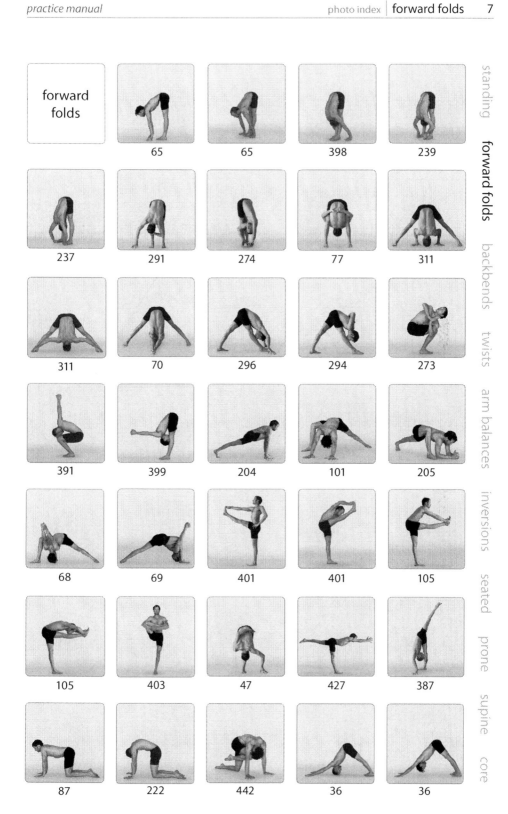

forward folds

65   65   398   239

237   291   274   77   311

311   70   296   294   273

391   399   204   101   205

68   69   401   401   105

105   403   47   427   387

87   222   442   36   36

standing   forward folds   backbends   twists   arm balances   inversions   seated   prone   supine   core

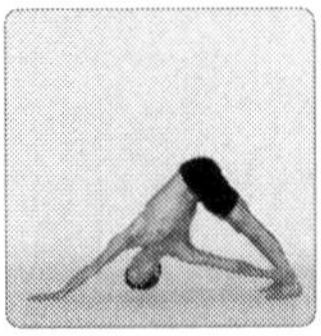

249

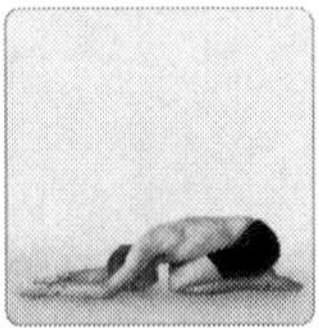

82

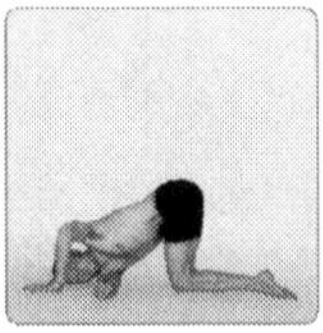

278

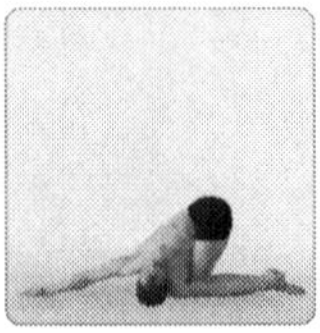

252

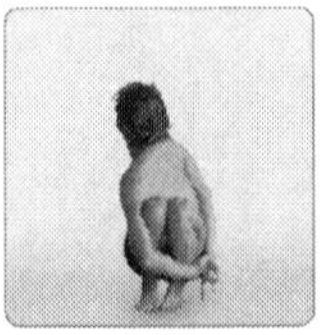

303

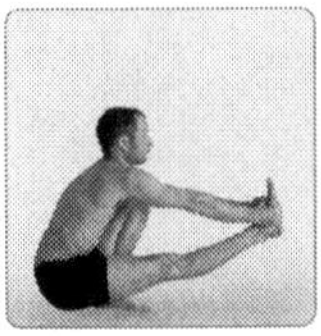

175

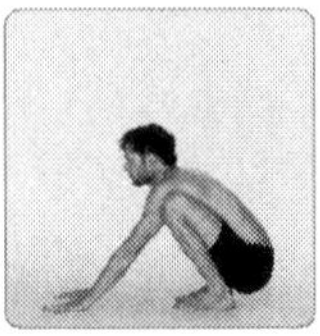

212

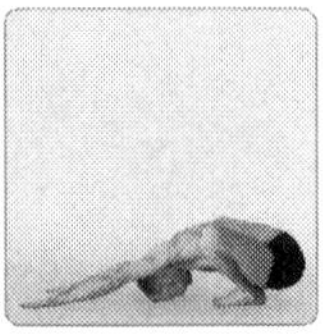

212

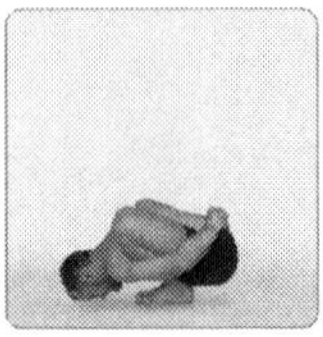

213

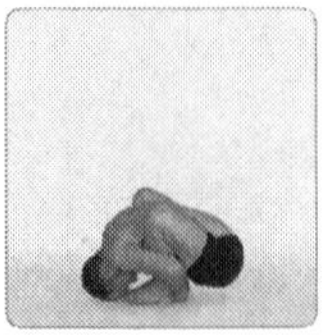

214

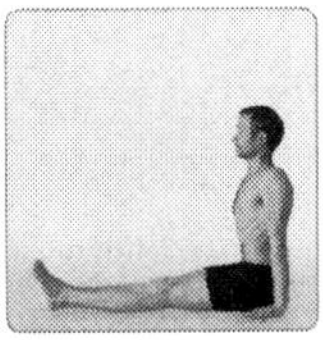

97

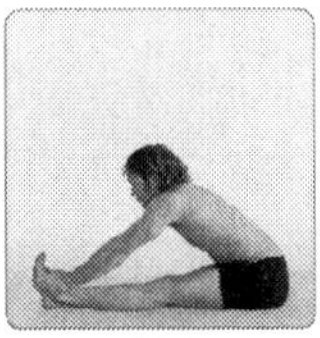

304

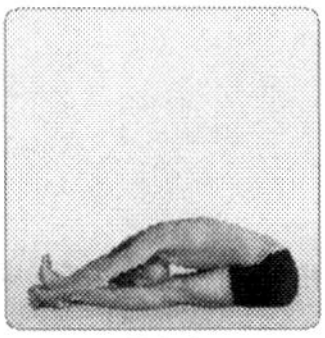

304

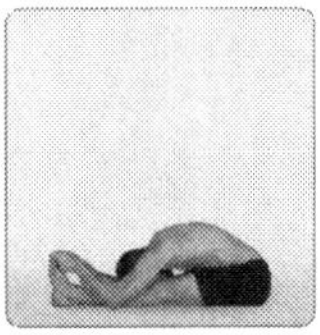

304

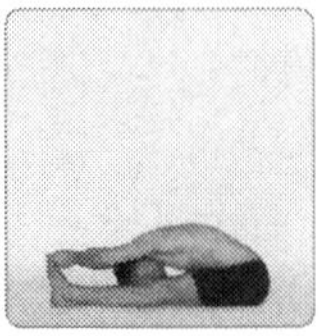

304

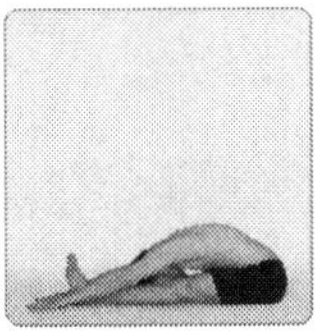

304

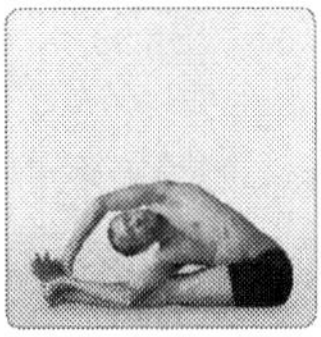

264

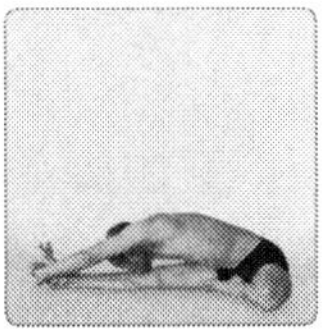

179

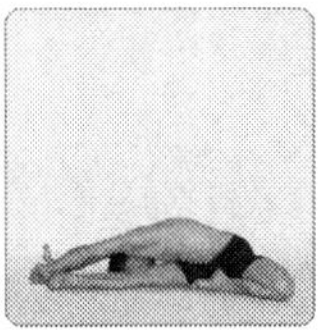

179

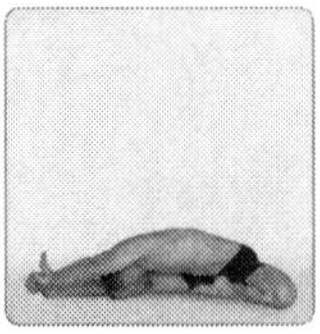

179

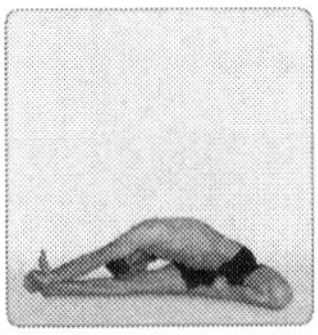

179

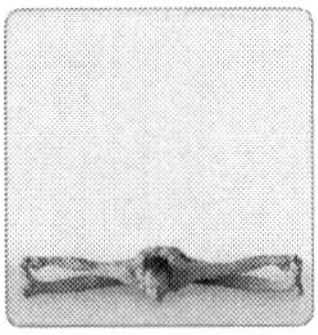

373

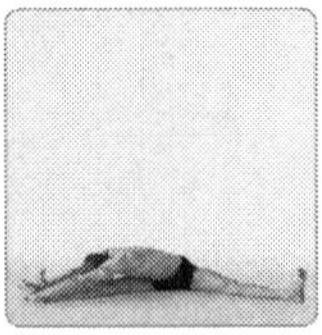

289

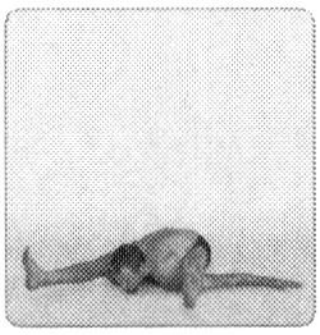

199

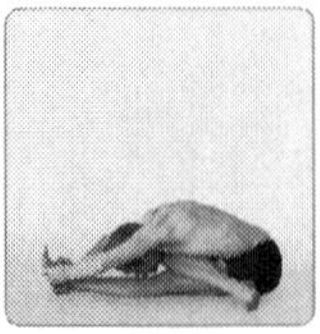

124

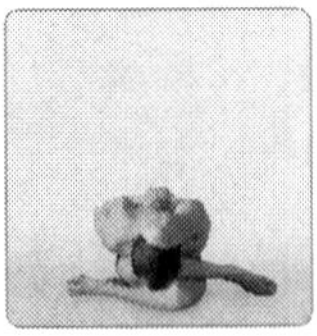

166

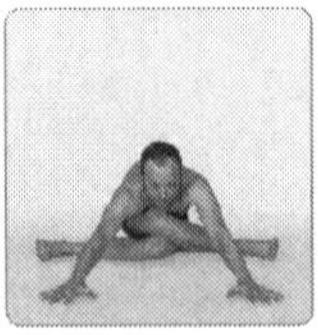

100

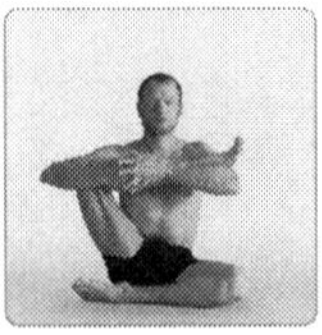

176

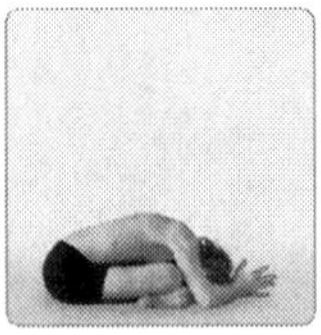

38

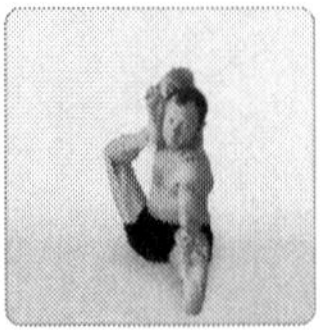

40

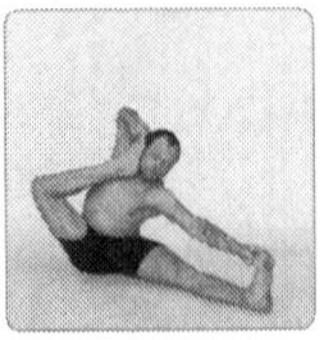

40

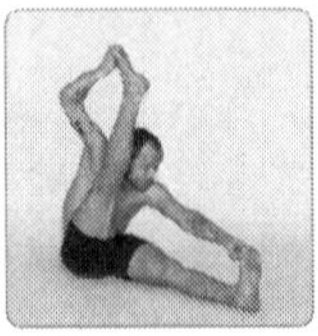

41

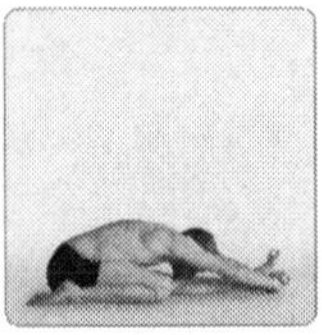

369

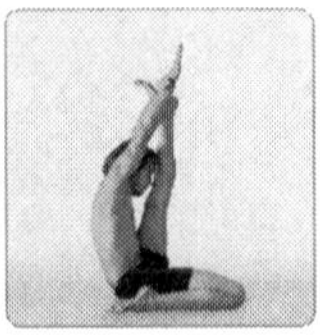

197

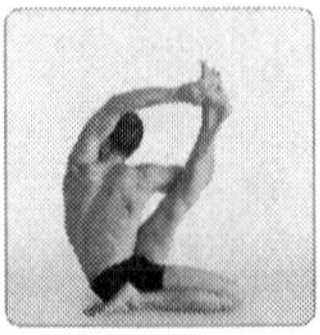

257

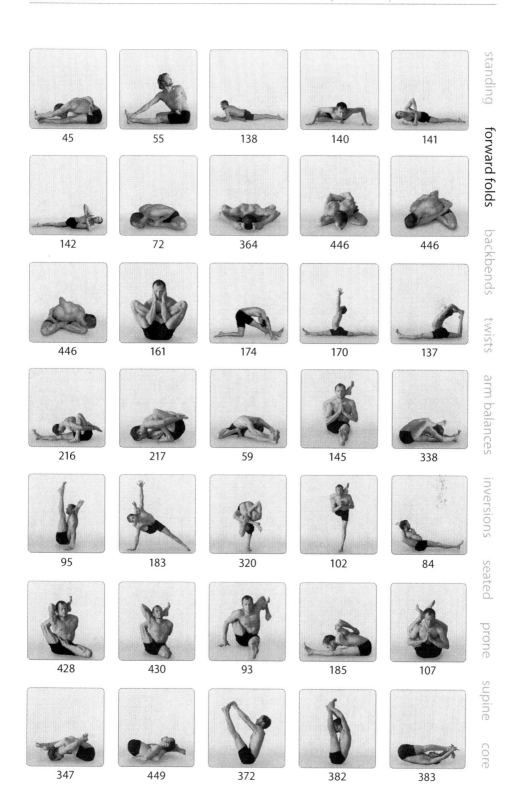

standing   **forward folds**   backbends   twists   arm balances   inversions   seated   prone   supine   core

45	55	138	140	141
142	72	364	446	446
446	161	174	170	137
216	217	59	145	338
95	183	320	102	84
428	430	93	185	107
347	449	372	382	383

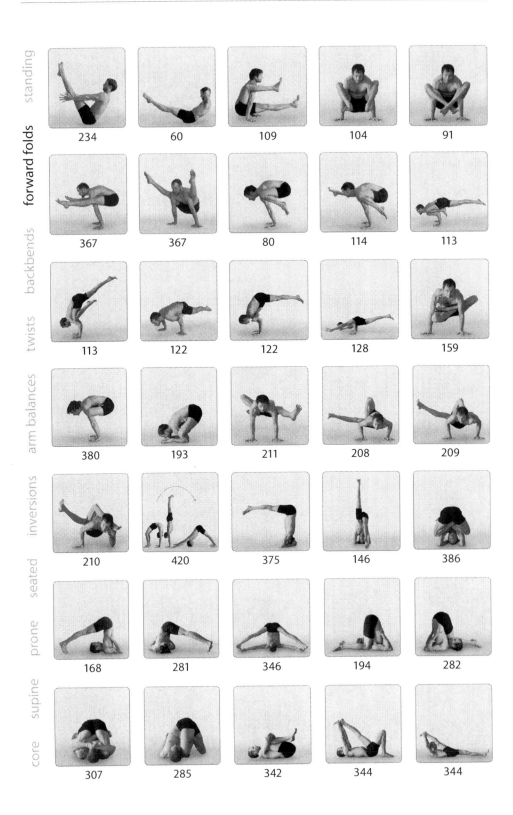

standing

forward folds

234   60   109   104   91

backbends

367   367   80   114   113

twists

113   122   122   128   159

arm balances

380   193   211   208   209

inversions

210   420   375   146   386

seated

prone

168   281   346   194   282

supine

core

307   285   342   344   344

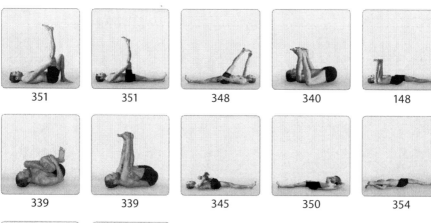

351   351   348   340   148

339   339   345   350   354

150   151

standing

forward folds

backbends

twists

arm balances

inversions

seated

prone

supine

core

standing

forward folds

backbends

twists

arm balances

inversions

seated

prone

supine

core

backbends

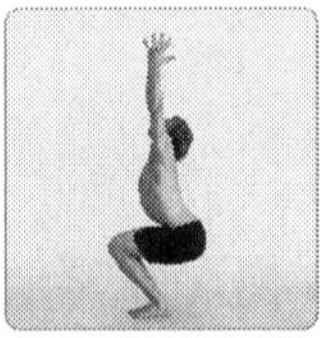

390	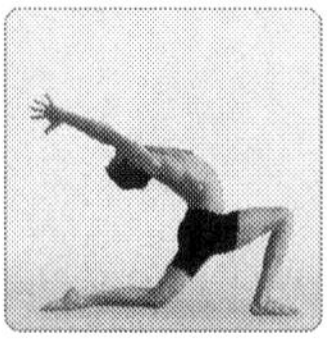 44	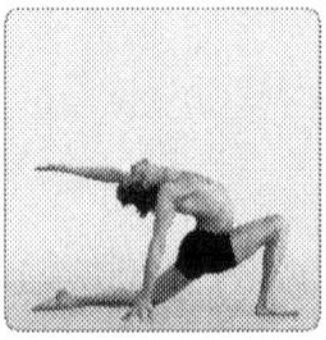 44	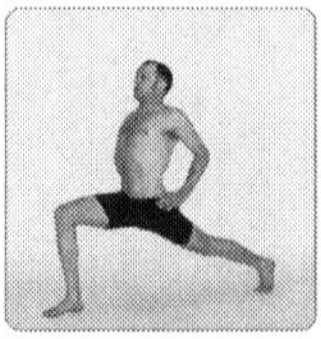 425

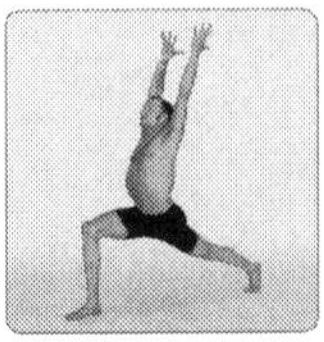

425	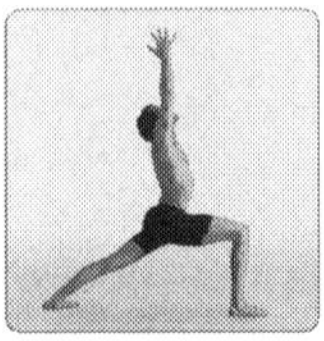 425	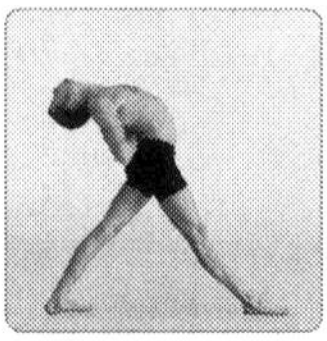 298	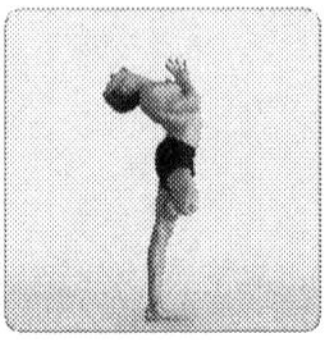 441	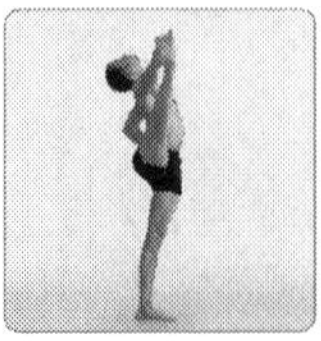 402

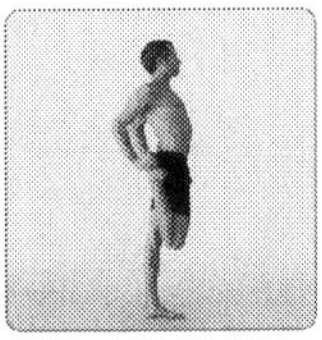

115	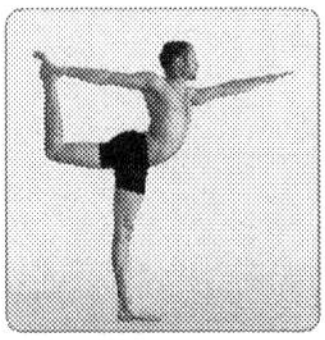 231	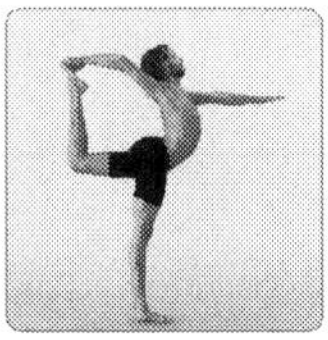 232	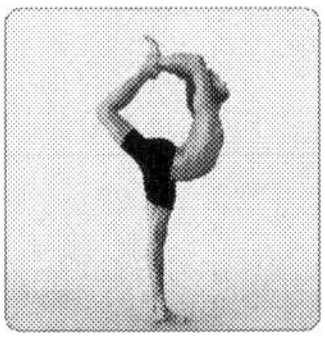 233	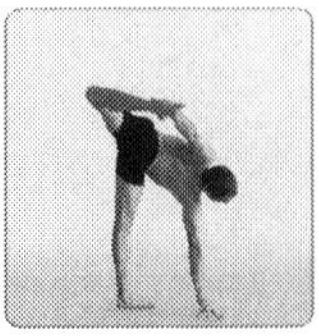 48

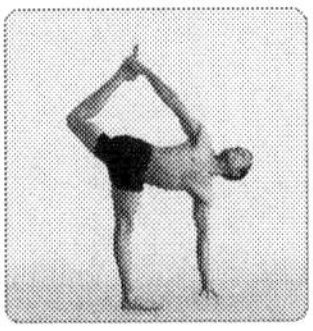

250	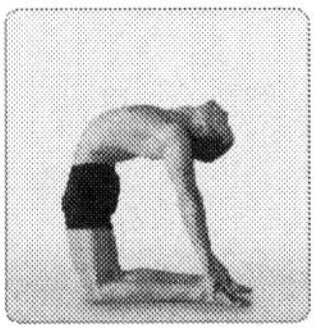 389	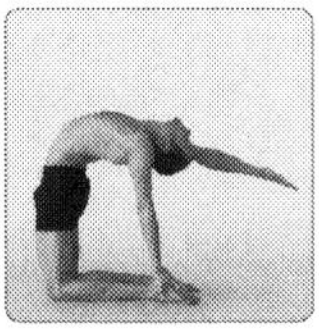 112	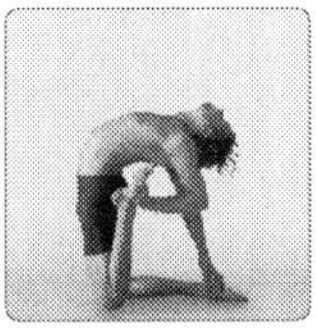 118	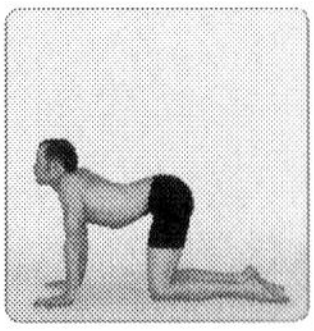 92

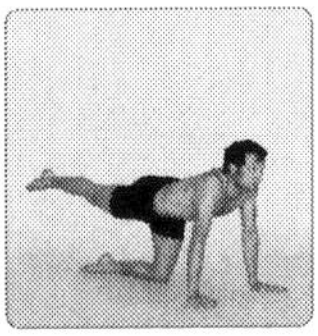

443	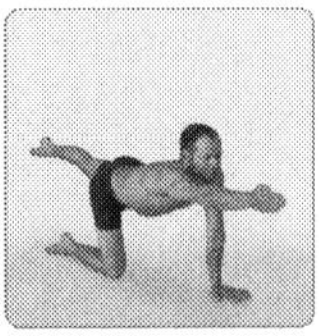 445	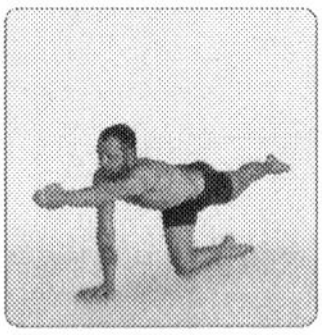 444	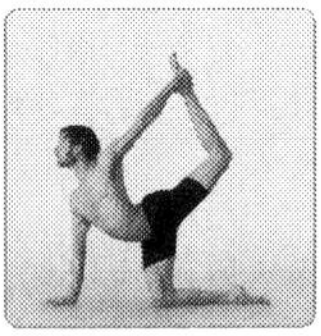 119	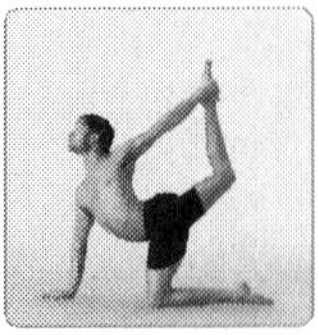 120

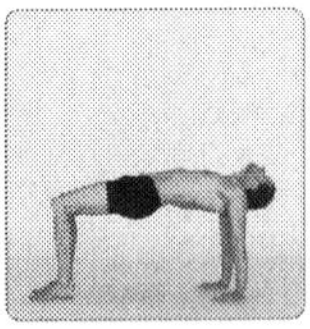

313	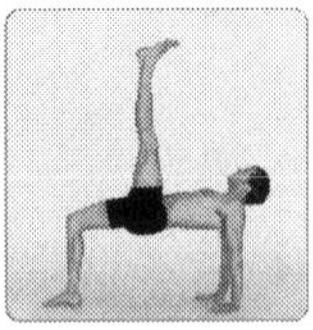 314	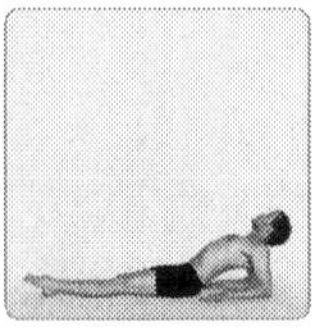 315	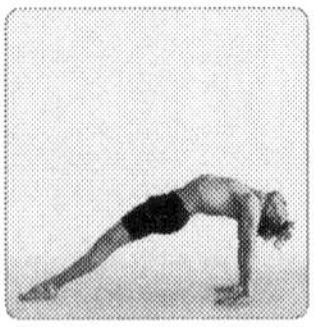 312	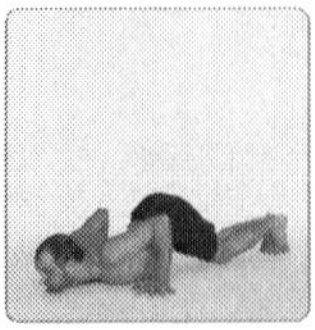 66

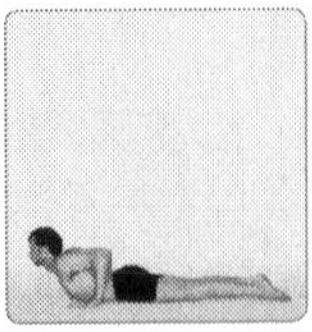

89	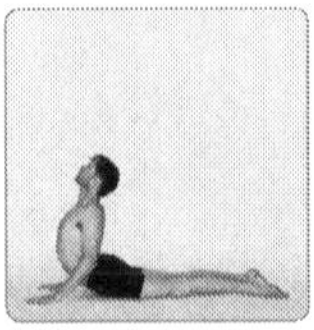 89	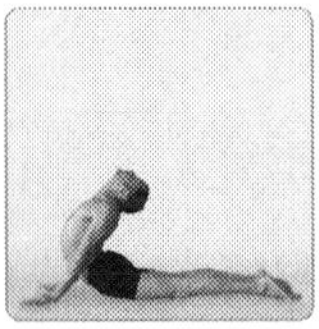 89	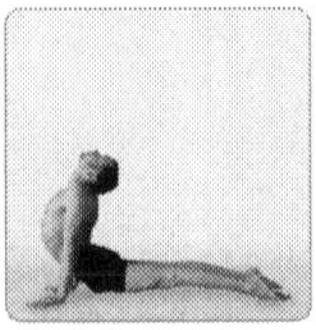 384	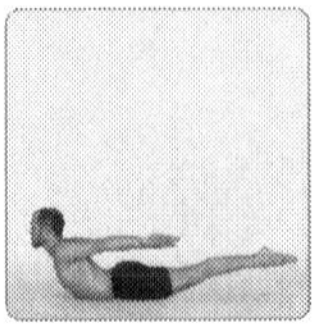 322

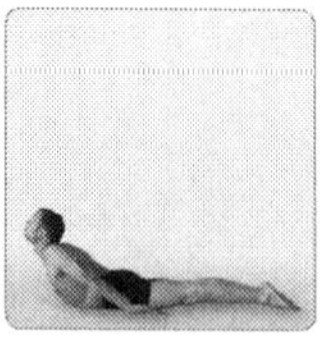

standing
forward folds
backbends
twists
arm balances
inversions
seated
prone
supine
core

322 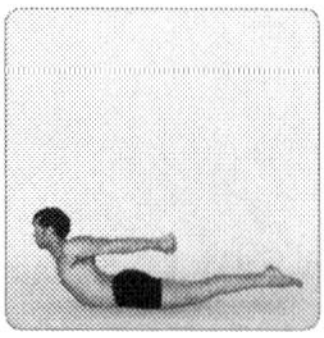   322 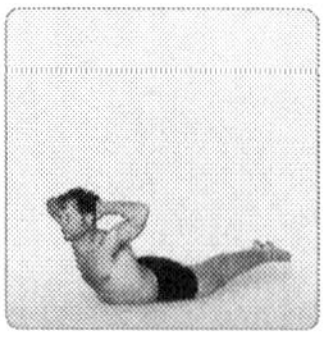   206 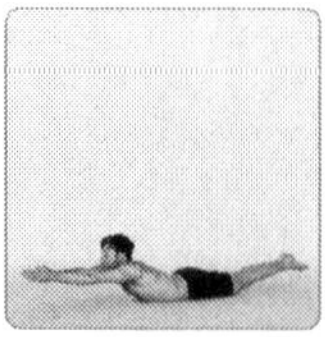   207 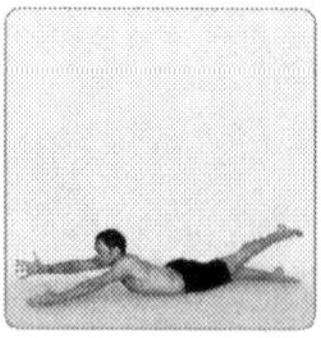   207

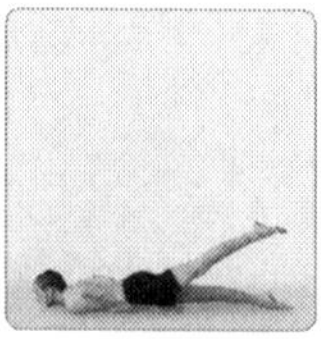

64 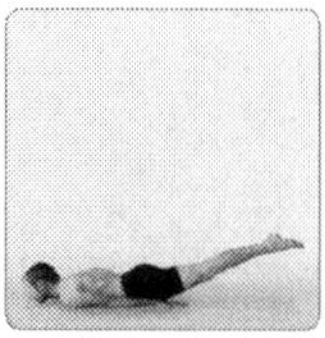   422 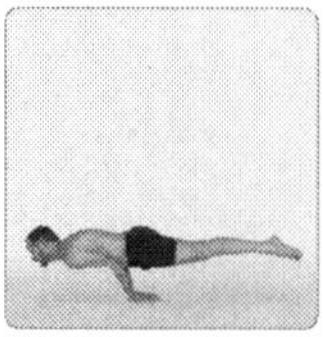   224 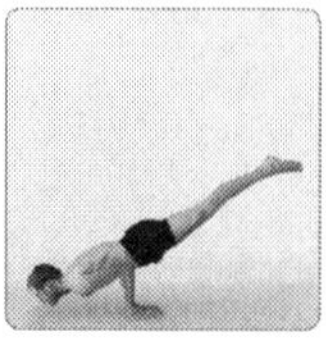   224 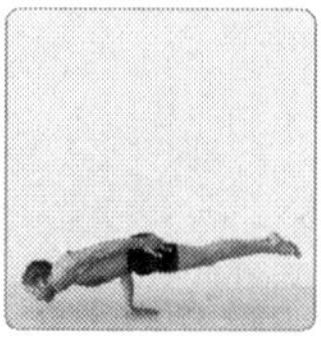   224

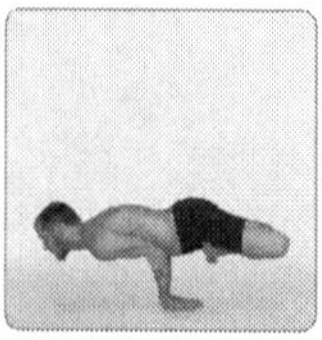

241 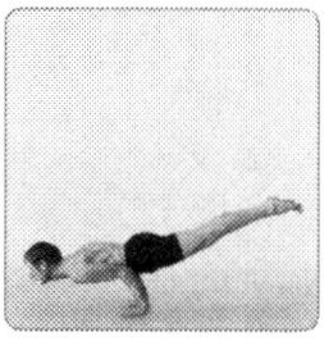   169 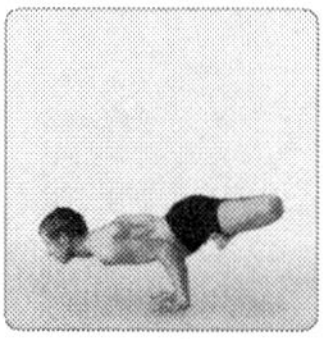   240 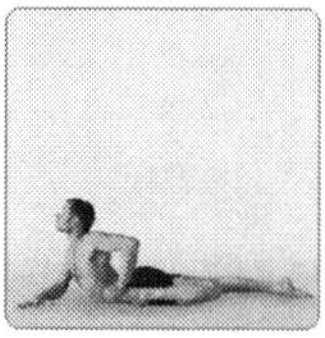   117 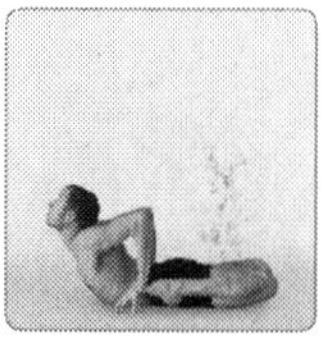   88

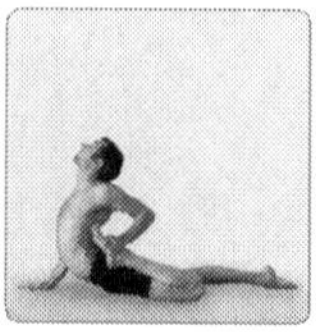

378 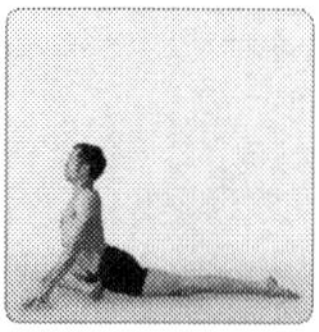   130 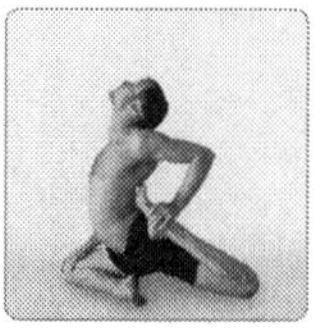   132 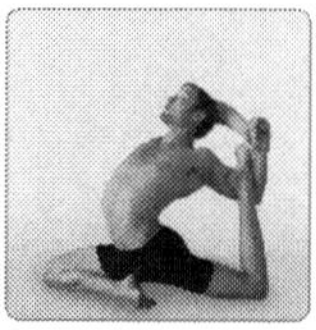   228 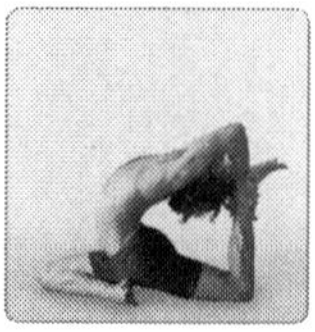   129

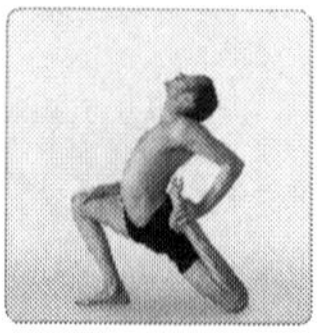

134 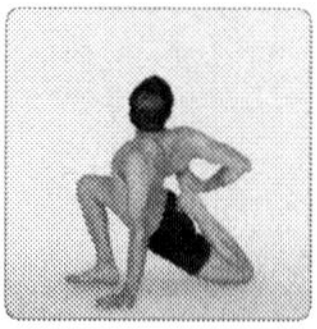   253 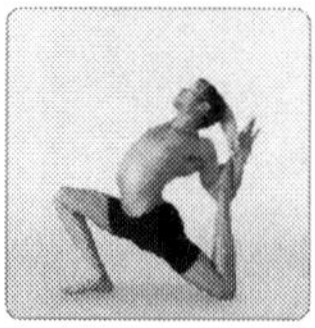   229 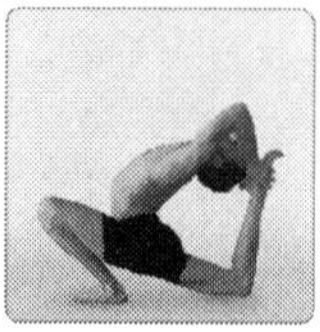   133 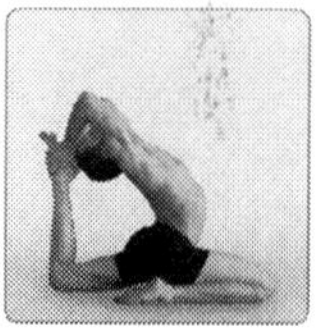   136

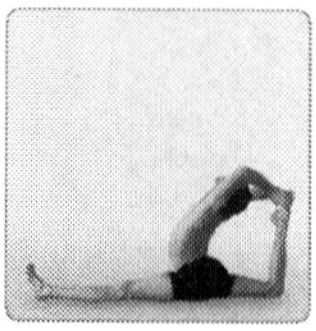

137 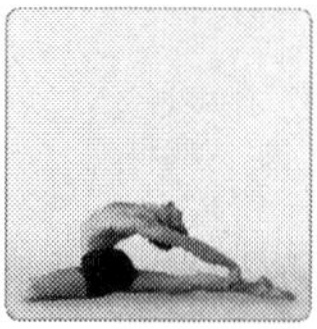   409 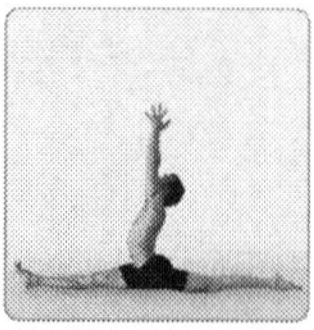   170 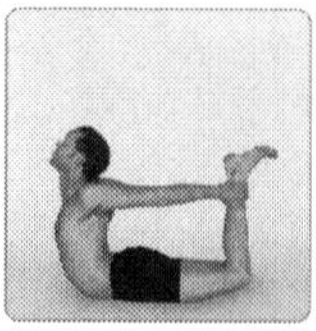   99 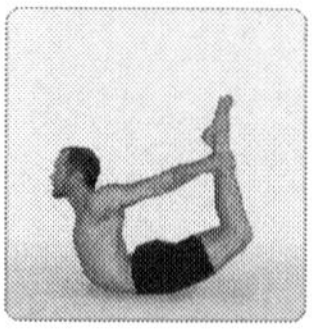   99

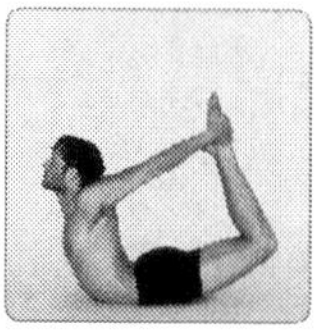

99 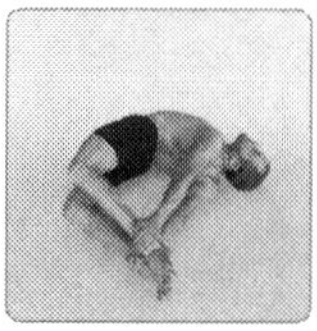   280 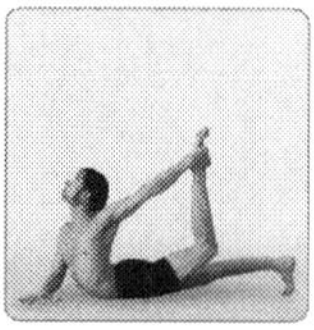   121 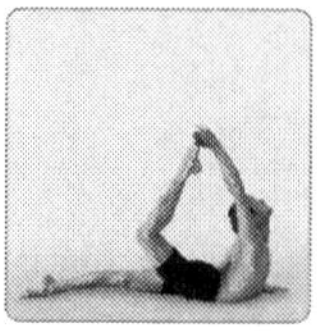   156 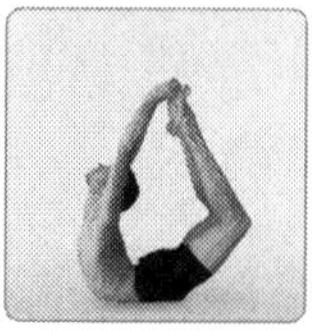   238

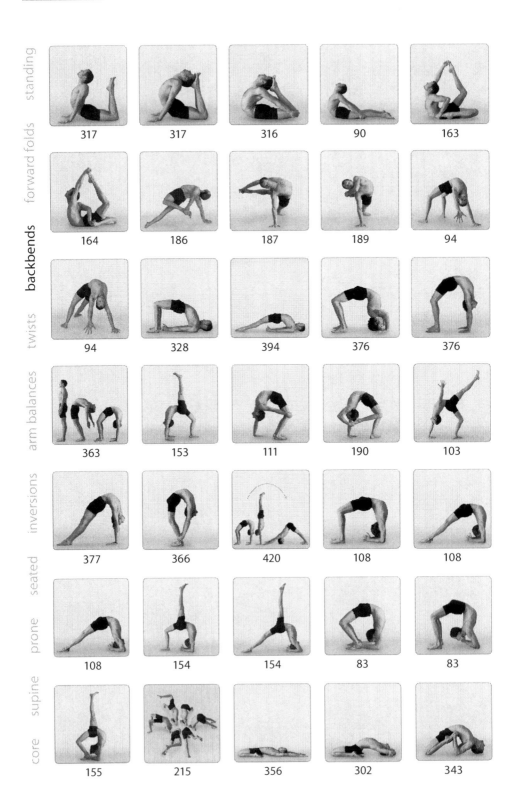

standing

317   317   316   90   163

forward folds

164   186   187   189   94

backbends

94   328   394   376   376

twists

363   153   111   190   103

arm balances

377   366   420   108   108

inversions

108   154   154   83   83

seated

prone

155   215   356   302   343

supine

core

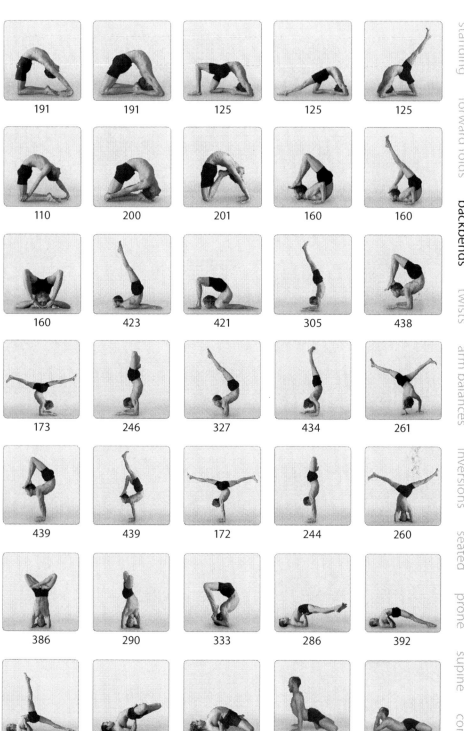

standing

191   191   125   125   125

forward folds

110   200   201   160   160

backbends

160   423   421   305   438

twists

173   246   327   434   261

arm balances

439   439   172   244   260

inversions

386   290   333   286   392

seated

prone

392   245   396   332   318

supine

core

standing

forward folds

backbends

twists

arm balances

inversions

seated

prone

supine

core

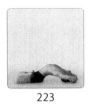 223

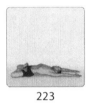 223

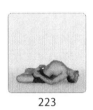 223

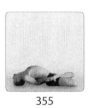 355

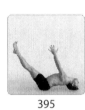 395

 329

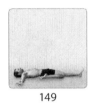 149

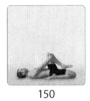 150

 151

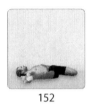 152

 365

twists

273

274

78

270

75

319

371

76

263

74

251

73

250

255

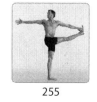

269

357

253

278

252

249

266

262

276

264

179

179

179

179

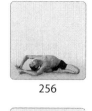
256

289

271

358

257

54

standing forward folds backbends **twists** arm balances inversions seated prone supine core

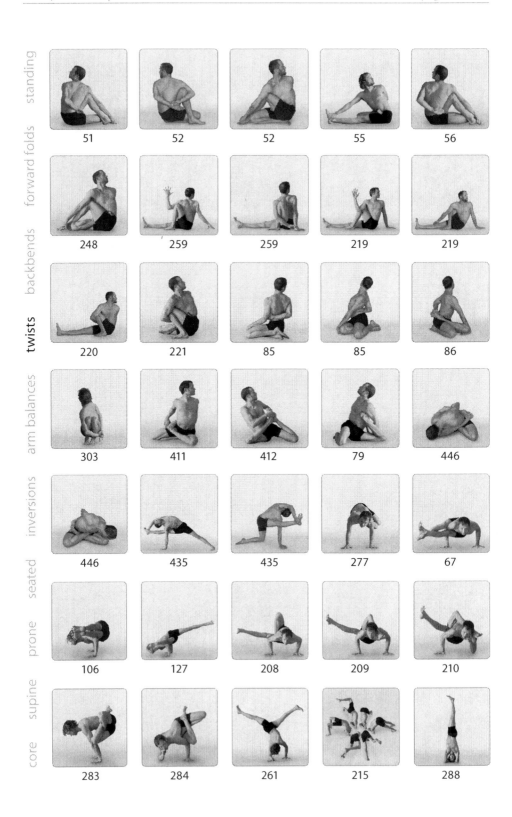

standing

51   52   52   55   56

forward folds

248   259   259   219   219

backbends

twists

220   221   85   85   86

arm balances

303   411   412   79   446

inversions

446   435   435   277   67

seated

prone

106   127   208   209   210

supine

core

283   284   261   215   288

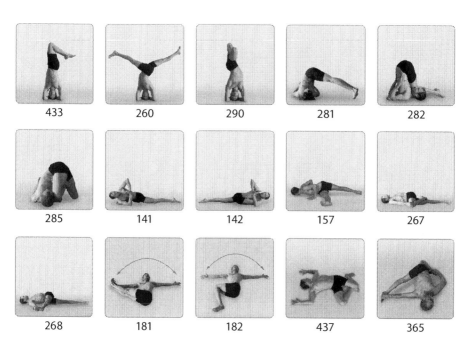

433   260   290   281   282

285   141   142   157   267

268   181   182   437   365

standing forward folds backbends **twists** arm balances inversions seated prone supine core

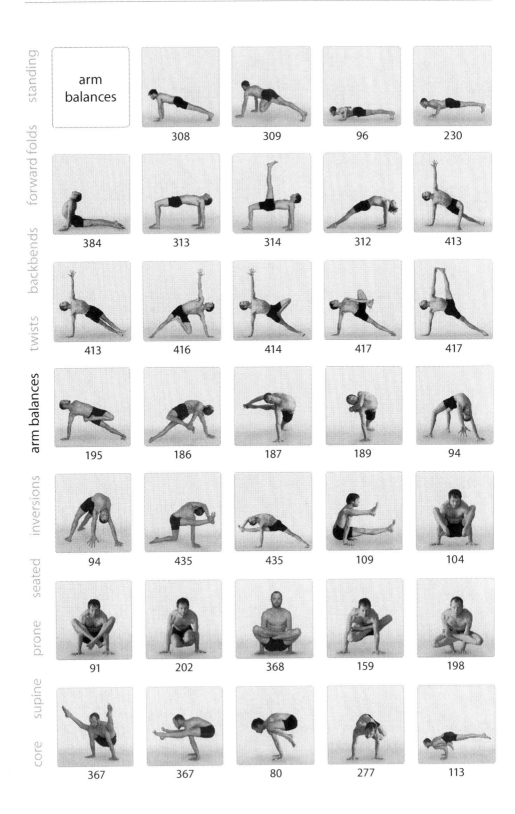

standing

forward folds

backbends

twists

arm balances

inversions

seated

prone

supine

core

arm
balances

308 309 96 230

384 313 314 312 413

413 416 414 417 417

195 186 187 189 94

94 435 435 109 104

91 202 368 159 198

367 367 80 277 113

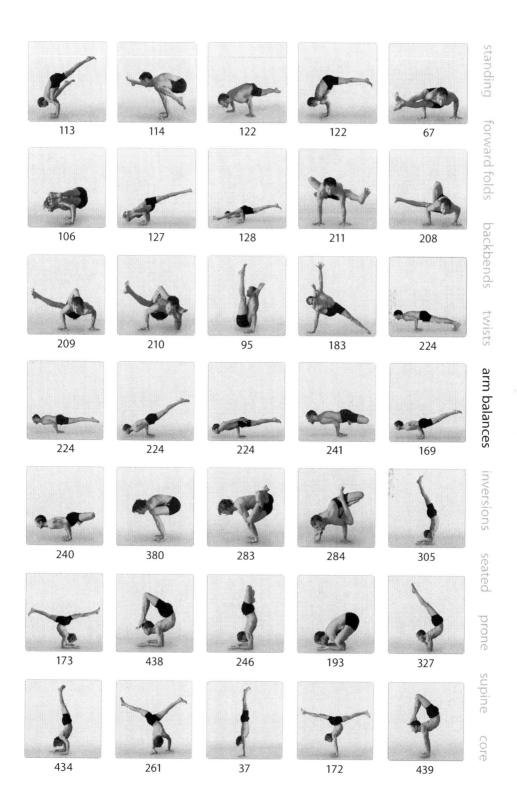

standing

forward folds

backbends

twists

arm balances

inversions

seated

prone

supine

core

113   114   122   122   67

106   127   128   211   208

209   210   95   183   224

224   224   224   241   169

240   380   283   284   305

173   438   246   193   327

434   261   37   172   439

standing

forward folds

backbends

twists

arm balances

inversions

seated

prone

supine

core

439

244

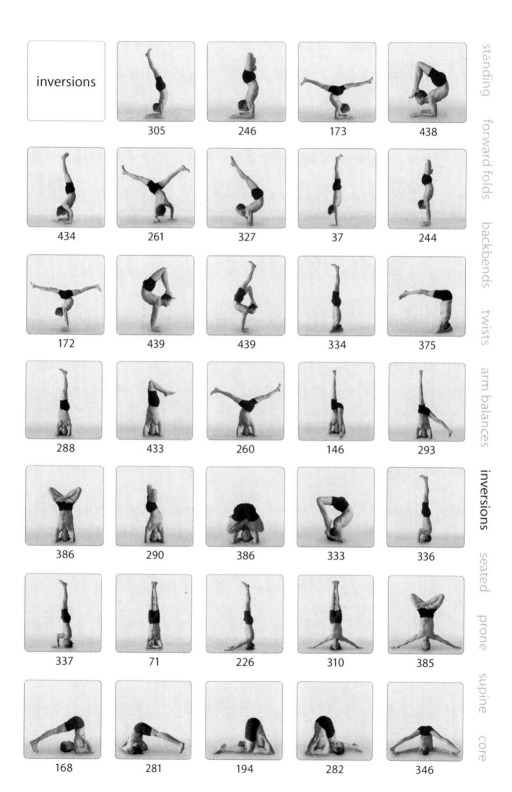

inversions

standing

305 246 173 438

forward folds

434 261 327 37 244

backbends

172 439 439 334 375

twists

288 433 260 146 293

arm balances

386 290 386 333 336

inversions

337 71 226 310 385

seated

prone

supine

168 281 194 282 346

core

standing

forward folds

backbends

twists

arm balances

inversions

seated

prone

supine

core

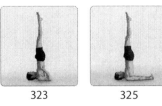

323

325

236

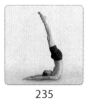

235

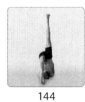

144

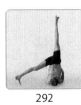

292

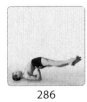

286

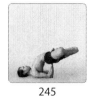

245

307

285

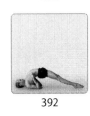

392

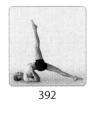

392

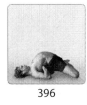

396

standing   forward folds   backbends   twists   arm balances   inversions   **seated**   prone   supine   core

seated

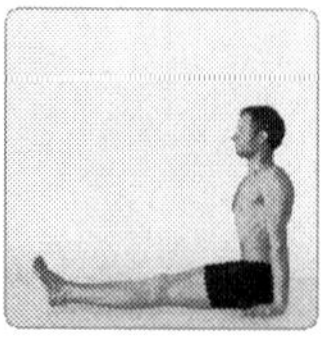

97 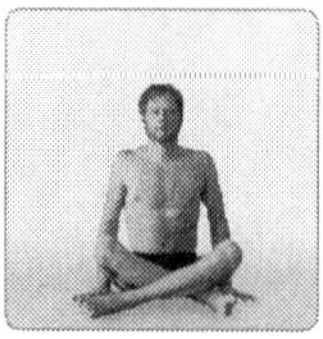   341 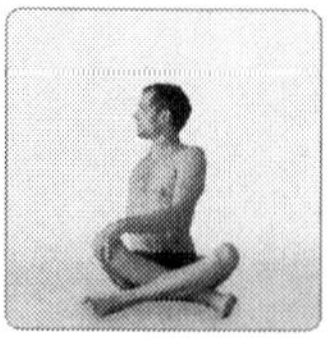   266 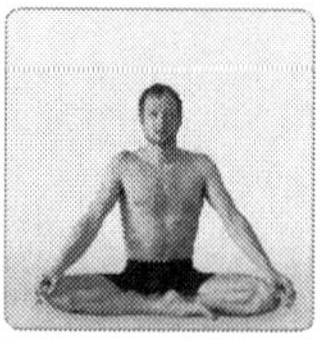   330

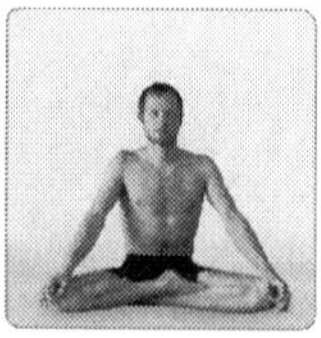

331 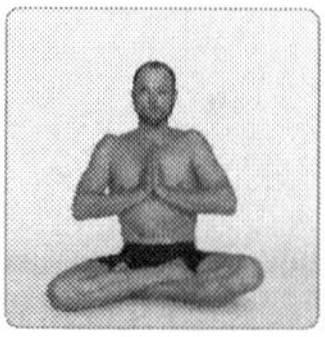   331 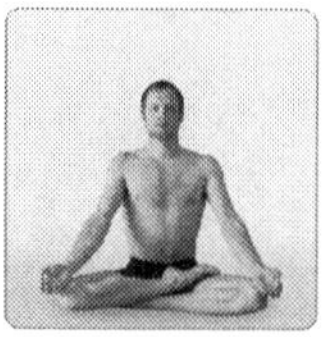   62 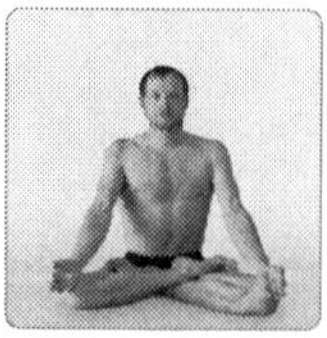   242 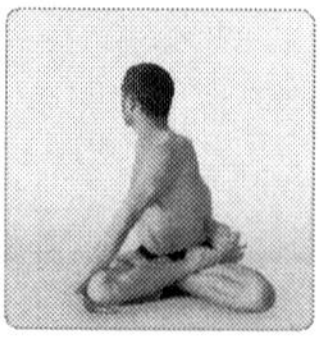   262

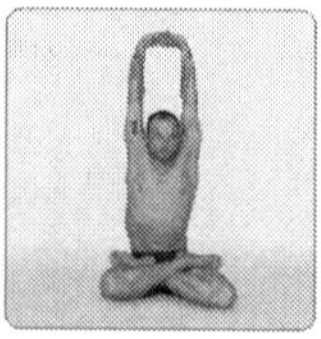

301 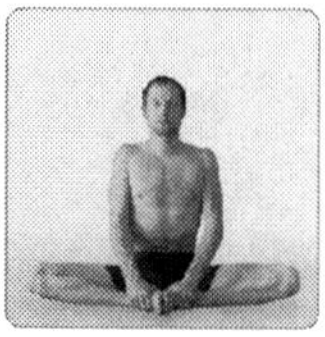   72 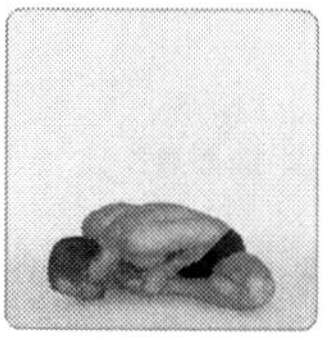   72 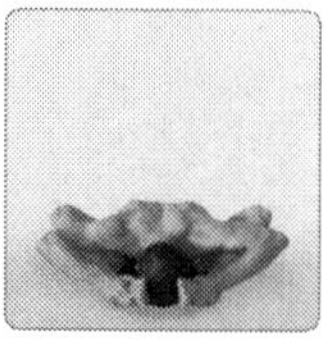   364 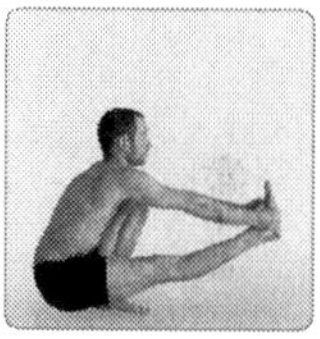   175

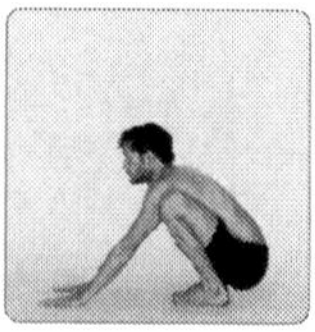

212 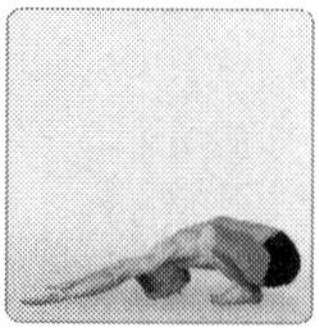   212 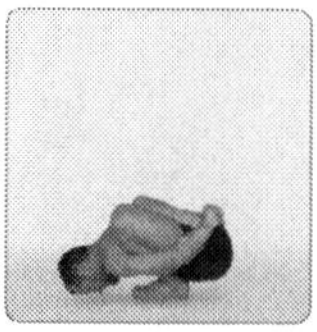   213 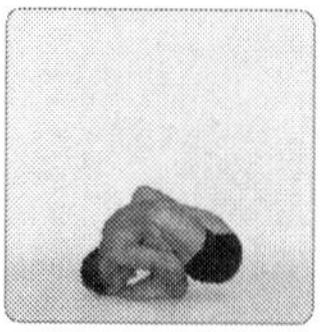   214 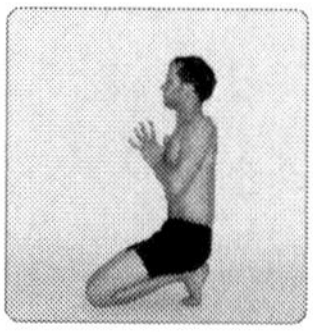   407

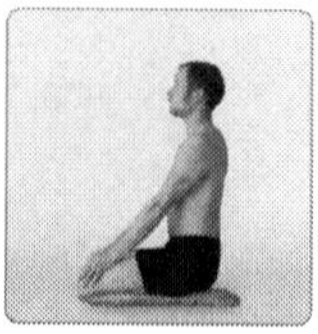

408 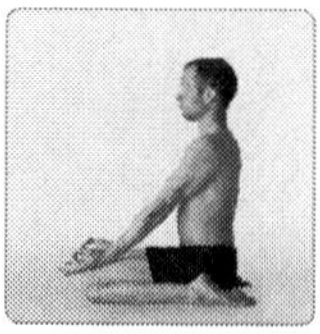   432 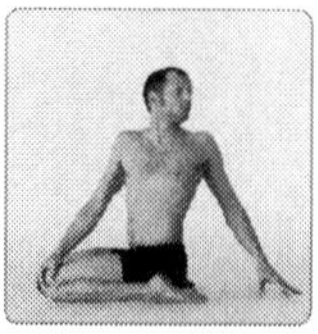   276 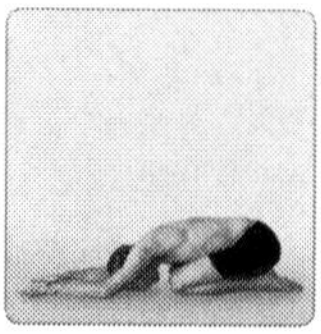   82 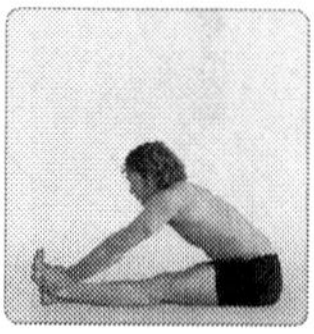   304

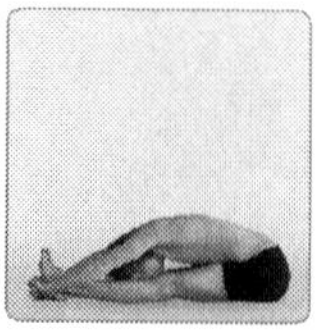

304 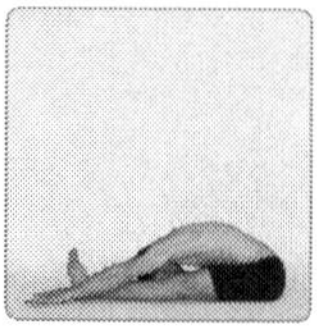   304 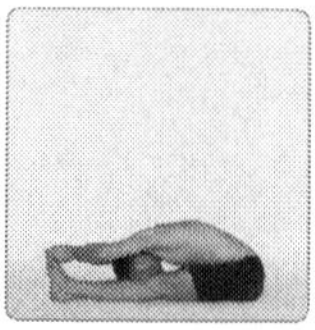   304 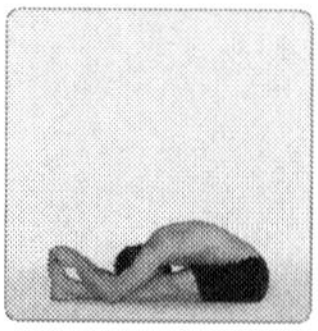   304 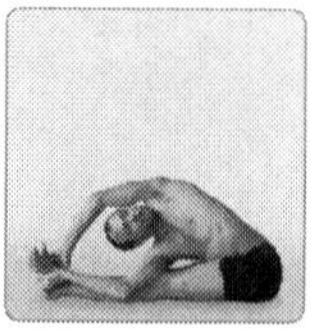   264

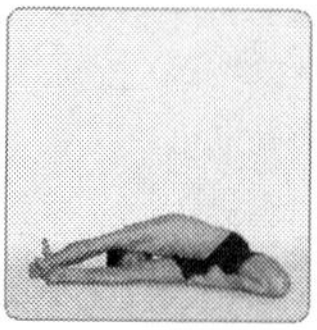

179 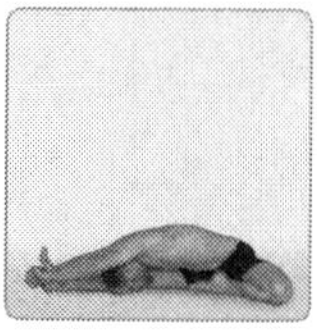   179 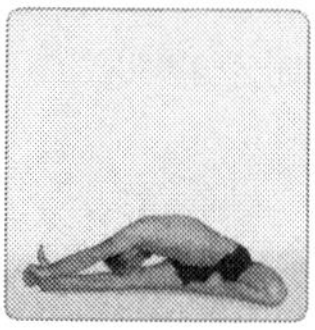   179 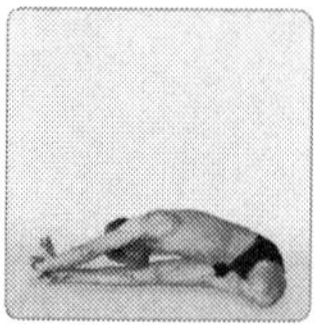   179 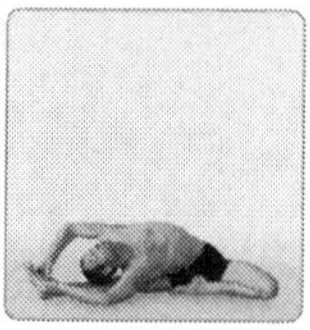   256

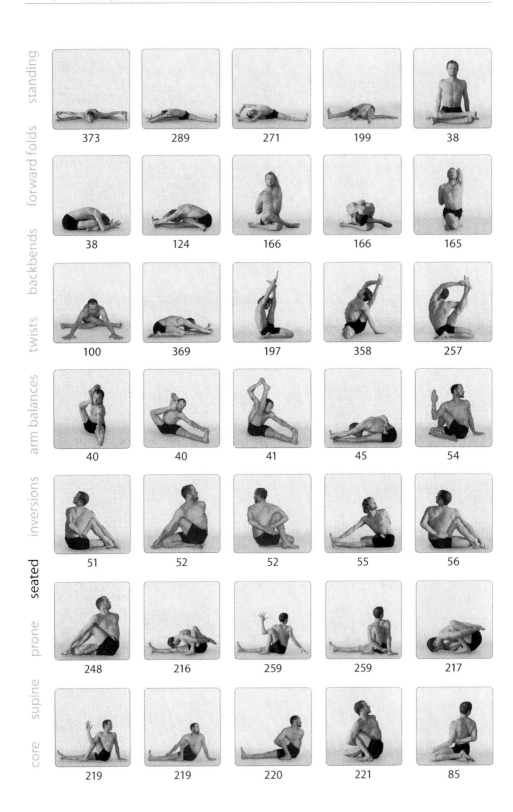

standing

forward folds

backbends

twists

arm balances

inversions

seated

prone

supine

core

373 289 271 199 38

38 124 166 166 165

100 369 197 358 257

40 40 41 45 54

51 52 52 55 56

248 216 259 259 217

219 219 220 221 85

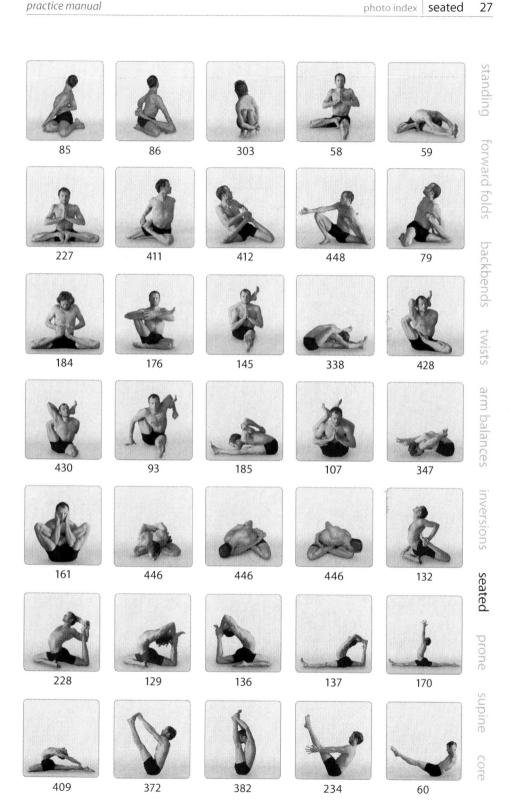

85   86   303   58   59

227   411   412   448   79

184   176   145   338   428

430   93   185   107   347

161   446   446   446   132

228   129   136   137   170

409   372   382   234   60

standing   forward folds   backbends   twists   arm balances   inversions   **seated**   prone   supine   core

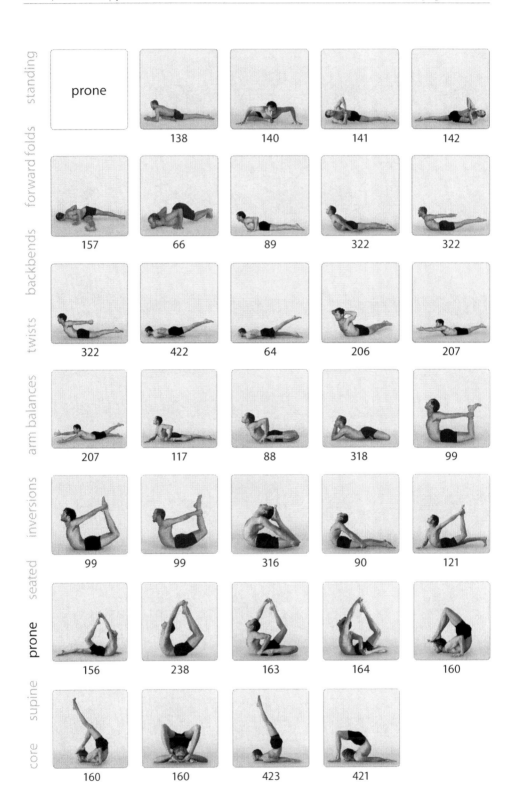

standing

forward folds

backbends

twists

arm balances

inversions

seated

prone

supine

core

prone

138

140

141

142

157

66

89

322

322

322

422

64

206

207

207

117

88

318

99

99

99

316

90

121

156

238

163

164

160

160

160

423

421

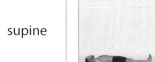

supine

353

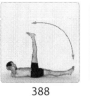
388

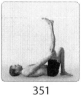
351

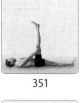
351

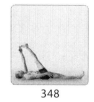
348

349

350

267

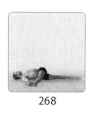
268

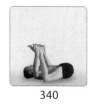
340

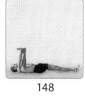
148

344

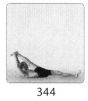
344

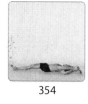
354

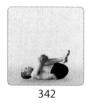
342

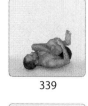
339

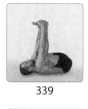
339

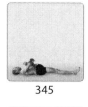
345

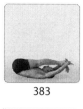
383

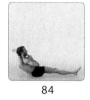
84

449

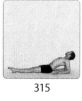
315

356

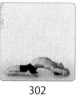
302

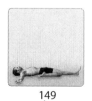
149

150

151

152

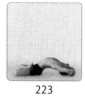
223

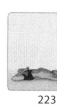
223

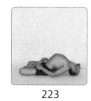
223

395

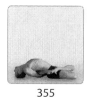
355

181

standing

forward folds

backbends

twists

arm balances

inversions

seated

prone

supine

core

standing

forward folds

backbends

twists

arm balances

inversions

seated

prone

supine

core

182

365

437

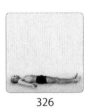

326

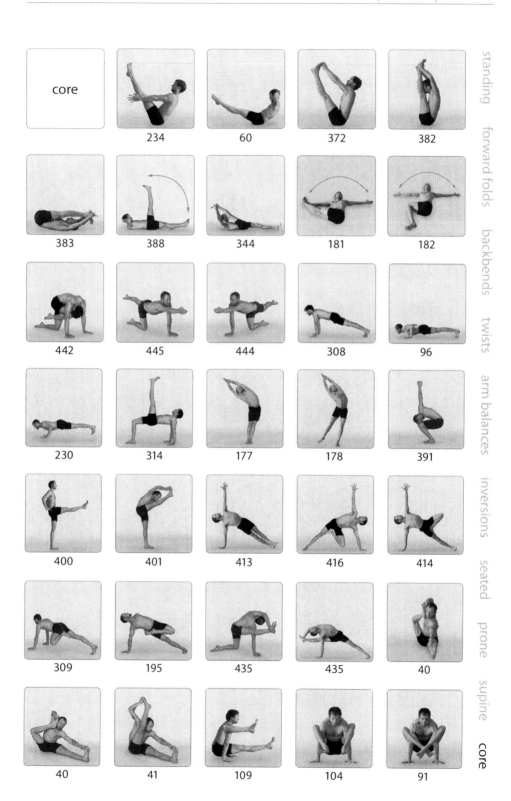

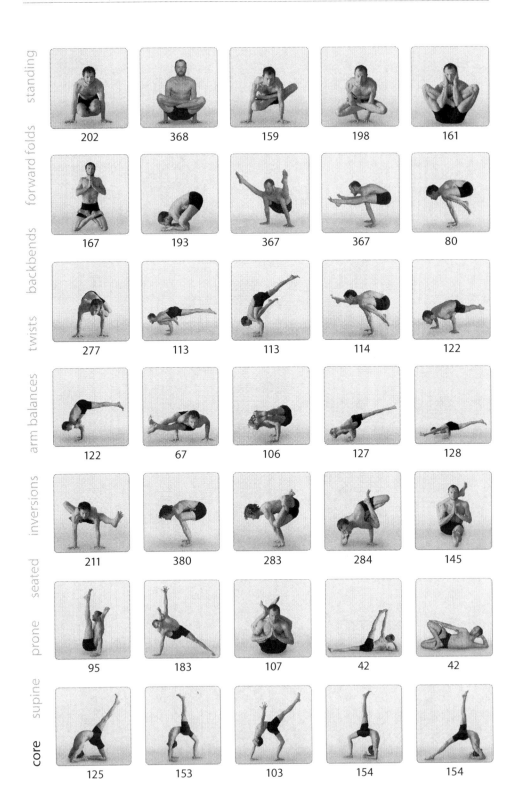

standing

202   368   159   198   161

forward folds

167   193   367   367   80

backbends

twists

277   113   113   114   122

arm balances

122   67   106   127   128

inversions

211   380   283   284   145

seated

prone

95   183   107   42   42

supine

core

125   153   103   154   154

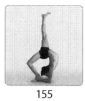
155

375

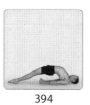
394

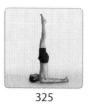
325

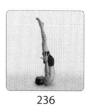
236

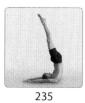
235

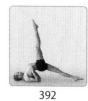
392

standing forward folds backbends twists arm balances inversions seated prone supine **core**

YOGA
resource

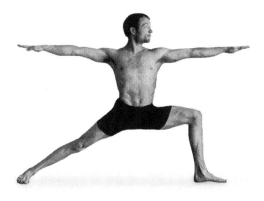

360 poses *featuring*

shape • safety • refinement **practice instructions**

arranged alphabetically by **Sanskrit name**

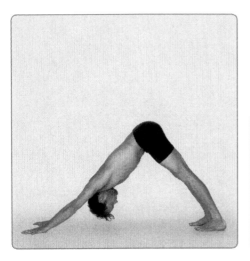
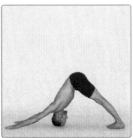

adho mukha svanasana
downward-facing dog pose

shape
(from *bharmanasana*)

1.   Move the knees back four to six inches and curl the toes under.
2.   Lift the knees and straighten the legs. Push the hands down and forward, and stretch the hips up and back.
3.   Relax the neck and gaze straight back. Hold the pose and breathe.
4.   To come out, bend the knees and place them on the floor. Bring the shoulders over the wrists and walk the knees forward until they are directly below the hips.

safety

*   Press the inner edges of the hands down and lift the inner shoulders.
*   Stretch the shoulders up, away from the hands.
*   If the shoulders are hyper-mobile and push the armpits/head of the arm bone down toward the floor, lift the armpits up slightly before lifting the inner shoulders and stretching back.
*   Point the biceps in and squeeze the elbows straight.
*   Lift the sit bones up, press the tailbone down.
*   Tone the legs—especially the quads and calves.
*   If the hamstrings are tight, the low back will round. To create a curve in the low back and length in the spine, bend the knees as much as necessary and stretch the spine. Keeping the knees bent, lift the sit bones up and curve the low back in. Do not straighten the legs if it causes the back to round.
*   Reach the heels toward/to the floor to stretch the back of the legs.

refinement

Adho mukha svanasana is an optimal warm up pose if you stretch your arms, spine, and legs to capacity. In a class or practice where this pose is done many times, it is easy to treat *adho mukha svanasana* like waiting in line. Waiting in line for the next pose that is. When waiting in line at a check-out counter, one isn't doing much of anything but standing there. *Adho mukha svanasana* is often practiced just like that. Perform *adho mukha svanasana* like you would any challenging standing pose. Give yourself completely to the practice and it will offer even more back.

A more advanced variation of *adho mukha svanasana* is to bring your head to the floor. Do not simply lower your head straight down to bring it to the floor. Bring your head to the floor by first stretching your shoulders, spine, and legs completely. This will bring your head down and back as opposed to straight down. When your head moves straight down to the floor, your shoulders stretch without strength, which can lead to strain. This variation of *adho mukha svanasana* is an excellent preparatory pose for learning the upper back, shoulder, and arm action in *urdhva dhanurasana*.

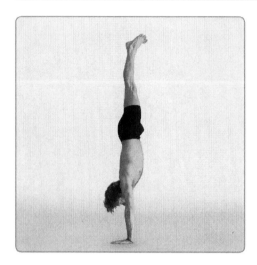

adho mukha vrksasana
downward-facing tree pose / handstand pose

shape
(from *adho mukha svanasana*)

1. Step the right foot forward—halfway to the hands.
2. Lift the left foot and straighten the leg. Straighten the arms.
3. Move the shoulders a few inches past the wrists.
4. Lower the upper spine between the shoulder blades so there is a divot in the upper back (as opposed to rounding in the upper back).
5. Inhale, press the right foot down and swing the left leg and torso up into a vertical position. Bring the right leg parallel to the floor.
6. Press the tailbone in. Join the legs and bring the feet halfway between a flexed and pointed position.
7. Look slightly forward between the hands. Hold the pose and breathe.
8. To come out, lower one leg and then the other. Step the feet back. Press the hands down and forward and push the hips up and back.

safety

- To avoid falling over backwards, practice *adho mukha vrksasana* against a wall.
- Before kicking up, shrug the shoulders forward and move the upper back toward the floor.
- To promote balance, once the right leg is parallel to the floor, move the inner edge of the left leg back.
- Press the fingertips and the perimeter of the palms down into the floor with equal pressure.
- Squeeze the elbows straight.

- Press the inner feet and knees together.
- Engage the legs and feet—flare the toes.
- Press the hands down to fully stretch the shoulders. Extend the spine, hips, and legs away from the floor.
- Reach the tailbone toward the heels and tone the low belly.
- To develop the balance required to stay in the pose, practice with one foot against the wall. Then bring both feet off the wall and balance for a few seconds. Increase the length of time in the balance. Eventually, practice in the middle of the room away from the wall.

refinement

In the beginning, as you learn to gain balance in the middle of the room, you may need to bring your top leg beyond vertical with both feet equidistant to the floor. This leg position is easier to balance in than when the legs are both vertical. Once you attain balance in this position, bring the feet together. Avoid attaining balance by repeatedly bending and straightening the elbows, which quickly becomes a difficult habit to break.

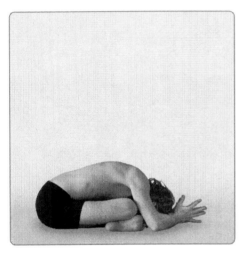
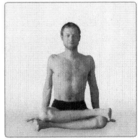

agnistambhasana
firelog pose

shape
(from *dandasana*)

1. Bend the left knee to a 90-degree angle—shin parallel to the top of the mat. Flex the foot so the sole of the foot points out.
2. Bend the right knee and place the right outer ankle on top of the left knee. Flex the foot and lower the right knee to the left ankle.
3. Place the hands next to the hips. Pause and breathe.
4. Inhale fully. Exhale, fold the torso over the legs. Rest the chest on the top shin.
5. Place the forearms on the floor and press the palms together. Look down. Hold the pose and breathe.
6. To come out, place the hands underneath the shoulders. Inhale, use the arms to lift the torso upright.

Repeat on the second side.

safety

- Before folding forward, if the top knee hovers at or above the level of the waist, place a folded blanket between the bottom ankle and top knee to support the top knee. Or, move the lower ankle closer to the sit bone.
- If the chest does not reach the legs, place one or more folded blankets between the chest and the legs, or rest the forehead on a block or the edge of a chair seat.
- Tilt the pelvis forward and the sit bones back.
- Isometrically lift the shins and push the inner edges of the feet out.
- Press the outer edges of the feet down; isometrically lift the ankles up.
- Point the toes forward. Flare the outer two toes.
- Lift the pelvic floor and draw the low belly in.

refinement

I do this pose every night before going to bed as a way to release stress and invoke deep relaxation. It is a funny thing for me to say considering a nickname for this pose is "agony-stambhasana." *Agnistambhasana* used to be relatively intolerable for me for the first few years of my practice. Then I began to hold each side for three minutes even though it was still agony-stambhasana for me; I could barely breathe. During those three minutes the only way I could relax my mind was to focus on my breath and to breathe deeply. With each inhale I connected to the tension in my hips. With each exhale I consciously released it. By the end of those six minutes, the tension in my hips felt completely dissolved. Although this is still a difficult pose for me, I have practiced it so consistently that I can release the tension in my hips in less than a minute. *Agnistambhasana* is a good preparatory pose for *padmasana, dirghasrngasana,* and *yogadandasana.*

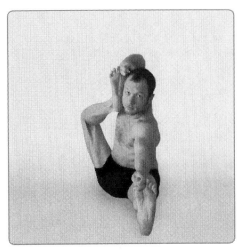
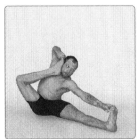

akarna dhanurasana 1
archer's pose 1

shape
(from *dandasana*)

1. Inhale fully. Exhale, lean forward and hold the big toes with the first two fingers and thumbs of each hand. Straighten the arms.
2. Keep the right leg straight and lift the right foot up as high as the head. Pause and breathe.
3. Bend the right knee and pull the inner edge of the foot to the ear with the right hand. Point the toes straight up and the soles of both feet straight ahead.
4. Look straight ahead. Hold the pose and breathe.
5. To come out, straighten the right leg and arm. Lower the leg and release the hands. Sit upright and place the hands next to the hips.

Repeat on the second side.

safety

- To reduce the intensity in the low back or hamstrings, place the left hand on the right heel and use both hands to pull the foot back toward the ear.
- Straighten and strengthen the extended leg. Press the heel and back of the knee down.
- Isometrically push the right heel down and flare the outer two toes of the right foot.
- Press the big toes into the fingers and pull the big toes back with the fingers.
- Lift the low back forward and up, even as it rounds.

refinement

Another variation of *akarna dhanurasana 1* is to bring the sole of the foot to the ear, which will sickle the ankle. Sickling the ankles does not compromise the knee if the foot is still engaged, like the foot-ankle position of the back foot in *trikonasana, virabhadrasana 2,* and *parsvakona-sana.* Whatever foot position the pose requires, practice with awareness so that your knee does not suffer negative consequences. *Akarna dhanurasana 1,* with the sole of the foot to the ear, is a good preparatory pose for *supta padangusthasana 3.*

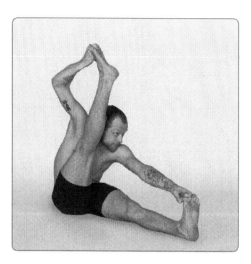

akarna dhanurasana 2
archer's pose 2

shape
(from *akarna dhanurasana 1*)

1. Without moving the right foot forward, straighten the right leg and bring the inner calf to the right ear.
2. Look forward. Hold the pose and breathe.
3. To come out, bend the knee and bring the foot to the ear.

Repeat on the second side.

safety
- If the hamstrings are tight, do not force the upper leg straight.
- Straighten and strengthen both legs. Tighten the knees and quads.
- Engage the toes to prevent cramping.
- Engage the abdomen. Lift the pelvic floor and low belly.
- Pull back on the top big toe and press the big toe into the hand.

refinement
This pose will require all of the strength and flexibility you have in your shoulders and upper back. If you hold the pose long enough, you will also develop strength in the fingers and hands. In *Light On Yoga*, B. K. S. Iyengar says *arkana dhanurasana 2* is "full of grace."[1]

---

[1]   B. K. S. Iyengar, *Light on Yoga* (New York: Schocken Books, 1977) p. 179.

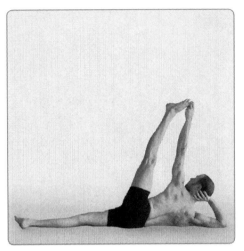
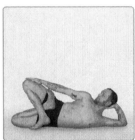

anantasana
endless pose

shape

1. Come onto the front body. Reach the right arm forward and straighten the arm.
2. Roll onto the right side of the body.
3. Lift the head and look up. Bend the right elbow and place the head into the hand.
4. Make a straight line from the right elbow to the hips and from the hips to the feet.
5. Balance on the right side body, lift the top leg, and bend the knee. Hold the big toe with the first two fingers and thumb of the hand.
6. Straighten the left arm and leg. Look up. Hold the pose and breathe.
7. To come out, exhale, bend the top knee and lower the leg. Place the upper hand on the outer left hip. Lift the head, straighten the right arm and return to the front body. Bring the arms by the sides.

Repeat on the second side.

safety

- To reduce the intensity of the hamstring stretch, bend the top knee.
- If the balance is difficult, lower the top leg, squeeze the legs together, and press the hand into the outer thigh. If the balance is still difficult, place the top hand on the floor in front of the chest.
- Lift and lengthen the back of the head with the lower hand.
- Tighten the knees, tone the thighs, and press the lower leg down toward the floor.
- Engage the right glutes.
- Press the outer edge of the bottom foot into the floor.
- Press the big toe into the fingers and pull the big toe with the fingers.
- Lengthen the tailbone down toward the heels and draw the low belly in.

refinement

Anantasana is a surprisingly difficult balancing pose, especially if you keep your hips perpendicular to the floor so the top hip is directly over the bottom hip. It is unique because the balance does not depend on the strength of a single standing leg like in most balancing poses. While the surface area of lying on the side body is larger than the surface area of the sole of the foot, it is more difficult to balance because the center of gravity is much lower. *Vasisthasana* is similar to *anantasana* except in *vasisthasana* the lower arm elevates the body and lifts the center of gravity. While it is more demanding for the wrists and upper back, *vasisthasana* is actually an easier balance. *Anantasana* can also be practiced with the legs in *padmasana* with the top hand on the top knee.

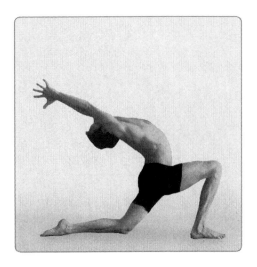 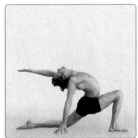

anjaneyasana
monkey lunge pose

shape
(from *lunge pose*)

1. Lower the back knee and top of the back foot to the floor.
2. Move the hips down and forward until the back thigh is at a 45-degree angle.
3. Inhale, lift the torso upright and the arms overhead—wrists above shoulders.
4. Press the palms together and squeeze the elbows in.
5. Exhale, curl the chest up and back.
6. Lift the chin and look up. Hold the pose and breathe.

To come out, inhale, bring the torso and arms vertical. Exhale, release the hands to either side of the front foot. Curl the back toes under, and lift the back knee.

Repeat on the second side.

safety
- Isometrically draw the back knee and front heel toward each other and draw the legs to the midline of the body.
- Press the back foot down and engage the back glutes.
- Press the tailbone down and draw the low belly in.
- Move the base of the sternum back and lift the chest.
- If looking up is too intense for the neck or jaw, look straight ahead.

refinement
Extend yo1ur hands up and back. Stretch your entire spine. To gain more power, interlace your fingers and release your thumbs and index fingers, or simply interlock your thumbs with hands in *anjali mudra*. For a more advanced variation, place your right fingertips to the floor directly below the shoulder and lift your left arm up and back—point the palm up.

Breathe consciously by using your breath to enhance the pose. There are certain actions that complement inhalations, and certain actions that complement exhalations, and it may be different for each person. Discover and differentiate how inhalations and exhalations affect your body in various poses. For some, the inhalations gather strength and stability, while exhalations create space and expansion. For others, it is the exhalations that stabilize and contain energy, while the inhalations create space and expansion. In *anjaneyasana*, use the inhalations to lengthen your spine and tone your low belly. Use the exhalations to curl and lift your chest and to deepen your backbend. Even though the exhalation calls for an action that can feel distinct from that of the inhalation, do not lose strength and stability on the exhalation. Doing one and not the other can cause injury or pain from either excessive flexibility or tightness due to overworked muscles. Yoga offers the opportunity to unify dualities by performing seemingly opposite actions simultaneously. When this is truly being done, you are practicing yoga.

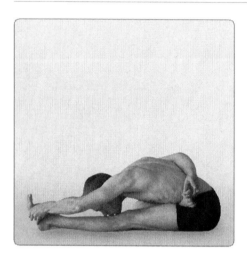

ardha baddha padma paschimottanasana
half bound lotus back stretched out pose

shape
(from *dandasana*)

1. Bring the right palm to the inner right knee.
2. Pull the knee as far right and back as possible so the legs come into an obtuse angle.
3. With the hands, lift the right foot and place the outer right foot on the upper inner left thigh at the crease of the groin. Point the right knee forward and lower the leg.
4. Press the heel into the low belly above and to the left of the pubic bone.
5. Lean to the left and place the left hand on the inner right thigh—fingers between the calf and thigh. As the hip lowers to the floor, spin the thigh down with the left hand and pull the right glutes back with the right hand. Repeat on the other side.
6. Inhale fully. Exhale, swing the right arm behind the back and hold the right big toe with the first two fingers and thumb. Square the torso toward the front of the mat.
7. Inhale, lift the left arm vertical. Exhale, fold the torso over the leg and hold the outer edge of the foot with the left hand.
8. Place the chin on the left shin. Look down. Hold the pose and breathe.
9. To come out, inhale, lift the head. Exhale, bring the front hand directly below the shoulder. Inhale, lift the torso. Exhale, release the back hand. Straighten the folded leg and place the hands next to the hips.

Repeat on the second side.

safety

- Before folding forward, use the hand to pull the front calf muscle out from under the leg. This will encourage the back of the knee to the floor.
- If the leg does not fold into *ardha padmasana*, do not fold forward.
- If the knee does not reach the floor in *ardha padmasana*, place a folded blanket below the thigh and knee for support.
- Press the outer edge/top of the right foot into the left thigh. Press the heel into the low belly.
- Engage the thigh of the extended leg. Press the back of the knee toward/to the floor.
- Press the front foot into the hand and pull the hand into the foot.
- If the forehead does not reach the shin, place the forehead on the edge of one or more blankets or blocks.
- Round the back evenly.

refinement

If you can do *ardha padmasana*, then all you need is to look at a photo to get you into the pose. If you cannot easily come into *ardha padmasana*, there are a few tricks that can help you reach what is otherwise impossible. One of these is what I call the "ratcheting technique." From *dandasana*, pull your right knee as far right and back as possible so that your legs come into an obtuse angle. With your left thumb, press down on your right big-toe mound so the top of your right foot rolls to the floor. Place your right hand on the floor behind your hips and point your left foot. Press your hand down, lift your hips slightly, move the top of your pelvis forward and your sit bones back. Lower your hips. Flex and point your foot in rapid succession to drag your hips forward. As you flex your foot, reach your heel forward and press your heel into the floor. Keep your heel pressing down and point your foot. Repeat several times to move your hips forward to capacity. The ratcheting technique is meant to internally rotate the legs and move the skin and muscles of the legs back. Once your legs are in position, continue into *ardha baddha padma paschimottanasana* with the above shape instructions. For me, the ratcheting technique is a very effective way to align the legs and hips in *janu sirsasana*, *paschimottanasana*, and *upavishta konasana*.

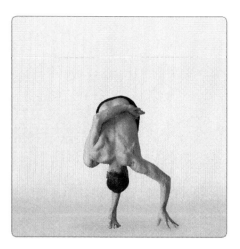

ardha baddha padmottanasana
half bound lotus stretched out pose

shape

(from *tadasana*)

1. Lift the right leg and hold the ankle with the right hand—arm to inside of the leg. Hold the top of the foot with the left hand.
2. Lift the knee higher than the hips and place the heel against the low belly just above the pubic bone.
3. Keeping the heel in place, continue to hold the right foot with the left hand and point the knee straight down.
4. Swing the right arm behind the back and hold the right big toe with the first two fingers and the thumb.
5. Inhale, lift the left arm vertical. Exhale, fold the torso over the standing leg.
6. Place the left fingertips on the floor 6 to 8 inches outside of the foot.
7. Round the back evenly and bring the chin toward/to the left shin. Hold the pose and breathe.
8. To come out, stretch the left arm forward. Inhale, lift the torso to stand. Release the right hand and lower the right leg. Bring the arms by the sides.

Repeat on the second side.

safety

*   If clasping the foot behind the back is not accessible, use a strap around the top of the lifted foot.
*   Flex the top foot and flare the outer two toes. Push the outer edge of the top foot into the groin.
*   Engage the thigh of the standing leg—lift the kneecap.
*   Move the tailbone down and draw the low belly in.
*   Lift the shoulders up away from the floor.
*   To reduce the intensity in the low back, place the lower hand on the hip before lifting to stand.

refinement

Point your bent knee straight down. Level your hips. For a more intense variation of this pose, hold the calf of your standing leg with your bottom hand.

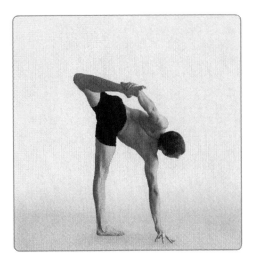

ardha chandrachapasana
half moon bow pose

shape
(from *ardha chandrasana*)

1. Exhale, look down.
2. Turn the lower hand toward the long edge of the mat.
3. Point the top foot, then flare the outer two toes.
4. Bend the top knee and hold the foot with the left hand.
5. Lift the knee slightly higher than the top hip. Point the knee back.
6. Rotate the top shoulder over the bottom shoulder.
7. Kick the top foot back and reach the chest forward. Curl the head and upper torso back. Look straight back. Hold the pose and breathe.
8. To come out, exhale, look down. Release the foot and straighten the leg. Lift the top arm vertical.

Repeat on the second side.

safety

- Point the standing foot forward.
- Strengthen the standing leg, especially the quads and hamstrings.
- Turn the standing thigh out until the kneecap points straight ahead.
- Move the tailbone down and draw low belly in.
- Engage the top foot—do not sickle the ankle.
- Point the lower bicep forward.
- If the torso and upper hip collapse toward the floor, place a block under the bottom hand and use a strap around the top foot. Keep the top arm straight by holding the strap as close to the foot as possible.
- If it is difficult to balance, prop the back foot up on a counter or table of appropriate height. Use the stability assist to discover the backbending action of the pose while reducing the risk of falling over.

refinement

Move your top shoulder back. Extend your top knee and chest away from your hips. If your back-bend is very deep, move the lower hand out so it remains underneath your shoulder. This will create more space to deepen the backbend in your chest and upper torso and will improve your balance. Slide the sides of your throat back and lift your chin.

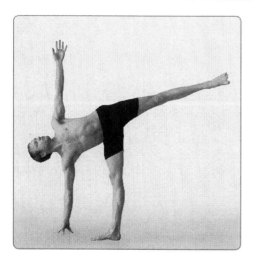

ardha chandrasana
half moon pose

shape
(from *tadasana*, facing long edge of mat)

1. Inhale, bend the knees.
2. Exhale, take a wide stance. Bring the arms parallel to the floor.
3. Turn the left foot in 30 degrees, right foot out 90 degrees.
4. Inhale fully. Exhale, bend the right knee, and place the right fingertips on the floor outside of the foot, left hand on left hip. Look down.
5. Step the back foot in half way and move the right hand forward 12 inches—hand below shoulder.
6. Keep the left leg straight and right knee bent. Lift the left foot slightly higher than the hip.
7. Rotate the left hip over the right hip, left shoulder over the right shoulder.
8. Exhale, straighten the right leg.
9. Lift the left hand vertical—thumb pointing forward.
10. Look up. Hold the pose and breathe.
11. To come out, exhale, look down. Bend the front knee and point the back foot. Reach the foot down to the floor and take a long stance. Hop the right hand back, next to the right foot. Inhale, lift the torso vertical. Straighten the front leg. Exhale, parallel the feet. Bring the feet together and lower the arms.

Repeat on the second side.

safety

- Engage the quads of the standing leg—lift the kneecap.
- Move the top thigh back and tailbone forward.

- Move the top foot forward in line with the hips.
- Engage the top glutes.
- Turn the thigh of the standing leg out until the kneecap points straight ahead.
- Rotate the abdomen and ribs up.
- Move the base of sternum back.
- Point the biceps toward the top of the mat.
- To reduce the intensity of the hamstring stretch, place the right hand on a block or chair, or slightly bend the right knee.
- If it is difficult to balance, place the back foot on a wall.
- If looking up is too intense for the neck or jaw, look down.

refinement

Press your bottom fingertips down and extend your top hand up. Extend your top foot and head away from your hips. Just as the moon lifts ocean tides, practice can uplift our mental and emotional state. It is said that the physical poses of hatha yoga move *prana* (subtle energy force) from the *ida* and *pingala nadis* (two of the side subtle energy channels, which are responsible for ignorant desire and ignorant dislike) into what is called *sushumna nadi* (the central energy channel). When this hatha-happens, a palpable sense of well-being occurs, which any practitioner of hatha yoga is likely familiar with. It is also said that the physical practice of hatha yoga prepares one for meditation. Another perspective is that the practice of hatha yoga creates an interest in meditation because the practitioner wants more of what hatha yoga offers. One place to find that is in meditation. Ready, sit, go!

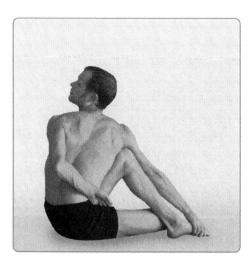

ardha matsyendrasana 1
half Lord of the Fishes pose 1

shape
(from *ardha matsyendrasana 1 prep*)

1. Look at the front foot.
2. Straighten the front arm and clasp the inner edge of the foot with the hand.
3. Swing the left arm behind the back and clasp the outer right thigh with the left fingers.
4. Inhale fully. Exhale, twist the torso to the left. Look over the left shoulder.
5. To come out, release the hands and place the hands next to the hips. Lean back and straighten the legs.

Repeat on the second side.

safety

- If the low back rounds, sit on one or more blankets and/or straighten the bottom leg.
- If the shoulder does not reach the outer knee, practice *ardha matsyendrasana 1 prep* instead.
- If the front arm hyperextends, push the elbow and back of the arm into the shin.
- Straighten and strengthen the front arm—engage the triceps.
- Press the front foot and hand into each other.
- Isometrically squeeze the back foot and sit bone toward each other.
- Press the front shoulder into the knee and the knee into the shoulder.
- Turn the abdomen to the left.
- Move both shoulders back.
- Lift the left elbow up and back.
- Lift the pelvic floor and tone the low belly.

refinement

Press your back fingers into your thigh and press the back wrist into your torso to deepen the twist. At first, it may be difficult to clasp your front foot with your hand. To make the clasp easier and prevent hyperextension, turn your front foot out 30 degrees toward your lower knee.

Hyperextension is not necessarily problematic if there is stability around the hyperextended joint. However, over time it may cause pain. Weight bearing on or through a hyperextended joint, even with relative stability, is not ideal. Hyperextension is not an injury or condition. It is a habit in which hyper-mobile joints push beyond straight. To retrain the tendency to hyperextend, stabilize the joint by consciously engaging the muscles surrounding the joint. This means that the joint may not appear bent to a spectator, but will likely feel bent to someone who is used to pushing past straight. While hyperextension may not reveal immediate discomfort, restrain from extending to capacity to avoid long-term damage.

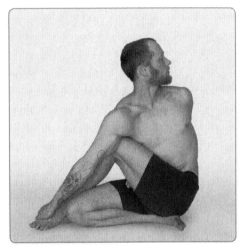
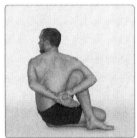

ardha matsyendrasana 1
half Lord of the Fishes pose 1

hips on feet, clasping front foot

shape
(from *purvottanasana* prep)

1. Look forward.
2. Lift the right leg parallel to the floor and point the foot.
3. Kick the right foot back underneath the hips and lower the knee. Point the toes to the left and bring the top of the foot to the floor. Point the right knee straight ahead.
4. Lower the sit bones onto the foot—right sit bone to inside of the heel, left sit bone to inside of the big toe mound.
5. Walk the hands forward and sit upright.
6. Bring the left foot to the outside of the right knee.
7. Place the left hand on the left thigh.
8. Inhale, lift the right arm vertical. Exhale, twist the torso to the left and bring the left shoulder to the outer left knee.
9. Look at the front foot and clasp the inner edge of the foot with the right hand.
10. Swing the left arm behind the back and press the fingertips into the outer right thigh.
11. Inhale, lengthen the spine. Exhale, twist the torso to the left and look over the shoulder. Hold the pose and breathe.
12. To come out, exhale, look forward. Release the hands and walk the hands back behind the hips. Lift the hips, uncross the legs, and place the feet on the floor hip-distance apart.

Repeat on the second side.

safety

- If the shoulder cannot reach the outer knee, practice *ardha matsyendrasana 1 prep* instead.
- If there is pain or discomfort from bearing weight on the bottom foot, engage the foot by pressing the toes down and apart. If there is still pain, place a blanket between the foot and the hips.
- If the front arm hyperextends, push the elbow and back of the arm into the shin.
- Straighten and strengthen the front arm—engage the triceps.
- Press the front foot and hand into each other. Isometrically squeeze the back foot and sit bone toward each other.
- Press the front shoulder into the knee and the knee into the shoulder.
- Turn the abdomen to the left.
- Move both shoulders back.
- Lift the left elbow up and back.
- Press the back wrist into the torso to deepen the twist.
- Lift the pelvic floor and tone the low belly.

refinement

Another variation is to bind your hands behind your back rather than extending your front arm and holding the foot. This is among my favorite poses to teach and practice. Maybe it is because Sage Matsyendra is regarded as one of the founding fathers of hatha yoga. The essence of the practice is held in this pose. Maybe, and maybe not. One thing is for sure: We all have our pose preferences. I once told my mom that I did not like practicing *parivrtta trikonasana*. She said, "Take that as a sign that it has something special to offer you." And sure enough, I now regard this pose as a national treasure—it continues to offer endless insights and benefits to me. Consider developing a penchant for the poses you avoid practicing (but not the ones that are beyond your physical capacity).

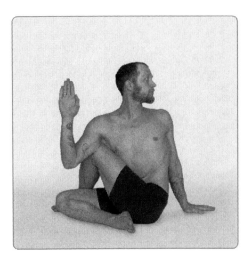

ardha matsyendrasana 1 prep
half Lord of the Fishes pose 1

shape
(from *dandasana*)

1. Bend the knees and place the soles of the feet on the floor.
2. Place the hands on the floor behind the hips.
3. Lean back and lift the shins parallel to the floor. Point the toes.
4. Place the right heel to the outer left hip. Lower the leg.
5. Place the left foot on the floor to the outside of the right knee.
6. Place the left hand on the left thigh.
7. Inhale, lift the right arm vertical. Exhale, twist the torso to the left and bring the right shoulder or upper arm to the outer left knee—bend the elbow and point the palm to the side.
8. Place the left hand on the floor a few inches behind the sacrum.
9. Inhale, lengthen the spine. Exhale twist the torso to the left. Look over the left shoulder. Hold the pose and breathe.
10. To come out, inhale, look forward and place the hands next to the hips. Lean back and lift the shins parallel to the floor. Lower and straighten the legs.

Repeat on the second side.

safety

*   If the low back rounds, sit on one or more blankets and/or straighten the bottom leg.
*   If the shoulder does not reach the outer knee, press the upper arm or outer elbow into the knee instead.
*   To gain more lift in the chest, bring the outer elbow to the knee before twisting.
*   Press the inner edge of the front foot and the top of the back foot down.
*   Press the front shoulder into top knee and push the knee into the shoulder.
*   Move both shoulders back and lift the chest.
*   Lift the pelvic floor and tone the low belly.

refinement

Lift your ribcage away from your waist to lengthen both sides of your torso. Isometrically push your lower hand down and out to twist even more. Gaze out of the corners of your eyes. This is a doable and effective way to warm up the knees, hips, and spine.

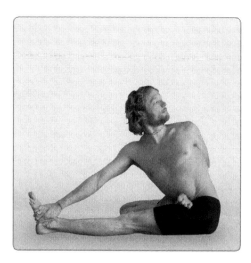

ardha matsyendrasana 2
half Lord of the Fishes pose 2

shape
(from *dandasana*)

1. Bring the right palm to the inner right knee.
2. Pull the knee as far right and back as possible so that the legs come into an obtuse angle.
3. With the hands, lift the right foot and place it on the upper inner left thigh at the crease of the groin. Point the right knee forward and lower the leg.
4. Press the heel into the low belly above, and to the left of, the pubic bone.
5. Lean to the left and place the left hand on the inner right thigh—fingers between the calf and thigh. As the hip lowers to the floor, spin the thigh down with the left hand and pull the right glutes back with the right hand.
6. Inhale fully. Exhale, swing the left arm behind the back and hold the top of the shin with the left hand.
7. Inhale fully. Exhale, lean forward and twist to the left to hold the outer edge of the left foot with the right hand. Straighten the right arm.
8. Turn the head and look past the left shoulder. Hold the pose and breathe.
9. To come out, inhale, look forward. Exhale, release the hands and straighten the leg.

Repeat on the second side.

safety

- If the low back rounds, sit on one or more blankets.
- If the back hand cannot reach the shin, hold the inner thigh instead.
- If the front hand cannot reach the front foot, use a strap to hold the foot. Straighten the arm.
- If the bent knee lifts off the floor, place a folded blanket beneath the knee.
- Press the outer edge/top of the foot into the thigh. Push the heel into the low belly.
- Engage the foot and thigh of the extended leg. Press the back of the knee into the floor.
- Press the back hand and top foot into each other.
- Lift the pelvic floor and tone the low belly.
- Move the base of the sternum back and lift the chest.

refinement

To deepen the twist, press the outer edge of your back wrist into the ribcage. What makes this pose difficult is clasping the shin with the hand behind the back. This will require you to lean forward rather than sit perfectly upright. This hand-to-leg position stretches the front of the shoulder. *Ardha matsyendrasana 2* is a good preparatory pose for *kasyapasana, paripurna matsyendrasana, yoga mudrasana,* and *supta vajrasana.*

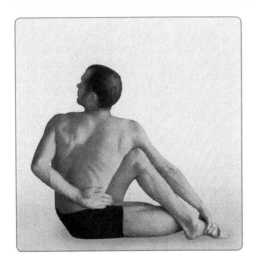

ardha matsyendrasana 3
half Lord of the Fishes pose 3

shape
(from *dandasana*)

1. Bring the right leg into *ardha padmasana.*
2. Keep the right knee on the floor and place the left heel just in front of the left sit bone—knee pointing up.
3. Place the left hand to the outside of the left hip. Lean onto the right hip and hold the left shin with the right hand.
4. Lift the left foot up and over the right knee. Place the foot on the floor outside of the knee.
5. In one quick movement, press the left hand into the left thigh and twist the torso to the left to bring the right shoulder to the outside of the left knee.
6. Straighten the right arm and hold the top of the left foot with the hand.
7. Inhale fully. Exhale, swing the left arm behind the back. Place the back of the hand just above the right hip at the waistline.
8. Inhale fully. Exhale, rotate the abdomen and head to the left and look straight back. Hold the pose and breathe.
9. To come out, inhale, look forward. Exhale, release the hands next to the hips. Release and straighten both legs.

Repeat on the second side.

safety

- If it is difficult to balance during or while coming into the pose, place a folded blanket under the lifted hip.
- Tighten all the joints in the *ardha padmasana* leg. Push the heel and big toe mound into the abdomen and push the top of the foot into the lifted thigh.
- Use the hands to make as much space as possible in the abdomen for the *ardha padmasana* foot.
- Do not practice deep twists or poses in which the foot or heel pushes the abdomen for many hours after eating.
- If the front hand does not reach the front foot, keep the heel down but turn the toes toward the lower knee before clasping the foot. Otherwise, use a strap around the front foot.
- Press the back hand into the torso.
- If there is pain in the back shoulder or if the back hand cannot reach the side waist, wrap a strap around the *ardha padmasana* foot before coming into the pose, and hold the strap with the back hand.
- Press the front arm and knee into each other to empower the twist.
- Reach the chest forward and lift the sternum.
- Lift the pelvic floor.

refinement

Ardha matsyendrasana 3 is a difficult pose because of the *ardha padmasana* leg position. Lift the *ardha padmasana* foot higher into your abdomen and point your knee as forward as possible in order to step the other foot over your knee. If this pose is too difficult, practice *ardha matsyendrasana 1* and *marichyasana 2* instead.

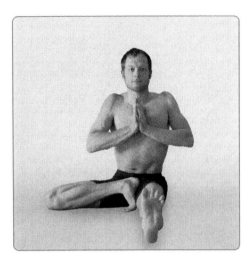

ardha mulabandhasana
half root lock pose

shape
(from *dandasana*)

1. Bring the right palm to the inner right knee.
2. Pull the knee back without moving the hips—outer leg and knee to floor.
3. Hold the right foot with the hands. Flex the foot and lift the foot and knee off the floor.
4. Place the right heel just above the pubic bone and bring the shin parallel to the floor.
5. Flex the toes back and lower the toe mounds to the floor just in front of the pubic bone.
6. Place the hands on the floor behind the hips. Inhale, lift the hips up and forward to push the foot vertical.
7. Place the right knee on the floor. Exhale, lower the hips to the floor.
8. Place the palms together in front of the chest. Look forward. Hold the pose and breathe.
9. To come out, release the hands and use the hands to release the foot. Straighten the leg.

Repeat on the second side.

safety
- If the low back rounds, if the foot in front of the pubic bone does not flex into a vertical position, or if there is pain or discomfort in the knee, sit on one or more folded blankets.
- Press the tips of the flexed toes down.
- Press the inner thigh of the bent leg down.
- Squeeze the bent knee to protect the knee.
- Engage the extended leg. Squeeze the leg straight and press the back of the knee into the floor. Point the toes up and push the mound of the big toe forward, pull the outer foot back.
- Move the base of the sternum back and lift the chest.
- Lift the pelvic floor and tone the low belly.

refinement
Elevated *vajrasana* can prepare the toes for this intense pose. If there is a sense of bulkiness in your calf as you come into the pose, use your hand (on the same side as the bent leg) to lift your calf muscle up as you bend your knee. Bringing the foot into a vertical position requires a great range of external rotation. To create more space around your hip joint, lean forward and pull

your glutes back from underneath your sit bone of the bent leg. Reach your hand on the same side as your bent leg between your groin and shin and pull the inner edge of your foot back. This will bring your toe mounds directly below your heel. Allow the knee of your bent leg to move forward if necessary. Eventually, reach your knee directly out to the side.

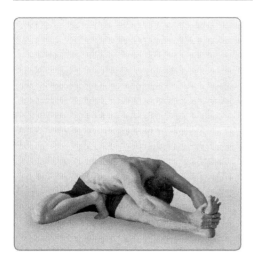

ardha mulabandhasana
half root lock pose

forward fold

shape
(from *ardha mulabandhasana,* upright)

1. Inhale, lift the spine. Exhale, fold the torso forward and hold the front foot with both hands.
2. Inhale, lift the chin and look up.
3. Exhale, fold the torso over the extended leg and place the forehead on the knee. Hold the pose and breathe.
4. To come out, inhale, lift the head and torso. Exhale, release the hands to the floor directly below the shoulders. Push the hands into the floor to lift the torso upright. Use the hands to release the foot. Straighten the leg.

Repeat on the second side.

safety
- If the low back rounds, if the foot in front of the pubic bone does not flex into a vertical position, or if there is pain or discomfort in the knee, sit on one or more folded blankets.
- Press the tips of the flexed toes down.
- Press the inner thigh of the bent leg down.
- Squeeze the bent knee to protect the knee.
- Engage the extended leg. Squeeze the leg straight and press the back of the knee into the floor. Point the toes up and push the mound of the big toe forward, pull the outer foot back.
- Push the foot into the hands and pull the foot with the hands. Extend the elbows out.
- Lift the pelvic floor and tone the low belly.
- Stretch the entire spine and round the back evenly.

refinement

Certain poses can rekindle and inspire your practice. I remember seeing a photo of Sharon Gannon, co-founder of Jivamukti Yoga, in *yogadandasana*. I had never seen the pose before and I decided to try it that day during practice. I realized quickly that in order to get into *yogadandasana* I would need more flexibility in my hips. My desire to get into *yogadandasana* inspired a much more intensive hip opening practice for the next several weeks. I hope *ardha mulabhandasana* inspires a similar response in you!

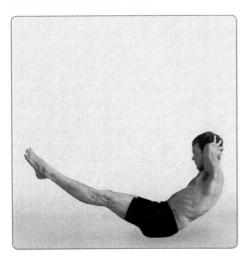

ardha navasana
half boat pose

shape
(from *dandasana*)

1. Slide the hands a foot and a half back—fingers pointed forward.
2. Bend the elbows and lean the torso back until the shoulders are directly above the hands.
3. Point the feet.
4. Lift the feet off the floor and press the feet and legs together. Pause and breathe.
5. Lift the feet higher until they are in line with the face.
6. Interlace the hands behind the head. Look straight ahead. Hold the pose and breathe.
7. To come out, release the hands, lower the legs, and lift the torso upright. Place the hands next to the hips.

safety

- If this pose is too difficult, keep your hands on the floor underneath the shoulders.
- Engage the legs fully. Straighten the legs and lock them into a straight position.
- Engage the glutes to help lift the feet.
- Lift the pelvic floor and tone the low belly.
- If the legs or abdomen begin to quiver or shake, come out of *ardha navasana* immediately.

refinement

"The cure for pain is in the pain," said the 13th century mystical poet Rumi.[1] This practice puts us into stressful situations for the sake of stress destruction. Oftentimes it is the more challenging classes that leave us feeling the most calm and relaxed. Challenge, by the way, has nothing to do with degree of difficulty, but rather depth of practice. To benefit from *ardha navasana,* keep your face, eyes, and jaw relaxed. Breathe slowly and deeply, and smile. See how difficult it is to have a bad time with a smile on your face. This is how yoga works. By shifting your shape, the shape shifts your state. The next time you are angry, frustrated, or overwhelmed, practice one of the most advanced asanas there is: smile.

[1] Jalal al-Din Rumi, Coleman Barks (translator), *The Essential Rumi* (San Francisco: Harper Collins, 1995) p. 205.

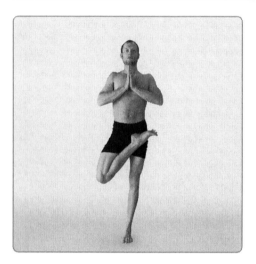

ardha padmasana
half lotus pose

standing

shape
(from *tadasana*)

1. Lift the right leg and hold the ankle with the right hand—arm to inside of leg. Hold the top of the foot with the left hand.
2. Lift the knee higher than the hips and place the heel against the low belly just above the pubic bone.
3. Keeping the heel in place, continue to hold the right foot with the left hand and point the knee down.
4. Bring the palms together at the middle of the sternum.
5. Look straight ahead. Hold the pose and breathe.
6. To come out, use the hands to lower the right foot. Bring the arms by the sides.

Repeat on the second side.

safety

- Flex the top foot and flare the outer two toes.
- Push the outer edge of the top foot into the groin.
- Engage the thigh of the standing leg—lift the kneecap.
- Move the tailbone down and draw the low belly in.
- Move the base of the sternum back and lift the chest.
- Shrug the shoulders up and back.
- If there is pain in the knee, come out of the pose immediately.

refinement

For a more intense variation, bring your bent knee toward your standing leg until your thigh is perfectly vertical. *Ardha padmasana* requires flexibility in the hips and the ability to externally rotate the thighs. Using half lotus as a way to open your hips is possible yet precarious. Generally, it is safer to open the hips with other poses and then come into *ardha padmasana*. In my public classes, I never teach half lotus. I only teach it in workshop settings because it is a very sophisticated pose that requires detailed alignment instructions. Many students have injured their knees attempting to get into half or full lotus. I call getting into full lotus at the expense of the knees "fool lotus."

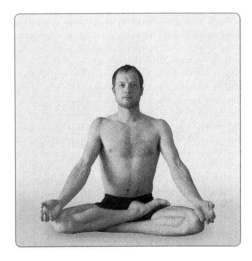

ardha padmasana
half lotus pose

shape
(from *dandasana*)

1. Bend the left knee and place the left heel against the perineum. Lower the top of the foot and shin to the floor.
2. Bend the right knee and point the foot.
3. Hold the right ankle with the right hand and the top of the foot with the left hand.
4. Lift the right foot, knee, and hip off the floor. Place the outer right foot on the upper inner left thigh at the crease of the groin.
5. Keeping the right foot in place, lower the right hip and knee to the floor.
6. Press the inner left big toe and toe mound between the right calf and thigh.

7. Place the hands on the knees. Join the tips of the thumbs and index fingers together and turn the palms up.
8. Look straight ahead. Hold the pose and breathe.
9. To come out, release the fingers and hold the right foot with the right hand. Slowly slide the foot to the floor and straighten the leg. Straighten the left leg and join the legs and feet. Place the hands by the sides.

Repeat on the second side.

safety

- Press the outer edge/top of the right foot into the thigh/groin to resist sickling the foot.
- Press the outer edge of the bottom foot down.
- Tilt the pelvis forward and curve the low back in.
- Lift the pelvic floor. Tone and lift the entire abdomen.
- Move the base of the sternum back and lift the chest.
- Level the shoulders and center the crown of the head over the pelvic floor. Lift the chin slightly.

refinement

Any pain in your knees is problematic if ignored. Some poses appear to depend on the flexibility of the knees to achieve the final forms. The knee, however, is a fragile joint that should never be stretched or strained to come into these poses. These types of poses, like *ardha padmasana*, require flexibility in the hips, legs, and ankles. Once this is achieved, there will be no pain or discomfort in the knee. To prepare for *ardha padmasana* or *padmasana*, practice hip and quad stretches regularly in your practice, and then return to this pose. Sometimes the safest way to get into a pose is through other poses. Other times, the best way to get into a pose is through the pose itself.

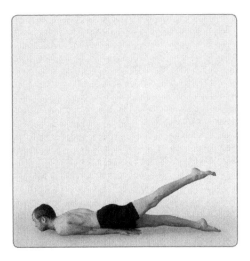

ardha salabhasana
half locust pose

shape

1. Bring the front body and chin to the floor.
2. Extend the arms alongside the body with the palms facing down.
3. Move the knees forward slightly and lift the hips.
4. Bring the outer edges of the hands together underneath the legs.
5. Slide the elbows underneath the torso.
6. Lower the hips onto the arms and straighten the legs. Bring the inner edges of the feet together.
7. Inhale, lift the left leg to capacity. Look forward. Hold the pose and breathe.
8. To come out, exhale, lower the lifted leg. Lift the hips to release the hands.

Repeat on the second side.

safety

- Press the fingertips and the perimeter of the palms into the floor with equal pressure.
- Lock both legs into a straight position.
- Press the bottom foot down and tighten the knee.
- Point the kneecap of the lifted leg straight down and engage the glutes.
- Bring the feet halfway between a pointed and flexed position. Spread the toes.
- To reduce pressure on the elbows, point the palms up instead of down.
- If there is pain or discomfort in the neck, place the forehead on the floor and look down.
- If there is pain or discomfort at the front of the shoulders, widen the hands.

refinement

Ardha salabhasana stretches the front of the neck, the upper back, shoulders, and elbows. It strengthens the low back, glutes, and legs. *Ardha salabhasana* is a good alternative if *viparita salabhasana prep* is too intense.

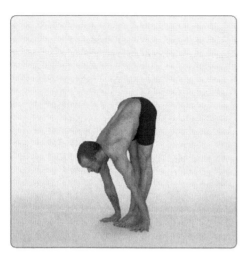
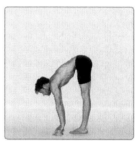

ardha uttanasana
half forward fold pose

shape
(from *tadasana*)

1. Inhale fully. Exhale, fold the torso over the legs.
2. Place the hands next to the feet—fingers in line with the toes.
3. Inhale, keep the hands on the floor and lift the torso. Straighten the arms, lift the chin, and look up. Hold the pose and breathe.
4. To come out, exhale, fold forward to *uttanasana*. Inhale, lift the torso to stand.

safety

- Squeeze the feet and legs together.
- Engage the legs, especially the thighs.
- Lift the kneecaps up.
- Lock the legs into a straight position.
- Press the tops of the feet down to engage the calves.
- Move the tailbone down and the low belly in.
- To reduce strain in the low back and hamstrings, separate the feet outer hip-width apart and bring the hands directly under the shoulders. Place the fingertips on the floor or on blocks, and bend the knees slightly.

refinement

This pose is found twice in *surya namaskar A*. Like *indudalasana,* this pose can become a dynamic movement by moving into and out of it with your breath. Inhale to *ardha uttanasana.* Exhale to *uttanasana.* Repeat this several times with your breath to warm up the body. While this pose may seem simple, try to access a back-bending aspect in this forward fold.

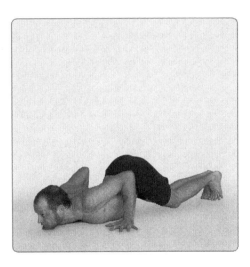

astangasana
eight angle pose

shape
(from *plank pose*)

1. Separate the hands slightly wider than shoulder-distance apart—middle of the wrists in line with the outer shoulders.
2. Separate the fingers and point the index fingers straight ahead.
3. Inhale, keep the hips elevated. Exhale, lower the knees, chest, and chin to the floor. Bring the wrists directly below the elbows and the chest between the hands.
4. Look straight ahead. Hold the pose and breathe.
5. To come out, lift the torso and knees.

safety
- Do not put any weight on the chin.
- Press the fingertips and the perimeter of the palms into the floor with equal pressure. Especially press the inner hands down and squeeze the shoulder blades together on the back.
- Lift the shoulders to capacity.
- Tone the pelvic floor, press the tailbone down, and lift the low belly.

refinement
Astangasana is among the most effective warm up poses. I often practice and teach it in place of *chaturanga dandasana* during *surya namaskar*. For a slightly more intense variation, lift the hands a few inches off the floor and hold for 20 to 30 seconds.

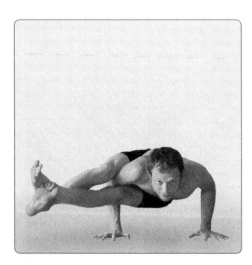

astavakrasana
eight crooks pose

shape
(from *eka hasta bhujasana*)

1. With the right knee bent, bend the left knee and cross the left ankle over the right ankle. Flex both feet and press the tops of the feet into each other.
2. Bend the left arm slightly.
3. Squeeze the legs and ankles together. Pause and breathe.
4. Bend the elbows 90 degrees so the forearms are vertical and the upper arms are parallel to the floor. Extend the legs to the right while lowering the torso parallel to the floor. Straighten the legs to capacity.
5. Look to the right, left, or straight ahead. Hold the pose and breathe.
6. To come out, exhale, straighten the arms, and lift the torso and legs. Release the top ankle and extend the top leg forward.

Repeat on the second side.

safety

- Press the fingertips and the perimeter of the right hand evenly into the floor—press the mound of the index finger down and lift the outer wrist up.
- Resist the tendency to let the shoulders collapse toward the floor. Lift and level the shoulders. The shoulder bearing the weight of the legs tends to drop.
- Squeeze the elbows in.
- Spin the thigh of the bottom leg out to press the bottom hip back.

refinement

This arm balance may be easier than you think. Once you have developed the strength and flexibility for *eka hasta bhujasana*, you have what it takes to perform this pose.

To make *astavakrasana* more accessible, begin in *eka hasta bhujasana*, then lower your hips and extended leg to the floor. Lean back on your hips and cross your left ankle over your right ankle. Lean forward, press your right knee into your right arm and lift your hips up. Bend your elbows to 90 degrees, lower your torso parallel to the floor, and squeeze the legs together while straightening your legs to the right.

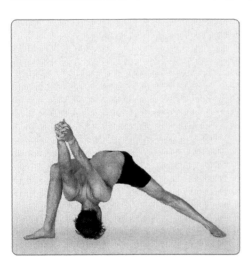

baddha hasta parsvakonasana
bound hands side angle pose

shape
(from *lunge pose*)

1. Pivot the back heel down and turn the foot in 60 degrees.
2. Interlace the fingers behind the sacrum.
3. Bend the elbows. Bring the shoulder blades together on the back.
4. Inhale, lift the torso slightly and straighten the arms.
5. Exhale, lower the head toward/to the floor inside the front foot. Keep weight off the head if it reaches the floor.
6. Stretch the arms up and overhead.
7. Tilt the front shin out slightly. Hold the pose and breathe.
8. To come out, inhale, lift the head and torso. Exhale, release the hands to either side of the foot. Lift the back heel.

Repeat on the second side with the alternate clasp.

safety
- Squeeze the feet toward each other.
- Press the back foot down.
- Move the right hip back until the front thigh is parallel to the long edge of the mat.
- If there is discomfort in the back inner knee, tone the thigh, lift the kneecap, and lift the hips slightly.
- Move the tailbone down and lift the low belly.
- If the shoulders are tight, keep the elbows bent.
- Lift the shoulder blades up.

refinement
Extend your hands forward to fully stretch your shoulders. To deepen the shoulder stretch, press your palms together.

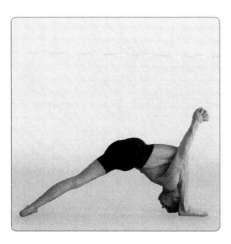

baddha hasta parsvakonasana
bound hands side angle pose

variation

shape
(from *lunge pose*)

1. Pivot the back heel down and turn the foot in 60 degrees.
2. Bring the right hand to the inside of the right foot. Inhale fully. Exhale, fold the torso to the inside of the front thigh.
3. Bring the right shoulder underneath the right knee.
4. Place the back of the right hand against the outer right hip.
5. Swing the left arm back behind the torso.
6. Interlace the fingers and straighten the arms. Press the palms together or pull the wrists apart.
7. Place the forehead toward/to the floor to the inside of the front foot. Hold the pose and breathe.
8. To come out, release the hands to the floor. Lift the torso up from under the leg. Bring both hands to the floor. Lift the back heel.

Repeat on the second side with the alternate clasp.

safety
- Squeeze the feet toward each other.
- Press the back foot down. Move the right hip back until the front thigh is parallel to the long edge of the mat.
- Move the tailbone down and lift the low belly.
- If the shoulders are tight, keep the elbows bent.
- Move the shoulders away from the head.

refinement
What is interesting to me about this pose is that I have never actually done it in a practice. The only time I've ever done it in my life is for the photo to be taken. So I will be practicing it soon to research its benefits. That is a practice I recommend: Look through this book to find a pose you rarely or never practice. Mix it into your practice several times to see what it has to offer and how it affects your practice and perspective. Try it. I dharma-dare you. I dharma-double-down-dog-dare you!

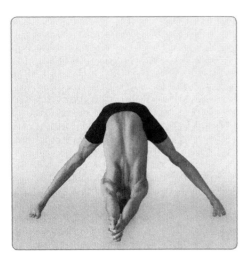

baddha hasta prasarita padottanasana
wide legs forward fold pose

hands bound

shape
(from *tadasana*, facing long edge of mat)

1. Place the hands on the hips.
2. Inhale, bend the knees. Exhale, take a wide stance and straighten the legs.
3. Interlace the fingers behind the sacrum.
4. Bend the elbows; squeeze the shoulders together on the back.
5. Straighten the arms. Press the palms together.
6. Inhale, lengthen the spine.
7. Exhale, fold forward—bring the top of the head toward/to the floor.
8. Extend the hands overhead, toward the floor. Hold the pose and breathe.
9. To come out, place the hands on the hips. Inhale, lift the torso to stand. Exhale, bring the feet together and lower the arms.

safety
- To reduce the intensity of the stretch, keep the knees and elbows bent, or place the forehead on a block.
- Engage the calves, quads, hamstrings—lift the kneecaps up.
- Simultaneously stretch the shoulders toward the floor and lift the shoulder blades up toward the ears.
- If there is pain or discomfort in the shoulders, pull the wrists apart.
- Do not put any weight on the head.

refinement
Extend your hands away from your torso. Press your feet down and apart. For a deeper variation, engage your abdomen, lengthen your spine, place the back of your head on the floor between your feet, and look up.

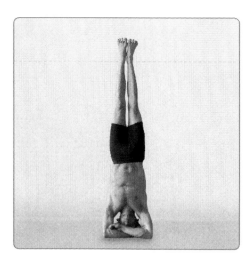

baddha hasta sirsasana
bound hands headstand pose

shape
(from *sirsasana* 2)

1. Extend down through the head and in one movement, bring the forearms to the floor in front of the forehead.
2. Hold the left elbow with the right hand. Hold the right elbow with the left hand. Look forward. Hold the pose and breathe.
3. To come out, bend the elbows and place the hands on the floor in front of the face shoulder-width apart.

Repeat on the second side—switch the cross of the arms.

safety

- Press the forearms down and lift the shoulders up.
- Stretch up through the legs and feet.
- Press the inner feet, ankles, and knees together.
- Engage the glutes and abdomen.
- Move the base of the sternum back and press the tailbone forward.
- If the balance is difficult, practice against or near a wall.

refinement

Of all the *sirsasana* arm variations, you will most likely lose your balance coming into *baddha hasta sirsasana*. My strategy in keeping my balance is to close my eyes as I bring the forearms to the floor in front of my face. Once in *baddha hasta sirsasana,* however, it is relatively easy to balance.

If moving from *sirsasana* 2 into *baddha hasta sirsasana* proves to be too difficult, start in *vajrasana*. Any of these headstand variations can also be approached from *sirsasana 1* or *2*.

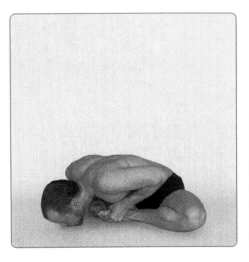
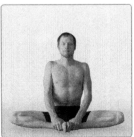

baddha konasana
bound angle pose

forward fold

shape
(from *dandasana*)

1. Bend both knees out to the sides and bring the soles of the feet together.
2. Bring your heels in line with your knees. Lower the knees to the floor.
3. Lift the torso upright.
4. Lean onto the left sit bone and hold the inner right thigh with the left hand, outer right thigh with the right hand. Roll the inner thigh down and pull the flesh from underneath the right sit bone out. Keeping the right hip back, lower the right sit bone to the floor. Repeat on the second side.
5. Keep the outer edges of the feet joined and separate the soles of the feet. Point the soles of the feet up.
6. Inhale fully. Exhale, fold the torso over the legs and lower the forehead to the floor. Bring the tip of the nose and chin to the floor.
7. Round the back evenly. Hold the pose and breathe.
8. To come out, lift the head and look forward. Inhale, lift the torso upright. Bring the hands to the outer knees and draw the knees together. Place the hands next to the hips and straighten the legs.

safety

- If the inner edges of the knees are higher than the waistline or the low back is rounded before folding forward, sit up on one or more blankets.
- If the knees do not reach the floor with the torso upright, do not fold forward. Practice *tarasana* instead.
- Press the feet together and squeeze them toward the hips to extend out through the knees.
- Turn the skin of the inner ankles forward, skin of the outer ankles backward.

refinement

Instead of pushing your knees down, isometrically lift your feet up. *Baddha konasana* is also an excellent way to prepare the nervous system for *savasana* after backbends.

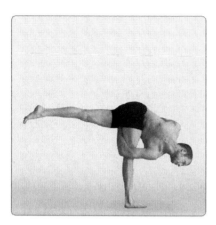

baddha parivrtta ardha chandrasana
bound revolved half moon pose

shape
(from *lunge pose*)

1. Place the right hand on the upper right thigh.
2. Inhale, lift the torso and left arm vertical.
3. Exhale, twist the torso to the right and place the left shoulder on the outer right knee.
4. Swing the left hand underneath the hips and place the back of the hand on the left side of the torso.
5. Swing the right arm behind the back. Hold the right wrist with the left hand.
6. Look down at the front foot and step the back foot halfway toward the front foot.
7. Shift the weight forward and lift the back leg parallel to the floor. Straighten the front leg.
8. Rotate the top shoulder over the bottom shoulder.
9. Look down for balance. Hold the pose and breathe.
10. To come out, bend the standing leg and lower the back foot to a long stance. Release the hands to the floor on either side of the front foot.

Repeat on the second side.

safety

- If the shoulder does not reach the knee, do not proceed further into this pose. Instead press the palms together and perform twisted lunge pose.
- Straighten the standing leg and lift the kneecap.
- Turn the thigh of the standing leg out until the kneecap points straight ahead.
- Point the kneecap of the lifted leg straight down.
- Move the tailbone down and draw the low belly in.
- Turn the abdomen and ribs up.
- Move the base of the sternum back.
- Shrug and move the shoulders back.
- Press the right wrist into the hand and pull the wrist with the left hand.
- Pull the right hip back and keep the torso parallel to the long edge of the mat.
- If the balance is lost when lifting the back leg, press the back foot into a wall before straightening the front leg.

refinement

If you have (or want to) develop exceptional balance, look up. Yoga requires strength, flexibility, balance, and overall agility. This requirement is its offering.

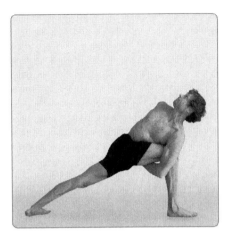

baddha parivrtta parsvakonasana
bound revolved side angle pose

shape
(from *lunge pose*)

1. Pivot the back heel down and turn the foot in 60 degrees.
2. Hold the upper right thigh with the right hand—thumb on top of thigh, fingers on outer quads.
3. Inhale, lift the torso and left arm vertical.
4. Exhale, twist the torso to the right and place the left shoulder on the outer right knee.
5. Swing the left arm under the right thigh and place the back of the hand onto the left side of the torso.
6. Swing the right arm around the back. Hold the right wrist with the left hand.
7. Look down at the front foot.
8. Move the right hip back until the thigh is parallel to the long edge of the mat.
9. Rotate the right shoulder over the left shoulder.
10. Straighten the top arm. Look up. Hold the pose and breathe.
11. To come out, look down and gently release the bind. Place both hands on either side of the front foot. Lift the back heel.

Repeat on the second side.

safety
- If the shoulder cannot reach the knee, do not proceed further into this pose. Instead, press the palms together and practice twisted lunge pose.
- Another way to reduce the intensity of the pose is to lift the back heel. Practice the pose with the back heel lifted until there is increased ease in the twist.
- Shrug and move the shoulders back. This minimal movement creates maximum stability for shoulder.
- Press the back foot down and engage the left glutes.
- Press the tailbone down and lift the low belly.
- If looking down is too intense for the neck or jaw, look down.

refinement
Extend your head away from hips. Lengthen your spine. Move the head back. Hold the pose without holding your breath. Instead of holding your breath, breathe to fuel and refine your effort.

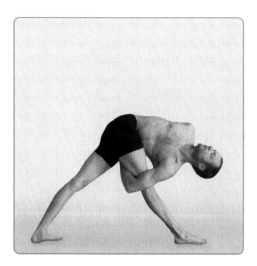

baddha parivrtta trikonasana
bound revolved triangle pose

shape
(from *lunge pose*)

1. Hold the upper right thigh with the right hand—thumb on middle of thigh, fingers on outer quads.
2. Inhale, lift the torso and left arm vertical.
3. Exhale, twist the torso to the right and place the left shoulder on the outer right knee.
4. Bring the right hand to the crease of the right hip. Pull the right hip back and down.
5. Swing the left arm underneath the right thigh and the right arm behind the back. Hold the right wrist with the left hand or vice versa.
6. Look down. Step the back foot forward slightly. Pivot the back heel down, turn the foot in 60 degrees.
7. Move the right hip back until the thigh is parallel to the long edge of the mat.
8. Straighten the front leg.
9. Turn the abdomen and ribs up, rotate the right shoulder over the left shoulder.
10. Look up. Hold the pose and breathe.
11. To come out, look down, bend the front knee and release the hands to either side of the front foot. Step the right foot back and lift the back heel.

Repeat on the second side.

safety

- If the shoulder does not come to the knee, do not proceed further into this pose. Instead, press the palms together and perform twisted lunge pose.
- Before straightening the front leg, shrug and move the bottom shoulder back. This minimal movement creates maximum stability for the shoulder.
- As the leg straightens, press the left elbow and front knee together. Lift the torso up.
- Press the back foot down.
- Tone and tighten the thighs—lift the kneecaps.
- Move the tailbone down and the low belly in.
- Squeeze the shoulder blades toward the spine.
- To reduce the intensity of the shoulder and hamstrings stretch, bend the front knee slightly.
- If looking up is too intense for the neck or jaw, look down.

refinement

Press your feet down and apart. Extend your head away from your hips. Although *baddha parivrtta trikonasana* is a standing pose, consider performing it as the apex pose in an intense forward folds and twists sequence.

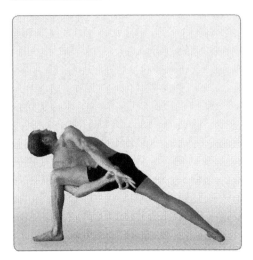

baddha parsvakonasana
bound side angle pose

shape
(from *lunge pose*)

1. Pivot the back heel down and turn the foot in 60 degrees.
2. Bring the right hand to the inside of the right foot. Fold the torso to the inside of the front thigh.
3. Bring the right shoulder under the right knee.
4. Place the back of the right hand against the outer right hip.
5. Swing the left arm back behind the torso.
6. Clasp the left wrist with the right hand or vice versa.
7. Turn the abdomen up and rotate the left shoulder over the right shoulder.
8. Straighten the top arm.
9. Look up. Hold the pose and breathe.
10. To come out, release the clasp and place the hands on either side of the front foot. Lift the back heel.

Repeat on the second side.

safety

- Keep the front knee over the heel and press the back foot down.
- Move the tailbone down and low belly in.
- Move the base of sternum back, stretch up through the chest.
- Engage the arms and move the bottom shoulder back. Although that action will not move the shoulder much, it will stabilize the shoulder.
- If the hand cannot clasp the wrist, bind the hands or hold a strap with the hands as close together as possible.

- If it is too intense to twist and rotate the torso with straight arms, keep the upper arm bent, or even work on rotating and opening the chest and shoulders without the clasp.

refinement

Reach your elbows apart. Extend your head away from your hips to lengthen your spine. This pose is great preparation for arm balances such as *visvamitrasana, eka hasta bhujasana, astavakrasana, tittibhasana,* and *eka pada koundinyasana 2.*

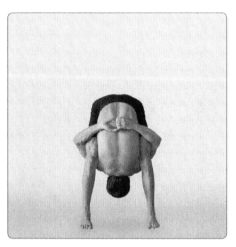

baddha tittibhasana
bound firefly pose

shape
(from *tadasana*)

1. Bring the outer edges of the feet in line with the outer edges of the mat.
2. Inhale fully. Exhale, fold the torso over the legs.
3. Bend the knees to bring the shoulders lower than the knees.
4. Widen the knees beyond the ankles.
5. Swing the arms back between the legs and hold the backs of the calves. Place the thumbs on the widest part of the calves—fingers around the outer shins.
6. Move the shoulders behind the legs. If the shoulders cannot come behind the legs, do not proceed further.
7. One at a time, place the backs of the hands on the outer hips.
8. Bend the knees a little more. Squeeze the arms in and clasp the hands behind the back.
9. Keeping the hands clasped, straighten the legs and look back or even up. Hold the pose and breathe.
10. To come out, release the hands to floor and walk the feet in until they are hip-width apart. Pause in *uttanasana*. Inhale, lift the torso to stand.

safety

- Straighten and strengthen the legs.
- Extend the inner edges of the knees back as the legs straighten.
- Press the hands into the hips, move the shoulders back.
- Extend the elbows out to the sides to take pressure off the sternum.
- Move the tailbone down and the low belly in.

refinement

This pose is an optimal preparation for *supta kurmasana*. The stance of this pose will likely feel too narrow. And yet, it is the only way to get the clasp behind the back. If you are unable to clasp your hands behind your back, try using a strap.

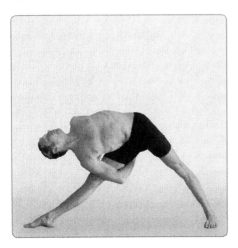

baddha trikonasana
bound triangle pose

shape
(from *lunge pose*)

1. Pivot the back heel down and turn the foot in 30 degrees.
2. Place both hands on the floor inside the front foot.
3. Inhale fully. Exhale, fold the torso inside the front thigh.
4. With the right hand, hold the back of the right calf.
5. Bring the right shoulder underneath the right thigh, top of the shoulder to back of the calf.
6. Place the back of the right hand on the outer right hip.
7. Swing the left arm up and behind the torso—hold the left wrist with the right hand or vice versa.
8. Rotate the left shoulder over the right shoulder. Look down.
9. Straighten the right leg.
10. Lift the torso parallel to the floor—press the knee into the arm and the arm into the knee so the torso and knee isometrically move in opposite directions.
11. Turn the abdomen and ribs up. Look up. Hold the pose and breathe.
12. To come out, look down. Bend the front knee. Release the bind and place the hands on either side of the foot. Lift the back heel.

Repeat on the second side.

safety

* Before straightening the front leg, engage the arms. Shrug and move the bottom shoulder back.
* Press the left wrist into the right hand and lift the right shoulder toward the right ear.
  If the hand cannot clasp the wrist behind the back, hold the fingers or use a strap.
* Squeeze the shoulder blades toward the spine.

- Press the top of the front foot down—engage the calf.
- Tone and tighten the thighs—lift the kneecaps up.
- Engage the upper, outer quads of the front leg.
- Pressing the inner edge of the front foot down, turn the front thigh out until the kneecap lines up with the top of the front foot.
- Press the back foot down, engage the left glutes.
- Engage the abdominal muscles; move the base of the sternum and shoulders back.
- To reduce the intensity of the stretch, bend the front knee slightly.
- If looking up is too intense for the neck or jaw, keep the gaze down.

refinement

Press your feet down and apart. Extend your head away from your hips. Stretch your spine fully. In order to perform *baddha trikonasana* safely, you must have already developed strong, supple shoulders. Preparatory poses that open the shoulders are: *parsvottanasana, utkatasana* (hands bound), *baddha parsvakonasana, gomukhasana,* and *parivrtta marichyasana 1. Baddha trikonasana* is a good preparatory pose for *svarga dvijasana.*

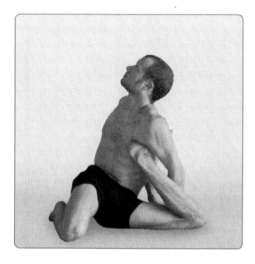

baddha yogadandasana
bound yoga staff pose

shape
(from *dandasana*)

1. Inhale fully. Exhale, lean and twist the torso to the right. Bend the left knee and bring the arch of the left foot to the left armpit. This may take several attempts.
2. Lower the top of the left thigh to the floor.
3. With momentum, swing the left hand behind the back above the left knee. Place the left palm flat on the floor underneath the left thigh.
4. Stay here for a few breaths. Then in one movement keep the knee pointing forward and bring the right foot to the outer right hip.
5. Inhale fully. Exhale, turn the torso to the right and clasp the left wrist with the right hand.
6. Lift the chin and look between the eyebrows. Hold the pose and breathe.
7. To come out, release the hands and the top leg. Straighten both legs.

Repeat on the second side.

safety

- Do not attempt this variation until you can safely perform *yogadandasana*.
- When bringing the foot to the armpit, lift the foot by pushing the back of the upper arm into the foot. Hold the lifted foot with the right hand and reach the left arm forward to bring the armpit toward the foot.
- Do not reach the left arm behind the back until the foot is in the armpit.
- Engage and flex the lifted foot. Push the foot into the armpit and the armpit into the foot.
- Isometrically pull the top heel down to engage the hamstrings.
- Roll the thigh of the lower leg out and allow the right sit bone to lift.
- Lift the pelvic floor and tone the low belly.

refinement

After teaching this pose in class using these instructions, a student asked me, "Was that meant to be an extremely challenging way to get into this pose? Was it supposed to make it more difficult?" I happened to be in an irascible mood that day and sarcastically replied, "Yes exactly. I'm trying to make the difficult more difficult!" The student said, "I just think this pose is much easier if you start with one leg in *virasana*." Some nodded their heads in agreement. Others shook their heads in disagreement. We all have our practice preferences. Try both and see which works better for you.

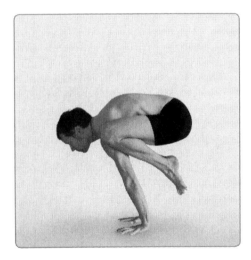

bakasana
crane pose

shape
(from *malasana 1*)

1. Place the hands directly below the shoulders—elbows pointing back. Firmly press the legs into the arms.
2. Stay low and lean forward to come up onto the toes. Transfer the weight of the body onto the hands.
3. Lift the feet off the floor. Press the inner edges of the feet together.
4. Squeeze the elbows in so the forearms are parallel to each other.
5. Inhale, round the back.
6. Exhale, straighten the arms.

7. Look straight ahead. Hold the pose and breathe.
8. To come out, exhale, lower the feet to the floor.

safety

- Press the fingertips and the perimeter of the palms into the floor evenly.
- While squeezing the inner edges of the feet together, lift the heels toward the hips. Spread the toes.
- As the arms straighten, move the hips down and forward.
- To reduce the pressure on the wrists, place the heels of the palms on the mat and the knuckles and fingers off the mat. (This will only be effective if you have a thick mat.)
- If there is still pain or discomfort in the wrists, keep the elbows bent and bring the shoulders directly over the wrists to reduce the angle of the arms.
- If it is difficult to lift the feet and hips, place a block underneath the feet in *malasana 1* before coming into the pose.

refinement

This pose often will bring up the fear of falling/failing. First try lifting one foot at a time. Then try lifting both feet at once. You may wish to place a soft blanket on the floor just in front of your hands to serve as a "crash pad." Chances are you won't need it, but the feeling of safety that it provides might give you the confidence necessary to attempt the pose. Interestingly, arm balances are often thought of as a way to build confidence!

Advanced practitioners can jump into *bakasana* from *adho mukha svanasana*. Or to start from *sirsasana 2*, keep your legs straight and lower your toes just above the floor. Extend your elbows forward—toward your feet—then bend and place your knees onto your outer shoulders. Move your elbows forward to capacity. Lift your head and come into *bakasana* for five breaths. Lower your head and lift back into *sirsasana 2*. Drop your feet over into *urdhva dhanurasana* prep. Exhale, straighten the arms to lift into *urdhva dhanurasana 1* and hold for five breaths. From *urdhva dhanurasana 1*, kick your feet up and over into *adho mukha svanasana* or stand up into *tadasana*. In *Light On Yoga*, B. K. S Iyengar gives essentially the same sequence as above for "advanced pupils." He says, "After one has mastered *viparita chakrasana* it is a soothing exercise after practicing *urdhva dhanurasana*."[1]

Another way to move from *bakasana* into *urdhva dhanurasana 1* is to float from *bakasana* into *adho mukha vrksasana* and drop over from there.

---

[1]   B. K. S. Iyengar, *Light on Yoga* (New York: Schocken Books, 1977) pp. 316–317.

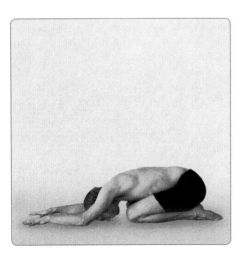

balasana
child's pose

shape
(from *bharmanasana*)

1. Separate the knees slightly wider than the torso. Keep the tops of the feet on the floor and bring the big toes together.
2. Inhale fully. Exhale, lower the hips to the heels. Relax the feet.
3. Stretch the arms forward. Place the forehead and forearms on the floor.
4. Close the eyes. Hold the pose and breathe.
5. To come out, lift the hips over the knees and bring the shoulders over the wrists.

safety
- If the sit bones do not reach the heels, place one or more blankets between the calves and thighs.
- If the sit bones reach the heels but the back is over-rounding or if placing the head on the floor strains the neck, place the forehead on the edge of a block.
- If there is pain or discomfort in the hip flexors, lift the torso upright and hold the tops of the thighs with the hands—thumbs on the hip creases and fingers on the outer quads/hips. Press the thighs down and spin the thighs away from the pubic bone. Use the hands to keep the legs in this position. Inhale, lengthen the spine. Exhale, fold the torso forward between the legs. Release the hands and stretch the arms forward.

refinement
Balasana can be one of the most relaxing and rejuvenating poses in hatha yoga. It is a great pose to rest and pause in during a strong yoga practice, especially in an arm balancing sequence. My colleague Christina Sell often begins her classes with *balasana* because it gives students a chance to soften and turn their attention inward before an intense practice. *Balasana* is also an ideal pose to learn the alignment principles of the more advanced arm balances in which all or much of your body weight is held in the wrists and hands. To experience this, straighten your arms and stretch your hands forward until your elbows lift off the floor. Press your hands down and forward, especially the roots of your index fingers, and spin your biceps up. Lift your inner shoulders toward your ears to experience external rotation of the shoulders. Practice this hand, biceps, and shoulder position in this relatively easy pose so that the alignment comes naturally to you when you begin bearing weight on your hands and wrists.

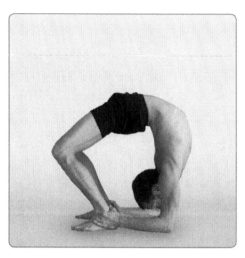
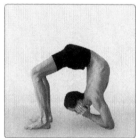

bandha chakrasana
bound wheel pose

shape
(from *urdhva dhanurasana 1*)

1. Bend the elbows and place the top of the head on the floor.
2. Lower the elbows to the floor shoulder-width apart. Interlace the fingers behind the head—thumbs pointing up.
3. Press the forearms down and lift the head. Reach the shoulders back and the chest forward until the upper arms are vertical. Look back at the heels.
4. Keeping the feet outer hip-width apart, walk the feet back toward the head and clasp the ankles with the hands.
5. Look down. Hold the pose and breathe.
6. To come out, release the hands and walk the feet away from the head. Place the hands near the head and straighten the arms.

safety

- Press the forearms down.
- Press the feet down. Move the hips up and away from the shoulders.
- Extend the inner edges of the feet down. Rotate the inner thighs down.
- Flare the outer two toes and squeeze the shins in.
- Engage the glutes and abdomen and lift the tailbone.
- Move the base of the sternum back and stretch the entire spine.
- Do not hold the breath.

refinement

Bandha chakrasana is both a preparatory and prerequisite pose for *eka pada viparita dandasana 2*. Do not attempt *eka pada viparita dandasana 2* until you can hold *bandha chakrasana* for 20 to 30 seconds with proficient alignment. The more advanced backbends can either help you develop nerves of steel or blow your fuse box, so to speak. For a more intense variation of this pose, look forward and lift your hands to your chin.

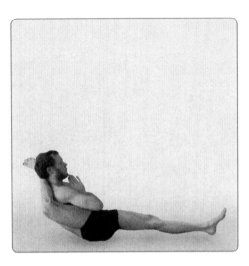

bhairavasana
formidable pose

shape
(from *eka pada sirsasana*)

1. Bend the knee of the extended leg and place the heel near the sit bone. Roll onto the back.
2. Place the hands on the floor next to the hips and straighten the left leg—toes pointing up.
3. Place the palms together in front of the sternum. Look up. Hold the pose and breathe.
4. To come out, release the hands to the floor next to the hips and bend the knee of the extended leg. If possible, rock back up to a sitting position.

Repeat on the second side.

safety
- Engage both feet, especially the top foot.
- Isometrically bend the top knee to engage the hamstrings.
- Flare the outer two toes of the top foot.
- Press the shoulder and neck into the top ankle.
- Straighten and strengthen the extended leg. Lift the left kneecap and reach as much of the backside of the leg to the floor as possible.
- If there is pain or discomfort at the top of the thigh, keep the knee of the extended leg bent.
- Lift the pelvic floor and tone the low belly.

refinement
All of the leg-behind-the-head poses can be done as a sequence. Go from one to the other without coming out. Then switch sides. If you hold the poses for thirty seconds each, your leg will be behind your head for a total of three and half minutes. However, if you cannot hold your leg behind the head for three and a half minutes, it is possible to come into *bhairvasana* and the other leg-behind-the-head poses from *dandasana* or *eka pada sirsasana* rather than move through the entire sequence. Although the shape of the upper body is the same in all of these poses, changing one or two minor variables can dramatically intensify or highlight a different aspect of the pose. If it is too difficult to do the entire sequence, build up to it slowly. The head and neck are in a precarious position and moving and adjusting the body with the leg behind the head must be done carefully.

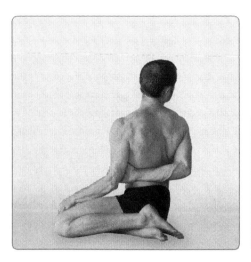
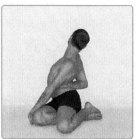

bharadvajasana 1
Sage Bharadvaja's pose 1

shape
(from *vajrasana*)

1. Lift the hips slightly and sit on the floor just outside of the right foot—feet to the outside of the left hip.
2. With the left hand, lift the left foot off the floor. Point the right foot out to the side and place the base of the left shin in the arch of the right foot. Point left foot back.
3. Bring the right arm behind the back and hold the left biceps with the right hand.
4. Inhale fully. Exhale, twist the torso to the right and hold the outer right knee with the left hand.
5. Look over the right shoulder. Hold the pose and breathe.
6. To come out, inhale, look forward. Exhale, release the hands next to the hips. Lift the hips slightly and slide the feet underneath the sit bones. Bring the ankles together and point the feet back.

Repeat on the second side.

safety

- Lift the pelvic floor and tone the low belly.
- Move the base of the sternum back and lift the chest.
- Lengthen the left side of the torso.
- Move the right shoulder and elbow back.

refinement

Point both knees forward and keep your thighs parallel. To deepen the twist, press your right hand into your left biceps and your left biceps into your hand. Press your left hand into your right knee. Advanced practitioners can place the back of the left hand on the right knee. Straighten your left arm and slide your left palm under your knee to the floor. After a few breaths, turn your head in the opposite direction. Tilt your head to the left and look down at your feet. This head variation provides a deep stretch along the opposite side of the neck.

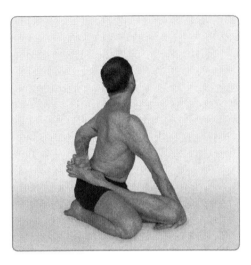

bharadvajasana 2
Sage Bharadvaja's pose 2

shape
(from *dandasana*)

1. Bend the right knee and place the inner ankle against the right outer hip—shin and top of foot on floor. Point the foot back.
2. Lean to the left and pull the right glutes back with the right hand. Repeat on the other side.
3. Bend the left knee and point the foot.
4. Hold the left ankle with the left hand and the top of the foot with the right hand.
5. Place the outer left foot on the upper inner right thigh at the crease of the groin.
6. Keeping the left foot in place, lower the left knee to the floor.
7. Bring the back of the right hand underneath the left knee. Press the hand down.
8. Swing the left arm behind the back and hold the left big toe with the first two fingers and thumb.
9. If optimal, bring the knees closer together so both knees point forward toward the top of the mat.
10. Inhale fully. Exhale, turn the torso to the left and look over the left shoulder. Hold the pose and breathe.
11. To come out, inhale, look forward. Exhale, release the hands and straighten the legs.

Repeat on the second side.

safety

- If it is not possible for the legs to fold into *ardha padmasana* and/or *virasana*, sit on one or more folded blankets to bring ease to the leg in *virasana*, bring the top shin parallel to the front of the mat, or hold the top leg in *hindolasana* to bring ease to the leg in *ardha padmasana*.
- For the leg in *virasana*, point the toes straight back and squeeze the ankle into the hip.
- For the leg in *padmasana*, press the top of the foot and toes into the thigh. Push the heel into the low belly.
- Isometrically squeeze the knees toward each other.
- Lift the back shoulder and elbow up and back.
- Lift the pelvic floor and low belly.

refinement

Instead of using *dandasana* as the origin pose, another way to come into *bharadvajasana 2* is from *ardha baddha padma paschimottanasana* with your torso upright. With your left leg in *ardha padmasana*, lean to the left and swing your right leg back into *virasana*. Lower your right hip to the floor. Press the *virasana* foot into your outer hip. With proper alignment, this entry into *bharadvajasana 2* can reduce the lateral pressure on the *ardha padmasana* knee.

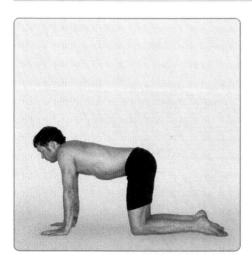

bharmanasana
table pose

shape

1. Come onto the hands and knees—wrists below shoulders, knees below hips.
2. Separate the hands slightly wider than the shoulders and line up the middle of the wrists with the outer shoulders.
3. Turn the hands out so the index fingers point straight ahead. Separate the fingers. Point the biceps forward.
4. Separate the knees hip-width apart—shins parallel.
5. Press the tops of the feet into the floor. Point the toes straight back and draw the outer ankles in until the heels are vertical.
6. Bring the spine to a neutral position—do not round the back or drop the belly.
7. Lift the chin slightly and look forward. Hold the pose and breathe.

safety

- Press the fingertips into the floor.
- Press the roots of the index fingers down so there is an even amount of weight along the perimeter of the palms.
- Press the tailbone down and lift the low belly.

refinement

Familiarize yourself with the alignment of this basic pose and it will benefit you in many other poses, especially those that bear weight on the hands. Any insight you gain in one pose applies to the full gamut of your practice.

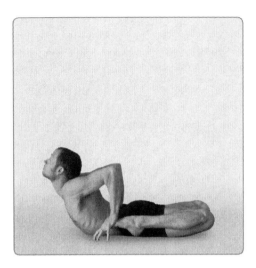

bhekasana
frog pose

shape

1. Lower the front body to the floor—legs straight and feet outer hip-width apart. Place the forehead on the floor.
2. Bend the knees so the heels are as close to the glutes as possible.
3. Place the backs of the hands on the tops of the feet with the wrists against the arches of the feet.
4. Bend the elbows and point them up.
5. Press the feet down with the hands and lift the head. Place the palms on the tops of the feet with the thumbs in and fingers out. Pause and breathe.
6. Inhale fully. Exhale, spin the hands to point the fingers forward. Wrap the fingers around the toes and lower the heels to the outer hips.
7. Lift the chin and look up. Hold the pose and breathe.
8. To come out, lift the feet and release the hands. Straighten and lower the legs.

safety

- Point the toes straight ahead and squeeze the ankles in.
- Engage the glutes.
- Press the tailbone and hips down. Tone the low belly.
- Press the hands down and lift the shoulders up and back.
- If there is pain or discomfort in the knees, widen the knees slightly. If there is still pain, discontinue the pose.

refinement

Advanced practitioners can press the tips of the fingers onto the floor. Another way to come into *bhekasana* is from *dhanurasana*. Keeping your left leg in *dhanurasana* bring your right leg into *eka pada bhekasana*. Lift your head as high off the floor as possible, and then bring your other leg into *bhekasana*. Coming into *bhekasana* from *dhanurasana* reduces the stretch required in the shoulders, which is often what is difficult for many practitioners.

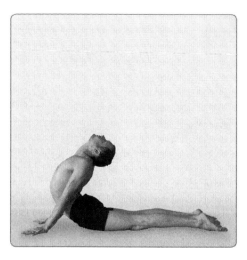 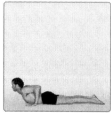 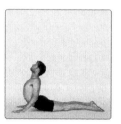

bhujangasana 1
cobra pose 1

shape

1. Bring the front body to the floor.
2. Straighten the legs, bring the feet outer hip-width apart, and point the toes straight back.
3. Place the hands on the floor outer shoulder-width apart with the wrists directly below the elbows—forearms vertical.
4. Separate the fingers and point the index fingers straight ahead.
5. Inhale, look forward and lift the chest to bring the shoulders as high as the elbows—upper arms parallel to the floor. Pause and breathe.
6. Inhale, lift the chest and straighten the arms. Curl the head back. Look between the eyebrows. Hold the pose and breathe.
7. To come out, exhale, bend the elbows and lower the torso to the floor.

safety

- If there is any pain or discomfort in the low back, engage the legs and abdomen, and bend the elbows as much as necessary.
- Separate the fingers. Press the entire perimeter of the palms down, especially the mounds of the index fingers.
- Press the feet down and toward each other. Isometrically squeeze the heels in.
- Lock the legs into a straight position so the knees lift off the floor.
- Point the kneecaps straight down.
- Press the tailbone down, tone the low belly, and contract the glutes.
- Isometrically press the hands down and back.
- Lift the shoulders up, back, and in toward each other.
- Engage the upper back muscles and press the shoulder blades into the upper back.
- Stretch the entire spine and extend the chest up.
- During menstruation, place a bolster below the front of the ribcage to lift the torso. This will reduce the upper back and core strength required while providing a stretch in the upper back.

refinement

For several years I never taught the final form of *bhujangasana 1* in any of my public classes. For the sake of students' low backs and shoulders, I taught *bhujangasana 1* with elbows bent instead. Recently I realized that in doing so I was holding several students back who would benefit from performing the final form. It also occurred to me that many students did not know what the full form of *bhujangasana 1* looked like. I now make it a point to educate students on what the final form of each pose looks like. Ideally a modification leads toward, rather than obscures, the final form of that pose. *Bhujangasana 1* is an important preparatory pose for many of the more advanced backbends such as *bhujangasana 2*, *rajakapotasana*, and *ganda bherundasana*.

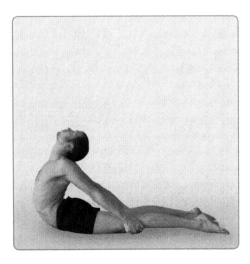

bhujangasana 2
cobra pose 2

shape
(from *dhanurasana*)

1. Deepen the bend in the right knee and slide the right hand halfway down the shin toward the knee. Kick the right foot up and back until the shin is vertical to the floor. Repeat on the left side.
2. Slide the right hand further down to the bottom of the shin just below the knee. Repeat on the left side.
3. Straighten the legs and catch hold of the knees with the hands. Point the feet.
4. Inhale, lift the chest. Exhale, curl the head back.
5. Look between the eyebrows. Hold the pose and breathe.
6. To come out, inhale, lift the head. Bend the knees and walk the hands up the shins to clasp the feet or ankles.

safety

- Isometrically squeeze the heels in and flare the outer toes.
- Point the kneecaps down and engage the glutes.
- Press the hips and tops of the feet down.
- Tone the pelvic floor and low belly.
- Stretch and lengthen the entire spine.

refinement

Surprisingly the full form of *bhujangasana 1* is a deeper backbend than *bhujangasana 2*. However, *bhujangasana 2* puts more pressure on the low back and is much more difficult to get into. In other words, it's six of one and a half dozen of the other.

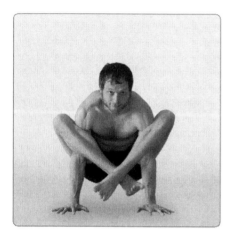

bhujapidasana
arm pressure pose

shape
(from *tadasana*)

1. Separate the outer edges of the feet as wide as the mat.
2. Inhale fully. Exhale, fold the torso over the legs.
3. Widen and bend the knees to lower the shoulders below the knees. Hold the backs of the calves with the hands.
4. Place the thumbs on the centers of the calves and fingers on the outer shins. Press the calves forward and in with the thumbs.
5. One at a time, bring the shoulders behind the knees.
6. Bend the knees and lower the hips. Place the hands on the floor shoulder-width apart behind the feet. Separate the fingers and point the index fingers straight ahead.
7. Squeeze the legs into the arms. Lean back and bring the weight into the hands to lift the feet off the floor. Straighten the arms.
8. Cross the left ankle over the right ankle. Flex the feet and flare the toes.
9. Look straight ahead. Hold the pose and breathe.
10. To come out, bend the elbows and lean forward to bring the feet to the floor. Release the arms and lift the torso to stand.

Repeat on the second side—switch the cross of the legs.

safety

- Press the fingertips and the perimeter of the palms into the floor with equal pressure. Do not collapse the weight of the body into the wrists.
- Lift the pelvic floor and tone the low belly.
- Move the shoulders back. Even though the *action* of the shoulders is back, the legs will *move* them forward.
- If the hips and legs cannot lift off the floor, place blocks underneath the hands.

refinement

Advanced practitioners can point the feet out to the side; lower the top of the head to the floor; take five deep breaths; and then return to *bhujapidasana*.

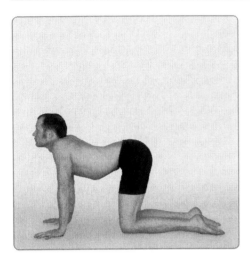

bitilasana
cow pose

shape

1. Come onto the hands and knees with the arms and thighs vertical—shoulders directly over the wrists, hips directly over the knees.
2. Separate the hands slightly wider than shoulder-distance apart.
3. Separate the knees and feet outer hip-width apart.
4. Bring the tops of the feet onto the floor. Point the toes straight back and squeeze the ankles in until the heels are vertical.
5. Inhale, lift the chest and extend the abdomen down toward the floor so that the entire spine moves into a slight backbend.
6. Lift the chin and tailbone. Look up between the eyebrows. Hold the pose and breathe.
7. To come out, exhale, return to a neutral spine.

safety

- Separate the fingers and point the index fingers forward. Press the entire perimeter of the palms down, especially the mounds of the index fingers.
- Lock the arms into a straight position.
- Press the knees, shins, and tops of feet down.
- Extend the chest forward and stretch the entire spine.
- Tone the low belly.
- For extra padding, place a blanket underneath the knees, shins, and feet.

refinement

Bitilasana warms up the spine and is most effective when done in tandem with *marjarasana*: Inhale, press your hands down, stretch your collarbones up and forward, and lift your sit bones up. Slide your head back in space before lifting your chin. Exhale, round your sit bones toward the backs of your knees and reach your chest up into the spine to round your back. At the end of your exhalation, stretch the back of your neck by reaching your chin into your chest. Repeat for several breaths before returning your spine to a neutral position.

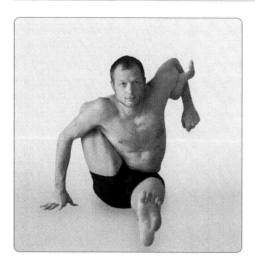

buddhasana
Buddha's pose

shape
(from *eka pada sirsasana*, right leg behind the head)

1. Lift the left arm parallel to the floor in front of the body. Make a fist with the left hand.
2. Bring the right elbow underneath the left arm and hold the right ankle with the right hand.
3. Pull the right foot down the back and lift the left elbow up and over the foot.
4. Once the elbow is over the top of the foot, flex and point the foot in quick succession to move the elbow toward the ankle.
5. Place the right hand on the floor outside of the right hip. Look straight ahead. Hold the pose and breathe.
6. To come out, use the right hand to hold the right foot. Lift the left elbow off the back foot.

Repeat on the second side.

safety

- Engage both feet, especially the top foot.
- Isometrically bend the top knee to engage the hamstrings.
- Flare the outer two toes of the top foot.
- Press the shoulder and neck into the top ankle.
- Little by little, use deep exhalations to move the top foot and shin down the back.
- If the top arm cannot hook over the top foot, continue to hold the foot with the hand and lift the left arm vertical. Push the left shoulder into the top foot.
- Lift the pelvic floor and tone the low belly.

refinement

It is easier to get into this pose if you are sweating profusely, which allows the top foot to slide down the back. It is likely that a hands-on adjustment from a skilled teacher will be required to get you into *buddhasana* for the first time.

My general recommendation for most practitioners is to not practice the advanced asanas. For most, it is simply not worth the risk. You can access all of the rewards of this practice with basic poses. That may seem like a contradiction considering I did all of the poses in this book. I did so because I couldn't not do so. It did not even occur to me to consider the perils of the practice. When I was 22 years old, my mom handed me B. K. S. Iyengar's *Light On Yoga*. After looking at the photos of B. K. S. Iyengar expressing these asanas with absolute grace and precision, I had a flash of inspiration. I said to myself, "One day I will be able to do all of these poses." At the time, I had no reason to think I could possibly succeed in fulfilling such an audacious task. Even so, 11 years later I fulfilled that goal. It was absolutely worth it despite the many prices I paid along the way. After performing the full gamut of these asanas, I can honestly say that I do not think the more advanced poses offer more than the basic ones. And yet, that will not stop some of you from attempting all of them. If practicing advanced asana turns hatha yoga into hurt-you yoga, don't do it!

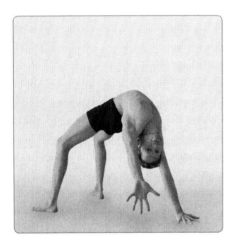 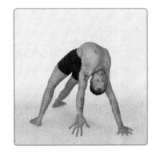

camatkarasana
wild thing pose

shape
(from *vasisthasana*, legs together)

1. With the right hand and foot on the floor, place the left hand on the hip and look down.
2. Step the left foot behind the right leg. Rotate the hips up—toward the ceiling—to bring the shin vertical.
3. Bend the right knee and bring the foot in line with the left foot—outer hip-width apart or wider. Point the toes straight back.
4. Lift the hips up and back and turn the front body up, toward the ceiling.
5. Curl the head back and extend the left arm forward and toward the floor. Straighten the arm.
6. Look back. Hold the pose and breathe.
7. To come out, bring the weight into the right hand and foot, and spin the hips to the right.

Repeat on the second side.

safety

- Press the bottom hand down.
- Separate the fingers of the bottom hand. Point the index finger and biceps straight ahead.
- Press the fingertips and the perimeter of the bottom hand evenly into the floor—press the mound of the index finger down and lift the outer wrist up.
- Press the inner edges of the feet down. Isometrically squeeze the feet in.
- Engage the glutes. Lift the tailbone up and tone the abdomen.
- In this pose, the hips must lift and the back must bend. If the hips drop and the spine remains straight, it will compromise the bottom shoulder.

refinement

In *camatkarasana* you can also straighten the right leg or both legs. To come into this pose from *adho mukha svanasana:* lift your right leg, bend your right knee and point your knee up, turn your torso to the right, and lift your right hand off the floor as you lower your right foot to the floor. When I know I will be teaching *urdhva dhanurasana 1* in a class, I will often teach *camatkarasana* after standing poses along with *vasisthasana* and *kapinjalasana prep*. Then I teach some hip openers and quad stretches to lead into *urdhva dhanurasana 1*.

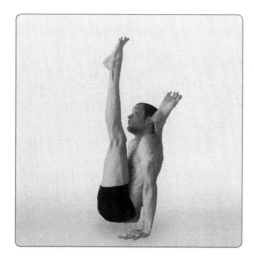

chakorasana
partridge pose

shape
(from *eka pada sirsasana*)

1. Place the hands on the floor beside the hips—shoulder-width apart.
2. Straighten the arms, lean the torso back, and lift the hips to lift the extended leg vertical to the floor.
3. Look up. Hold the pose and breathe.
4. To come out, exhale, lean forward and lower the hips and leg.

Repeat on the second side.

safety

- Push the hands down and squeeze the arms in toward the torso.
- Engage both feet, especially the top foot.
- Isometrically bend the back knee to engage the hamstrings.
- Straighten and strengthen the extended leg.
- Lift the pelvic floor and tone the low belly.

refinement

If your hips are extremely flexible, this pose will require more from your arms and abdomen. Interestingly, if your hips are tight (relatively speaking) it will be easier to get your straight leg vertical. If one of your hips is tighter than the other, you will notice that it's easier to do this pose on the tighter side.

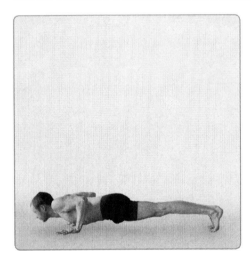

chaturanga dandasana
four-limbed staff pose

shape
(from *plank pose*)

1. Inhale, bend the elbows to a 90-degree angle—upper arms parallel to the floor, forearms vertical.
2. Keep the legs and spine straight.
3. Bring the heels directly above the toe mounds.
4. Lift the chin and look straight ahead. Hold the pose and breathe.
5. To come out, exhale, straighten the arms.

safety

- If supporting the body weight with the arms is not possible, place a block under the lower rib cage and a block under the pelvis. To gain strength, lift the body slightly above the blocks and hover.
- Separate the hands slightly wider than the shoulders. Separate the fingers. Point the index fingers straight ahead.
- Evenly press the fingertips and the perimeter of the palms into the floor.
- Tighten the knees. Tone the thighs.

- Press the tailbone down and lift the low belly.
- Move the base of the sternum up.
- Do not round the shoulders or lift the hips.

refinement

When performing *chaturanga dandasana,* many practitioners will round their shoulders to more easily support their body weight instead of keeping their shoulders at the height of their elbows. This is not necessarily problematic if you are holding *chaturanga dandasana* for five breaths and then resting. Rounding the shoulders when repeatedly moving from *chaturanga dandasana* into *urdhva mukha svanasana* during *surya namaskar* can lead to shoulder injury. If you cannot perform *chaturanga dandasana* in good form, be sure to rest your front body on the floor, and lift your shoulders up before moving into *urdhva mukha svanasana.*

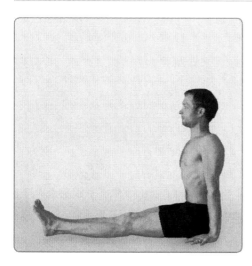

dandasana
staff pose

shape

1. Come into a seated position.
2. Extend the legs straight out. Bring the torso vertical.
3. Lean to the right and move the left glutes back with the left hand. Repeat on the other side.
4. Place the palms flat on the floor beside the hips. Straighten the arms.
5. Bring the inner edges of the feet together.
6. Point the kneecaps and toes straight up.
7. Push the inner edges of the feet forward, pull the outer edges of the feet back.
8. Look straight ahead. Hold the pose and breathe.

safety

- To reduce the intensity of the hamstring stretch, separate the feet outer hip-width apart or, if needed, as wide as the mat.
- If the palms do not reach the floor, bring the fingertips to the floor or place the hands on blocks.
- Lean to the right and move the left glutes back with the left hand. Repeat on the other side.

- Hold the right thigh with both hands and simultaneously rotate the thigh down, from the pubic bone to the knee, and pull the hamstring muscles out. Repeat on the other side.
- Lift the kneecaps toward the hips and press the backs of the knees down.
- Curve the low back in and tilt the top of the pelvis down and forward slightly. Feel the spine with the fingers to be sure the low back is curved in. If the low back rounds, sit up on one or more folded blankets.
- Lift the pelvic floor and tone the low belly.
- Press the hands down, lift the chest, and stretch the entire spine.

refinement

Notice that the geometry of the body in *adho mukha svanasana* is the same as in *dandasana*, but with arms lifted and hands and feet flexed. Even though they are the same in shape, the body's relationship to gravity in each pose will emphasize a different aspect of the pose. Because *adho mukha svanasana* bears weight on the hands and wrists, the pose can challenge one's upper body strength. Because *dandasana* is a seated position in which the demands of the upper body are minimal, the focus is on the legs and pelvis.

Even though the challenges differ, understanding what makes them similar can teach us how to apply the alignment of one pose to related poses. This means that if the legs are straight and the low back is rounded in *dandasana*, performing *adho mukha svanasana* with straight legs will only cause the back to round. If the priority of the asana is to maintain length in the spine (which it usually is), then practitioners with tight hamstrings and a tight low back should practice *adho mukha svanasana* with bent knees. This will help keep the spine long and the breath unrestricted.

Dandasana is an ideal pose to assess the flexibility of the hamstrings and low back and use it to understand other poses similar in shape. Advanced practitioners can come into *dandasana* from *adho mukha svanasana* in one movement. As you swing your legs through the arms, bend your knees and cross your ankles; work toward keeping your legs straight as they pass through your arms.

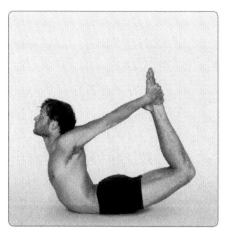 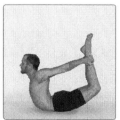 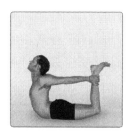

dhanurasana

bow pose

shape

1. Bring the front body to the floor.
2. Straighten the legs and bring the feet outer hip-width apart.
3. Bend the knees and clasp the outsides of the ankles or shins with the hands.
4. Look straight ahead and squeeze the shoulders toward the spine.
5. Bring the feet halfway between a flexed and pointed position and spread the toes.
6. Inhale, kick the legs into the hands, and lift the knees up and back to capacity.
7. Lift the chin slightly and look up. Hold the pose and breathe.
8. To come out, exhale, lower the torso and knees. Release the hands and lower the arms and legs.

safety

- Keep the knees outer hip-width apart or slightly wider.
- Lift the inner edges of the thighs up and press the tailbone down.
- Engage the glutes.
- Tone the pelvic floor and low belly.
- Stretch the spine and chest up.
- If there is pain or discomfort in the knees, hold the ankles and flex the feet.
- If there is pain or discomfort at the front of the hips, place a folded blanket below the hips for additional padding.

refinement

Advanced practitioners can hold the ankles and bring the inner edges of the feet, and even the heels, together. I believe *salabhasana* and preps, *makarasana* and variations, and *dhanurasana* offer the backbend essentials to most practitioners; the risk is low and the reward is hatha high!

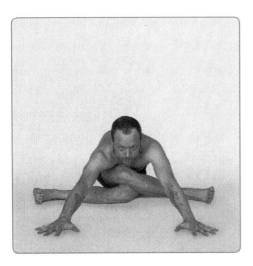

dirghasrngasana
long horn pose

shape
(from *dandasana*)

1. Bend the right knee and place the heel on the floor against the outer left hip. Flex the foot and point the toes out to the left. Lower the knee.
2. Bend the left knee and place the heel on the floor against the outer right hip. Flex the foot and point the toes out to the right. Lower the knee.
3. Place the hands behind the hips. Slide the feet forward until the shins are parallel to the front of the mat.
4. Inhale fully. Exhale, fold the torso over the legs.
5. Stretch and straighten the arms forward. Place the palms flat on the floor wider than the shoulders.
6. Look straight ahead. Hold the pose and breathe.
7. To come out, walk the hands back underneath the shoulders. Inhale, lift the head and use the hands to lift the torso upright. Place the hands by the hips and straighten the legs.

Repeat on the second side.

safety
- Engage the feet. Press the outer edges of the feet down.
- Isometrically pull the feet back.
- Lift the pelvic floor and tone the low belly.

refinement
Press your knees in toward each other so that your top knee is directly above your bottom knee. To turn this into a restorative pose, rest your forehead on the edge of a block and look down or even close your eyes. One of the benefits of this pose is stretching the hips, not straining the knees. If this pose strains your knees, practice *gomukhasana* instead.

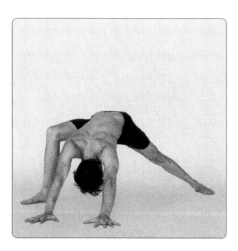

down dog lunge pose

shape
(from *lunge pose*)

1. Pivot the back heel down to the floor in line with the front heel.
2. Turn the front foot out 30 degrees. Tilt the front knee out so it is in line with the heel.
3. Place the palms flat on the floor inside the front foot—right hand next to right foot.
4. Fold the torso forward, to the inside of the front thigh—lower the torso below the thigh.
5. Walk the hands forward and straighten the arms.
6. Press the palms flat on the floor shoulder-width apart—separate the fingers.
7. Relax the neck.
8. Keep the right thigh parallel to the floor and to the long edge of the mat. The hips tend to lift and sway to the right and the front knee tends to fall in toward the center. If the right hip is higher than the right knee, take a longer stance via the back foot until the front thigh is parallel to the floor.
9. Bring the lower body into lunge pose and the upper body into *adho mukha svanasana*. Hold the pose and breathe.
10. To come out, lift the torso and walk the hands back until they are below the shoulders. Bring the hands to either side of the front foot.

Repeat on the second side.

safety
- Press the front big toe down, flare the outer two toes.
- Press the back foot down, lift the back thigh up.
- Engage the left glutes.
- Move the tailbone down and the low belly in.
- Keep the front knee above the heel.
- Press the hands down and lift the inner shoulders up.

refinement

Press your hands down and forward. Press your feet down and back. Isometrically extend your front knee and back heel away from the hips. Focus your eyes on your back big toe. Every pose has a *drishti*—a point of visual focus. This keeps the eyes still and steady, which promotes mental concentration. A steady gaze on a single point or object can naturally draw the attention inward. As Swami Chidvilasananda says, "Turning within is called yoga."[1]

[1]   Gurumayi Chidvilasananda, *The Yoga of Discipline* (South Fallsburg, New York: SYDA Foundation, 1996).

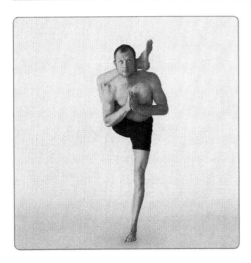

durvasasana
Sage Durvasas's pose

shape
(from *ruchikasana*)

1. Release the hands to the floor, directly below the shoulders.
2. Inhale, lift the torso vertical and place the palms together in front of the chest.
3. Stand as straight as possible.
4. Look between the eyebrows. Hold the pose and breathe.
5. To come out, release the hands, fold the torso, and place the hands directly below the shoulders.

safety

- Engage both feet, especially the top foot.
- Isometrically bend the top knee to engage the hamstrings.
- Flare the outer two toes of the top foot.
- Press the right shoulder and neck into the top leg.
- Straighten and strengthen the standing leg. Lift the left kneecap.
- Lift the pelvic floor and tone the low belly.
- If it is difficult to balance, separate the hands out to the sides.

refinement

To lift your torso vertical and come to stand, walk your hands up your legs. To get a feel for this pose, bend your standing leg slightly and place your hands on your thigh.

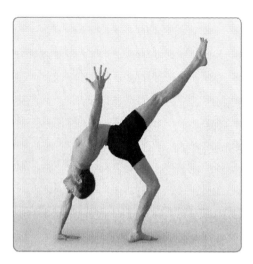

dwi anga urdhva dhanurasana
two limb upward bow pose

shape
(from *urdhva dhanurasana 1*)

1. Bring the inner edges of the feet together.
2. Keep the heels together and turn the toes out.
3. Inhale, lift and straighten the right arm and leg—bring them toward/to vertical.
4. Exhale, curl the head back. Look at the tip of the nose. Hold the pose and breathe.
5. To come out, exhale, lower the hand and foot to the floor—hands shoulder-width apart, feet hip-width apart.

Repeat on the second side.

safety

- Press the fingertips and the perimeter of the bottom palm down with equal pressure. Dig the thumb into the floor and squeeze it isometrically toward the palm.
- Lock both elbows into a straight position.
- Move the shoulder of the bottom arm back and the chest forward simultaneously.
- Move the inner thigh of the bottom leg back and down. Press the inner edge of the bottom foot down.
- Flare the outer two toes. Squeeze the shins in.
- Engage the glutes and abdomen. Lift the tailbone.
- Move the base of the sternum back and stretch the entire spine.

refinement

It is difficult to establish balance in *dwi anga urdhva dhanurasana*. You must be willing to fall over again and again. Practice *eka pada dhanurasana* (from all fours, same leg and arm) to help develop the balance needed in this pose.

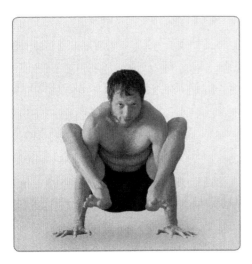

dwi hasta bhujasana
two hand and arm pose

shape
(from *tadasana*)

1. Separate the outer edges of the feet as wide as the mat.
2. Inhale fully. Exhale, fold the torso over the legs.
3. Widen and bend the knees to lower the shoulders below the knees. Hold the backs of the calves with the hands.
4. Place the thumbs on the centers of the calves and fingers on the outer shins. Press the calves forward and in with the thumbs.
5. One at a time, bring the shoulders behind the knees.
6. Bend the knees and lower the hips. Place the hands on the floor shoulder-width apart behind the feet. Separate the fingers and point the index fingers straight ahead.
7. Squeeze the legs into the arms. Lean back and bring the weight into the hands to lift the feet off the floor. Straighten the arms.
8. Press the feet toward one another. Flex the feet and flare the toes.
9. Look straight ahead. Hold the pose and breathe.
10. To come out, bend the elbows and lean forward to bring the feet to the floor. Release the arms and lift the torso to stand.

safety

-   Press the fingertips and the perimeter of the palms into the floor with equal pressure. Do not collapse the weight of the body into the wrists.
-   Engage the abdomen.
-   Lift the pelvic floor and tone the low belly.
-   Move the shoulders back.
-   If the hips and legs cannot lift off floor, place blocks underneath the hands.

refinement

Action and movement often oppose each other in poses. In *dwi hasta bhujasana*, for example, the action of the shoulders is backward. And yet, the weight of the legs will cause the shoulders to move forward. Being overzealous in your attempt to move the shoulders back will put them into a potentially dangerous position. Press the shoulders back—just enough to create stability—but do not force them back. The distinction between action and movement in hatha yoga is an important one. Once you can perform *upavishta konasana*, *kurmasana*, and *dwi hasta bhujasana*, you are ready to proceed onto *tittibhasana*.

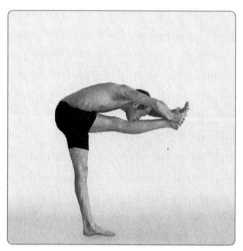 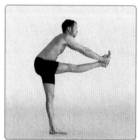

dwi hasta padasana
two hand foot pose

shape
(from *tadasana*)

1. Balancing on the left foot, lift the right leg and interlace the fingers around the sole of the foot.
2. Lift the right foot in line with the hip.
3. Round the back and bend both knees slightly.
4. Straighten the standing leg, then straighten the lifted leg.
5. Inhale fully. Exhale, fold the torso forward over the lifted leg—chin toward/to shin.
6. Bend the elbows out to the sides. Hold the pose and breathe.
7. To come out, inhale, lift the head and look forward. Exhale, release the leg and lift the torso to stand.

Repeat on the second side.

safety

- To reduce pressure on the low back, bend both knees and lift the top foot as high as the hips or use a strap around the lifted foot. Or, straighten the arms and keep the torso lifted.
- To strengthen the hamstrings, straighten the standing leg completely.
- Engage the lifted leg—pull the foot with the hands and push the foot into the hands.
- Isometrically pull the top foot down.

refinement

Move the hip of your lifted leg down. To improve your balance in this pose, gaze at a single point on the floor. *Dwi hasta padasana* is a challenging pose that intensely stretches and strengthens the spine and hamstrings. It also improves balance. In yoga, the purpose of challenge is to initiate the very change you seek.

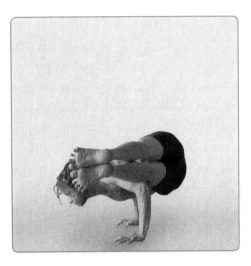

dwi pada koundinyasana
two leg Sage Koundinya's pose

shape

1. Come into a squat position—feet and knees together.
2. Place the hands on the floor behind the hips and lean back.
3. Inhale, squeeze the legs together and lift the left arm vertical.
4. Exhale, twist the torso to the right and place the left shoulder on the outside of the right knee.
5. Place both hands on the floor shoulder-width apart.
6. Separate the fingers and turn the hands out until the index fingers are parallel to each other.
7. Lift the heels and lean forward. Place the outer right leg against the upper arms and bring weight into the hands. Straighten the right leg out to the side—leg parallel to the floor.
8. Bend the elbows 90 degrees so the forearms are vertical.
9. Balancing on the hands, lift and straighten the left leg. Bring the inner edges of the feet together.
10. Tone the low belly and turn the abdomen away from the legs.
11. Look straight ahead. Hold the pose and breathe.

Repeat on the second side.

safety

- Press the fingertips and the perimeter of the palms down into the floor with equal pressure.
- Avoid rounding the shoulders down, toward the floor. Lift and level the shoulders.
- Stack the top hip over the bottom hip.
- Squeeze the inner feet, ankles, and knees together.
- Bring the feet halfway between a flexed and pointed position. Flare the toes.

refinement

Advanced practitioners can move into *dwi pada koundinyasana* from *sirsasana 2*. Keeping your legs straight, exhale, lower your feet just above the floor. In one swift movement, swing your feet to the left as you bring your outer right leg to your upper left arm. Inhale, lift your head off the floor and look straight ahead. After five breaths, exhale, lower the top of your head onto the floor and lift your legs to return to *sirsasana 2*. Repeat on the second side and after five breaths return to *sirsasana 2*. Exhale, bend your knees and lower your feet to the floor behind your head as you straighten your arms to come into *urdhva dhanurasana*. After five breaths kick your feet up and over into *adho mukha svanasana*.

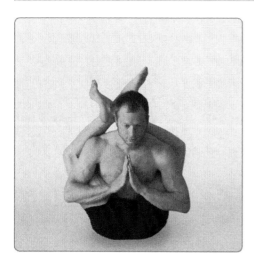

dwi pada sirsasana
two legs behind the head pose

shape
(from *dandasana*)

1. Bring the left leg behind the head as described in *eka pada sirsasana*. Pause and breathe.
2. Bring the right ankle to the top of the left toes. Flex the left foot to pull the ankles together. Pull both shoulders in front of the torso.
3. Balance on the hips and place the palms together in front of the chest.
4. Look down. Hold the pose and breathe.
5. To come out, release the hands to the floor. Lean the torso forward and one at a time, pull the legs off the back. Lower and straighten the legs.

Repeat on the second side.

safety

*   Press the head, neck, and shoulders into the legs.
*   Engage the feet. Flare the outer two toes of each foot.
*   Isometrically bend the knees to engage the hamstrings.
*   Lift the pelvic floor and tone the low belly.
*   If it is difficult to balance, practice the pose with the back against a wall and/or the hands on the floor.

refinement

If you can perform *eka pada sirsasana* on both sides, you are ready for this pose. Advanced practitioners can place the hands on the floor, straighten the arms and lift the hips away from the floor. Then lean forward, release your legs from behind the head and come into *tittibhasana*. In one fluid movement, lift up into *adho mukha vrksasana*. Drop over into *urdhva dhanurasana 1*. Hold for five even breaths. Then lower down and rest.

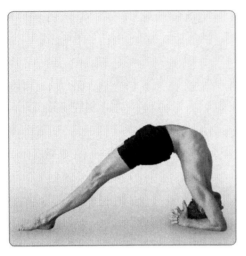
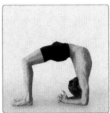
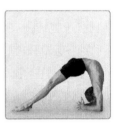

dwi pada viparita dandasana
two leg inverted staff pose

shape
(from *urdhva dhanurasana 1*)

1. Bend the elbows and place the top of the head on the floor.
2. Lower the elbows to the floor shoulder-width apart. Interlace the fingers behind the head—thumbs pointing up.
3. One at a time, slide the feet away from the head and straighten the legs.
4. Look straight ahead. Hold the pose and breathe.
5. To come out, exhale, walk the feet in toward the head until the feet are directly below the knees. Place the hands on the floor shoulder-width apart. Press the hands down and straighten the arms to lift the head and torso.

safety

- For a more accessible variation or to reduce the intensity of the shoulder stretch, lift the head and bring the upper arms vertical. If this is still too intense, bend the knees and walk the feet in toward the head.
- Press the wrists into the floor.
- Simultaneously move the shoulders back and extend the chest forward.
- Press the feet down and away from the hips.
- Extend the inner edges of the feet down. Rotate the inner thighs down.
- Flare the outer two toes and squeeze the shins in.
- Lock the legs into a straight position.
- Engage the glutes and abdomen. Lift the tailbone.
- Move the base of the sternum back and stretch the entire spine.
- Breathe evenly. Soften the eyes.

refinement

It is a common mistake to progress too quickly in backbends. I recommend you do not proceed beyond the basic belly-down backbends and *urdhva dhanurasana 1* for the first several years of your practice. Slow is the way to go. If you progress too fast it could turn your practice into a thing of the past. I am aware that I've already said essentially the same thing in other Refinement sections. Well, I've also said the same thing countless times in the Safety sections. Repetition is part and parcel of this practice.

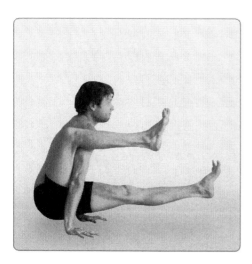

eka hasta bhujasana
one hand and arm pose

shape
(from *dandasana*)

1. Bend the right knee in toward the chest and hold the right heel with the left hand. Lift the shin parallel to the floor.
2. Hold the right calf with the right hand—arm to inside of the knee.
3. Bring the back of the right knee onto the right shoulder.
4. Place the right hand on the floor in front of the hips and slightly to the right. Place the left hand on the floor just outside of the left leg—hands parallel and shoulder-width apart.
5. Move the shoulders back and press the shoulder into the leg.
6. Push down through the hands to lift the hips and extended leg off the floor. Bring the lower leg and top shin parallel to the floor.
7. Look straight ahead. Hold the pose and breathe.
8. To come out, exhale, lower the hips and leg to the floor. Release the top leg to the floor.

Repeat on the second side.

safety

- Press the fingertips and the perimeter of the right hand evenly into the floor—press the mound of the index finger down and lift the outer wrist up.
- Squeeze the legs toward the midline of the body.
- Flex the feet and engage the toes.
- Strengthen the lifted leg—tone the thigh and lock the knee into a straight position.
- Engage the abdomen.
- Lift the pelvic floor and tone the low belly.

refinement

To work toward the full pose, begin by lifting your hips while keeping your lower heel on the floor. Hold this for several breaths. Lower the hips, then lift only the lower leg. Hold that for several breaths and then attempt the full form of *eka hasta bhujasana*.

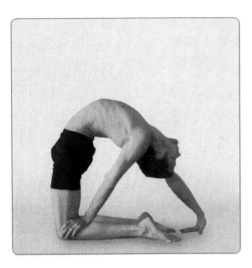

eka hasta laghuvajrasana
one hand graceful thunderbolt pose

shape

1. Come into an upright kneeling position—knees outer hip-width apart and shins parallel.
2. Bring the tops of the feet to the floor and point the toes straight back.
3. Inhale, lift the chest. Exhale, curl the torso and head back. Hold the backs of the knees with the hands.
4. Extend the right arm overhead and place the hand on the floor behind the feet.
5. Look between the eyebrows. Hold the pose and breathe.
6. To come out, walk the hands to the feet and hold the heels. Pause and breathe. Inhale, lift the torso. Once the torso is upright, lift the head.

Repeat on the second side.

safety

- Isometrically squeeze the knees and ankles in. Flare the outer two toes.
- Move the inner thighs back, engage the glutes, and extend the hips forward.
- Press the tops of the feet down, move the hips forward, and lift the chest.
- Keep the neck muscles engaged.
- Strengthen the arms and lock the elbows into a straight position.
- Extend the right shoulder down and back.

refinement

For a more doable variation of this pose, place your hands on the backs of the legs halfway between your hips and knees. Extend one arm overhead parallel to the floor.

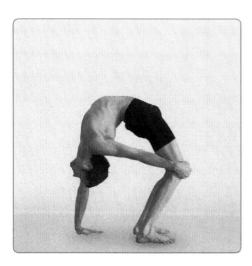

eka hasta urdhva dhanurasana
one hand upward-facing bow pose

shape
(from *urdhva dhanurasana 1*)

1. Shift the weight of the torso into the left hand.
2. Inhale fully. Exhale, clasp the right knee with the right hand.
3. Look at the tip of the nose. Hold the pose and breathe for 15 to 20 seconds.
4. To come out, exhale, place the right hand on the floor—hands shoulder-width apart.

Repeat on the second side.

safety
*   If the forearms are not vertical in *urdhva dhanurasana 1,* do not attempt this pose.
*   Press the fingertips and the perimeter of the bottom palm down. Dig the thumb down and squeeze it isometrically toward the palm.
*   Lock both elbows into a straight position.
*   Simultaneously extend the left shoulder back and the chest forward.
*   Press the inner edges of the feet down. Rotate the inner thighs down.
*   Flare the outer two toes. Squeeze the shins in.
*   Engage the glutes and lift the tailbone.
*   Lift the pelvic floor and tone the low belly.
*   Move the base of the sternum back and lengthen the spine.
*   Hold the pose, not the breath.

refinement
Eka hasta urdhva dhanurasana is a good preparatory pose for *bhujangasana 2.*

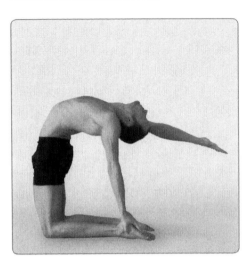

eka hasta ustrasana
one hand camel pose

shape
(from *ustrasana*)

1. Inhale, lift the right arm overhead with the upper arm in line with the right ear.
2. Straighten the right arm and point the palm up. Look between the eyebrows. Hold the pose and breathe.
3. To come out, exhale, release the top hand to the heel. Inhale, lift the torso. Once the torso is upright, lift the head.

Repeat on the second side.

safety
- Isometrically squeeze the knees and ankles in. Flare the outer two toes.
- Move the inner thighs back, engage the glutes, and extend the hips forward.
- Press the tops of the feet down and extend the chest up.
- Engage the pelvic floor and low belly.
- Keep the neck muscles engaged.
- Lock the elbows into a straight position.
- Extend the shoulder of the lifted arm down and back.

Refinement
Eka hasta ustrasana is a good preparatory pose for *eka hasta laghuvajrasana*. To strengthen your core, place your hand on your hip instead of on your heel. To deepen your backbend and strengthen your neck, hold the back of your head with your right hand and point your elbow up. Press your head into your hand, and lift the back of your head with your hand.

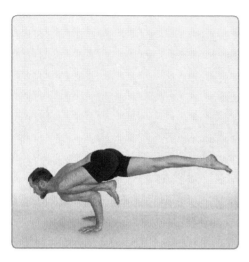
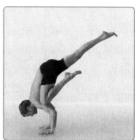

eka pada bakasana 1
one leg crane pose 1

shape
(from *malasana 1*)

1. Place the hands directly below the shoulders to rest the middle of the shins against the shoulders. Point the elbows straight back.
2. Lean forward, lift the heels, and transfer the weight to the hands.
3. Lift the feet off the floor. Keep the inner edges of the feet together.
4. Squeeze the elbows in so the forearms are parallel.
5. Round the back.
6. Isometrically squeeze both legs toward the midline and extend the right leg back—straighten it to capacity.
7. Lean forward and bend the elbows 90 degrees.
8. Bring the torso and back leg parallel to the floor. Point the feet.
9. Look straight ahead. Hold the pose and breathe.
10. To come out, exhale, bend the back knee and bring the foot below the hips. Lower the hips and feet.

Repeat on the second side.

safety

- Press the fingertips and the perimeter of the palms into the floor with equal pressure.
- Engage the abdomen and press the tailbone down.
- Strengthen the back leg. Engage the quads and back glutes.
- Point the back kneecap straight down.
- To reduce the pressure on the wrists, place the heels of the palms on the mat and the knuckles and fingers off the mat. (This will only be effective if you have a thick mat.)
- If there is still pain or discomfort in the wrists, keep the elbows bent and bring the shoulders directly over the wrists to reduce the angle of the arms.

refinement

Advanced practitioners can lift the torso and legs toward vertical for a challenging variation of this pose. It makes for a very unpleasant yet pose-productive experience!

Advanced practitioners can attempt the following sequence: from *sirsasana 2*, lower into *eka pada bakasana 1*, then transition into *astavakrasana*. Move from *astavakrasana* into *eka pada koundinyasana 2*. Bend your knees and come back into *sirsasana 2*. Repeat on the second side. Once complete, drop your legs back from *sirsasana* 2 into *urdhva dhanurasana* and hold for five breaths. From here, come onto your back for a well-earned rest.

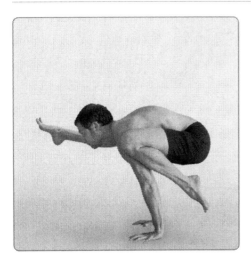

eka pada bakasana 2
one leg crane pose 2

shape
(from *malasana 1*)

1. Place the hands directly below the shoulders to rest the middle of the shins against the shoulders. Point the elbows straight back.
2. Lean forward, lift the heels, and transfer the weight to the hands.
3. Lift the feet off the floor. Keep the inner edges of the feet together. Point the feet and flare the toes.
4. Squeeze the elbows in so the forearms are parallel.
5. Sway the hips and feet to the right, slide the back of the right knee over the right arm, and extend the right leg straight ahead—leg parallel to the floor.
6. Round the back, straighten the arms, and look straight ahead. Hold the pose and breathe.
7. To come out, bend the right knee back. Pause and breathe in *bakasana*, and then lower the hips and feet.

Repeat on the second side.

safety

- Press the fingertips and the perimeter of the palms down into the floor with equal pressure.
- Pressing the hands down, lift the pelvic floor.
- Move the tailbone forward and engage the abdomen.
- Strengthen the extended leg. Bring the foot halfway between a flexed and pointed position.

- Squeeze both legs into the arms.
- To reduce the pressure on the wrists, place the heels of the palms on the mat and the knuckles and fingers off the mat. (This will only be effective if you have a thick mat.)
- If there is still pain or discomfort in the wrists, keep the elbows bent and bring the shoulders directly over the wrists to reduce the angle of the arms.

refinement

I have only injured myself in hatha yoga a few times. Each of these injuries occurred while doing a demo. For example, back in the day when I taught a class called "radical expansion," I demonstrated the final form of *kandasana*. During the demo, there was a sound like someone ripping a piece of paper. That sound was me spraining my ankle. Amazingly, no swelling occurred and I healed quickly, but you can imagine no one really wanted to attempt *kandasana* after that!

In B. K. S Iyengar's *Light On Yoga*, he gives the beneficial effects of 200 poses—beneficial if all goes according to plan, that is. Like in the instance of my *kandasana* demo, the potential benefit became immediate detriment. When injury occurs, that could be a reason to discontinue practice. Or, it could be the opportunity to continue practice in a different way.

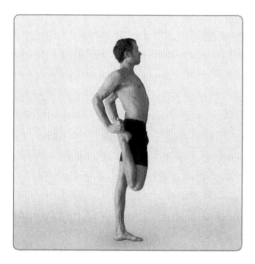

eka pada bhekasana
one leg frog pose

standing

shape
(from *tadasana*)

1. Place the left hand on the left hip. Reach the right arm back, palm facing out.
2. Kick the right foot back and hold the top of the foot with the hand—thumb across sole of foot.
3. Pull the heel toward the outer right hip. Rotate the arm by simultaneously pointing the elbow back and spinning the hand—thumb to arch, fingers to outer edge of foot. Flare the toes.
4. Point the knee straight down.
5. Look straight ahead. Hold the pose and breathe.
6. To come out, slowly release the foot and bring the arms by the sides.

Repeat on the second side.

safety

- If there is tightness in the shoulder, do not overcompensate by increasing the backbend in the low back. Keep the knee pointing down to the floor and tone the low belly. From this stable foundation, work the arm position little by little. Start by pulling the heel to the outer hip without rotating and spinning the arm. As the upper back, inner shoulder, and pectoral muscles begin to open, spinning the hand forward will become more accessible.
- Press the inner edge of the top foot toward/to the outer hip. If the top foot moves out/away from the hips, it can strain the knee.
- Engage the standing leg.
- Engage the glutes.
- Move the tailbone down and draw the low belly in.
- Move the base of the sternum back and lift the chest.
- Lift the shoulders up and back.

refinement

Simultaneously press both hands down and stretch your spine up. This pose is similar in shape to *eka pada bhekasana* prone variation (on the front body). The standing version adds an element of balance, which builds strength in the standing leg, while the prone version depends on the strength of the front arm to prop up the upper body, as well as flexibility at the top of the spine. Getting the arm into the proper position in order to pull the foot to the outer hip provides ample stretch in the inner shoulder. In both cases, the thigh stretch will only be as deep as the arm is strong, considering it is the strength of the arm that determines how much the thigh is stretched.

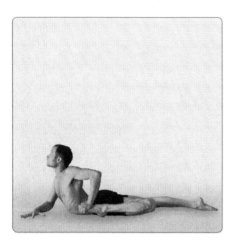

eka pada bhekasana
one leg frog pose

shape

1. Lower the front body to the floor—legs straight, feet outer hip-width apart.
2. Place the right forearm on the floor parallel to the top of the mat—elbow directly below shoulder.
3. Bend the left knee and hold the foot with the left hand. Bring the heel to the top of the left glutes. Pause and breathe.
4. Bring the hand to the inner edge of the foot and place the thumb around the arch of the foot—fingers around the outer edge of the foot.
5. Point the elbow up. Inhale fully. Exhale, lower the inner edge of the left heel to the outer left hip. Look straight ahead. Hold the pose and breathe.
6. To come out, release the hand and straighten the bent leg.

Repeat on the second side.

safety

- Lock the back leg into a strong and straight position.
- Tone and lift the inner thighs.
- Press the tailbone down, lift the low belly, and contract the glutes.
- Press the back foot and front forearm down. Pull the front forearm toward the hips to lift the chest up and forward.
- Extend the bent knee and chest away from the hips.
- Square the torso and shoulders to the top of the mat. Move both shoulders up and back.
- If there is pain or discomfort in the knee, widen the knee slightly. If there is still pain, discontinue the pose.
- If there is pain or discomfort in the low back, walk the front forearm forward until the elbow is in front of the shoulder and the torso and chest lowers.

refinement

Advanced practitioners can wrap the fingers around the toes and press the heel to the floor. In *eka pada bhekasana*, the less you stretch the quad, the more you will be required to stretch your shoulder; the more you stretch the quad, the less you will be required to stretch your shoulder. In either case, this pose does not require as much of a backbend in the spine compared to other backbending poses.

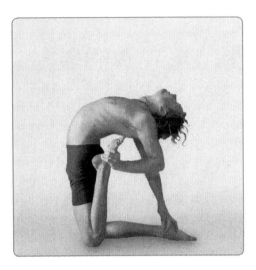

eka pada bhekasana in ustrasana
one leg frog in camel pose

shape

1. Come into an upright kneeling position—knees outer hip-width apart and shins parallel.
2. Bring the tops of the feet to the floor and point the toes straight back.
3. Lift the left foot and hold the top of the foot with the left hand. Wrap the outer edge of the left foot with the fingers and the arch of the foot with the thumb.
4. Inhale, lift the chest. Exhale, curl the torso and head back and place the right hand on the right heel.
5. Look between the eyebrows. Hold the pose and breathe.
6. To come out, inhale, lift the torso. Once the torso is upright, lift the head. Lower the foot to the floor.

Repeat on the second side.

safety

- Isometrically squeeze the knees and ankles in, and flare the outer two toes of both feet.
- Move the inner thighs back, engage the glutes, and extend the hips forward.
- Press the top of the bottom foot down and lift the chest.
- Press the inner edge of the lifted foot into the outer hip.
- Move the shoulders back and in toward the spine.
- Engage the pelvic floor and low belly.
- Keep the neck muscles engaged.
- If the hand cannot reach the foot, curl the bottom toes under and hold the heel.
- If curling the head back is too intense for the neck, look straight up or straight ahead.

refinement

Eka pada bhekasana in *ustrasana* is a good preparation for *supta bhekasana*.

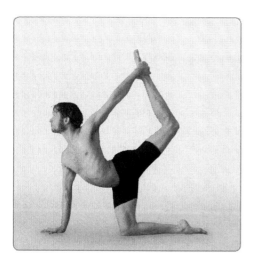

eka pada dhanurasana
one leg bow pose

from all fours, same leg and arm

shape

1. Come onto the hands and knees with the arms and thighs vertical—shoulders directly over the wrists, hips directly over the knees.
2. Separate the hands slightly wider than shoulder-distance apart. Straighten the arms.
3. Separate the knees and feet outer hip-width apart.
4. Bring the tops of the feet onto the floor. Point the toes straight back and squeeze the ankles in until the heels are vertical.
5. Inhale, lift the chin and the left leg parallel to the floor. Point the toes straight down.
6. Transfer the weight onto the right hand and right knee.
7. Keeping the left thigh parallel to the floor, bend the knee.
8. Clasp the outer edge of the left foot with the left hand and straighten the top arm.
9. Kick the top foot back and up to capacity. Look forward. Hold the pose and breathe.
10. To come out, release the top hand, and lower the arm and leg to the floor.

Repeat on the second side.

safety

- Separate the fingers of the bottom hand and point the index finger forward. Press the entire perimeter of the palm down, especially the mound of the index finger.
- Lock the elbows into a straight position.
- Press the lower knee, shin, and the top of the foot down.
- Move the hip of the lifted leg down to level the hips.
- Tone and lift the inner thigh of the lifted leg.
- Engage the glutes of the lifted leg.
- Point the lifted kneecap down.
- Press the top hand and foot into each other.
- Press the tailbone down and lift the low belly.
- Stretch the spine, and extend the chest and top knee away from the hips.
- If the balance is difficult, practice the pose against a wall (line up the side of the body with the planted hand and foot along the wall).

refinement

Eka pada dhanurasana is a good preparatory pose for *dhanurasana* and *kapinjalasana* prep. The elevated position of the torso yields a deeper and more doable backbend. Notice in the photo that the back knee is almost as high as the head. This is a much higher leg position than the knees in *dhanurasana*. Balancing on the same leg and arm makes for a unique and difficult balancing pose.

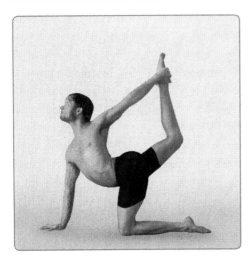

eka pada dhanurasana
one leg bow pose

from all fours, opposite leg and arm

shape

1. Come onto the hands and knees with the arms and thighs vertical—shoulders directly over the wrists, hips directly over the knees.
2. Separate the hands slightly wider than shoulder-distance apart. Straighten the arms.
3. Separate the knees and feet outer hip-width apart.
4. Bring the tops of the feet onto the floor. Point the toes straight back and squeeze the ankles in until the heels are vertical.
5. Inhale, lift the right leg parallel to the floor.
6. Keeping the thigh parallel to the floor, exhale, bend the knee.
7. Clasp the inner edge of the right foot with the left hand and kick the foot up and back to capacity.
8. Lift the chin and look straight ahead. Hold the pose and breathe.
9. To come out, exhale, release the top hand, and lower the lifted leg and arm.

Repeat on the second side.

safety

- Separate the fingers of the bottom hand and point the index finger forward. Press the entire perimeter of the palm down, especially the mound of the index finger.
- Lock the elbows into a straight position.
- Press the lower knee, shin, and top of the foot down.
- Move the hip of the lifted leg down to level the hips.

- Tone and lift the inner thigh of the lifted leg.
- Engage the glutes of the lifted leg.
- Point the lifted kneecap down.
- Press the top hand and foot into each other.
- Press the tailbone down and lift the low belly.
- Stretch the spine and extend the chest and top knee away from the hips.

refinement

Square your shoulders to the top of the mat. Lift the waist on the side of your lifted leg. Push your lower hand down and back to lift your collarbones. Point the toes of your lifted foot straight up. Spread your toes. *Eka pada dhanurasana* is a good preparatory pose for *parivrtta ardha chandrachapasana*.

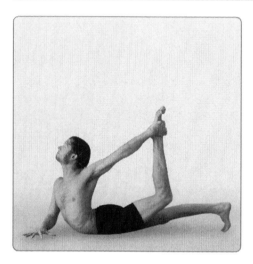

eka pada dhanurasana
one leg bow pose

shape

1. Bring the front body to the floor—legs straight and feet outer hip-width apart. Curl the toes under.
2. Place the right elbow slightly in front of the right shoulder and bring the forearm parallel to the top of the mat.
3. Bend the left knee and hold the outside of the foot with the left hand. Bring the foot halfway between a flexed and pointed position.
4. Inhale fully. Exhale, kick the left foot into the hand and lift the left knee and thigh.
5. Lift the chin and look up. Hold the pose and breathe.
6. To come out, exhale, release the foot and lower the arm and leg.

Repeat on the second side.

safety

- Strengthen the top arm and extended leg. Lock the elbow and knee into a straight position.
- Engage the feet. Flare the outer two toes of the top foot and press the toes of the bottom foot down.
- Press the tailbone and hips down. Tone the abdomen.

- Engage the glutes of the lifted leg.
- Isometrically pull the front forearm toward the hips to extend the spine forward and up.
- Lift the shoulders up and back.
- Lift the chest and extend the back of the head up.
- If there is any discomfort in the bent knee, hold the ankle and flex the foot.
- To reduce the intensity of the pose, place a bolster underneath the lower ribcage to elevate the torso. Place the hand out in front of the shoulder and straighten the arm.
- If the back hand cannot reach the top foot, use a strap. If there is pain or discomfort at the front of the hips, place a folded blanket below the hips for additional padding.

refinement

Square your torso and shoulders to the top of the mat. Soften your throat, jaw, and eyes. Hold the pose without holding your breath. Advanced practitioners can point the front hand forward toward the top of the mat and straighten the arm. This will lift the torso and chest, and increase the backbend.

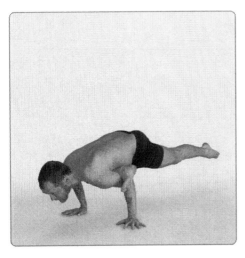
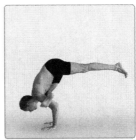

eka pada galavasana
one leg Sage Galava's pose

shape
(from *tadasana*)

1. Bend the knees slightly.
2. Place the right outer ankle just above the left knee. Lower the hips to the same height as the left knee.
3. Fold the torso forward and place the hands on the floor directly below the shoulders.
4. Separate the fingers and point the index fingers straight ahead.
5. Flex the right foot and hook the top of the foot around the left upper arm. Place the upper right shin on the upper right arm as high toward the armpit as possible.
6. Bend the elbows and lean forward until the forearms are vertical. Rest the chest against the top shin.
7. Transfer all of the body weight onto the hands and lift the left foot. Reach the leg back and straighten the leg. Bring the leg parallel to the floor.
8. Look forward. Hold the pose and breathe.

9. To come out, bend the back knee and swing the foot forward. Release the top leg and lift the torso to stand.

Repeat on the second side.

safety

- If it is too difficult to bring the body and back leg parallel to the floor, lean forward toward the face and lift the back leg higher than the hips.
- Press the fingertips and the perimeter of the palms down into the floor with equal pressure.
- Flex the front foot and pull the foot into the arm.
- Straighten and strengthen the back leg. Engage the glutes.
- Lift the inner edge of the back leg up. Point the back kneecap straight down.
- Press the tailbone down.

refinement

Advanced practitioners can enter into this pose from *sirsasana 2* and can exit by jumping into *chaturanga dandasana*. To enter from *sirsasana 2*, bend your knees and place your right ankle just above your left knee. Bend and lower your left knee. Bring the top of your right knee onto your upper right arm and the right ankle onto your upper left arm. Lower your hips and transfer your weight into the hands. Lift your head off the floor and extend the left leg straight back. Lower your torso, hips, and back leg parallel to the floor. Hold the pose for five breaths and then come back into *sirsasana 2*. Repeat on the second side.

Eka pada galavasana can also be entered from *adho mukha vrksasana*. Once in *eka pada galavasana* hold the pose for five breaths and then in one movement, return to *adho mukha vrksasana*. This is a difficult maneuver.

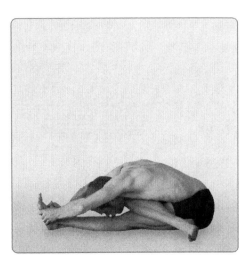

eka pada gomukha paschimottanasana
one leg cow face back stretched out pose

shape
(from *dandasana*)

1. Bend the right knee and place the right heel to the outer left hip. Flex the right foot and point the toes to the left. Lower the right knee to the left thigh.
2. Inhale fully. Exhale, fold the torso forward to hold the front foot with both hands.
3. Inhale, straighten the arms and lift the shoulders and chin.
4. Exhale, fold the torso over the legs and place the face on the shin. Look down. Hold the pose and breathe.
5. To come out, walk the hands back underneath the shoulders. Inhale, lift the head and look up. Use the arms to lift the torso upright. Straighten the right leg next to the left leg. Place the hands next to the hips.

Repeat on the second side.

safety

- If the low back rounds, sit on one or more blankets. Bring the hands to the floor shoulder-width apart. Fold forward part of the way and lengthen the spine.
- Press the left heel and knee down.
- Engage the left quads.
- Use the arms and abdomen to pull the face toward the shin.
- Lift the pelvic floor and tone the low belly.

refinement

The pressure of your right shin and knee on your left thigh will make it difficult to engage your left quads. However, if you do not engage your quads, the weight of the body will push the back of your extended knee down and may cause hyperextension in the knee. Instead of placing your right shin and knee on top of your left quads, you can squeeze the outer left quads up and in with the right calf as you bring the right heel to your outer left hip.

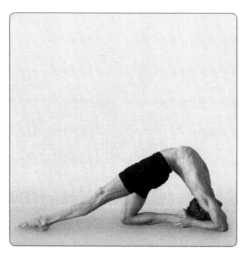 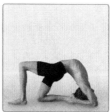 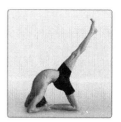

eka pada kapotasana
one leg pigeon pose

straight leg, foot to floor

shape
(from *supta virasana*)

1. Place the hands flat on the floor by the head—thumbs facing in. Point the elbows up.
2. Inhale, lift the hips and torso. Straighten the arms.
3. Walk the hands toward the feet until the thighs are vertical.
4. Place the inner edges of the feet together. Bring the elbows to the floor directly under the shoulders. Walk the hands toward the feet and clasp the right ankle with both hands.
5. Place the top of the head on the sole of the right foot.
6. In one movement, lift the left knee and bring the foot flat on the floor—knee bent to a 90-degree angle. Pause and breathe.
7. Slide the left foot forward and straighten the leg. Point the toes to bring the sole of the foot to the floor.
8. Keeping the leg straight, inhale, lift the left leg as high as possible.
9. Look straight back. Hold the pose and breathe.
10. To come out, exhale, lower the left shin and top of the left foot back to the floor. Walk the hands away from the feet and place the hands on the floor next to the feet—thumbs facing in. Keep the chest full and inhale, lift the torso vertical. Once the torso is upright, lift the head.

Repeat on the second side.

safety
- Flare the outer two toes.
- Press the top of the bottom foot down and move the hips forward.
- Move the inner thigh of the bottom leg down.
- Press the tailbone forward and engage the glutes.
- Lift the pelvic floor and tone the low belly.
- Press the wrists down.
- Expand the chest while simultaneously moving the shoulders back.
- Press the head and foot into each other.

• Strengthen the top leg.

refinement

Kapotasana and variations are, in many ways, more difficult to perform than *rajakapotasana* and variations. *Kapotasana* and variations can, however, be held for much longer and with much more comfort. *Rajakapotasana* and its variations require the spine to be upright, which makes it more difficult to extend the spine. In *kapotasana* and variations, the spine is basically inverted, which allows gravity to support the extension of the spine. In both cases, one of the biggest challenges is to breathe fully. It is a common mistake to hold one's breath when performing the more advanced backbends, which can bring excess internal pressure to the head. If you are holding your breath in any advanced pose, it is arguable that you are not really in the pose. Attaining the external form is just one of many aspects of each and every asana.

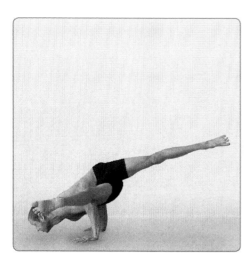

eka pada koundinyasana 1
one leg Sage Koundinya's pose 1

shape
(from *dwi pada koundinyasana*)

1. Simultaneously extend the left leg straight back and lower the head toward the floor.
2. Look forward. Hold the pose and breathe.

Repeat on the second side.

safety
*   Press the fingertips and the perimeter of the palms down onto the floor with equal pressure.
*   Avoid rounding the shoulders down toward the floor. Lift and level the shoulders.
*   Straighten and strengthen both legs. Bring the back foot halfway between a flexed and pointed position and flare the toes.

refinement
Eka pada koundinyasana 1 and *dwi pada koundinyasana* are both twisting arm balances. To properly prepare the body for *eka pada koundinyasana 1*, practice revolved lunge, fallen sage, and *eka pada rajakapotasana prep*, shoulder to knee. If you cannot come into *dwi pada koundinyasana*, enter *eka pada koundinyasana 1* from lunge pose. Place both hands on the floor outside of your front leg. Bend your elbows to lean forward, place your leg against your upper arm, and lift your front leg. Then lift your back leg. Straighten your legs and twist your navel away from your front leg. Advanced practitioners can move from one side of *eka pada koundinyasana 1* to the other in a single mid-air movement.

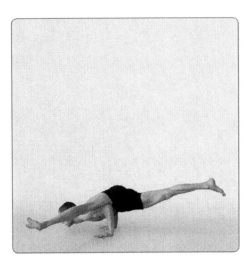

eka pada koundinyasana 2
one leg Sage Koundinya's pose 2

shape
(from *eka pada koundinyasana 1*)

1. Keep the back leg straight and bring the inner thigh to the upper left arm—just in front of the right leg.
2. Extend the right leg straight back.
3. Look forward. Hold the pose and breathe.
4. To come out, reach the top leg back into *chaturanga dandasana*. Move through *urdhva mukha svanasana* and *adho mukha svanasana*.

Repeat on the second side.

safety
- Press the fingertips and the perimeter of the palms down into the floor with equal pressure.
- Avoid rounding the shoulders down toward the floor. Lift and level the shoulders.
- Straighten and strengthen both legs. Engage the glutes.
- Lift the inner edge of the back leg up. Extend the outer edge of the front leg down.
- Press the tailbone down.

refinement
Dwi pada koundinyasana, eka pada koundinyasana 1, and *eka pada koundinyasana 2* can be practiced individually. I am putting them together as one sequence for those that are able. If you cannot come into *eka pada koundinyasana 2* from *eka pada koundinyasana 1,* start from lunge pose with your left foot forward. Lower your back knee and bring your left shoulder under your left knee. Place your hands on the floor shoulder-width apart. Bend your elbows and lean forward—toward your head—until your forearms are vertical. Straighten your front leg and lift your back leg.

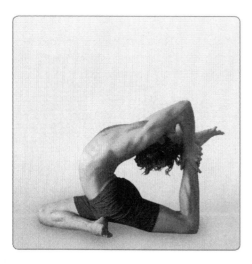

eka pada rajakapotasana 1
one leg king pigeon pose 1

shape
(from *adho mukha svanasana*)

1. Inhale fully. Exhale, bring the right knee to the floor to the right of and just behind the right hand—knee slightly wider than the right hip.
2. Lower the right sit bone and leg to the floor.
3. Point the right foot and press the right heel to the front of the left hip.
4. Inhale, lift the torso to a vertical position. Bend the back knee to lift the shin vertical.
5. Place the palms together behind the head, point the fingers straight back, and separate the elbows shoulder-width apart.
6. Inhale fully. Exhale, curl the head and torso back and clasp the foot with the hands. If possible, flex the foot and slide the hands down to the ankle.
7. Press the forehead into the heel. Look back. Hold the pose and breathe.
8. To come out, keep the chest full and inhale, release the hands and lower the back leg. Lift the torso upright and place the hands on the floor in front of the top shin. Separate the hands shoulder-width apart, curl the back toes under, and push the hands down and forward to push the hips up and back.

Repeat on the second side.

safety

- Move the left hip forward and the right hip back to square the hips.
- Press the outer edge/top of the front foot down and clamp the front knee closed.
- Isometrically squeeze the knees toward each other.
- Press the tailbone down, engage the back glutes, and lift the low belly.
- Move the base of the sternum back and stretch the spine and chest up.
- Extend the elbows up and move the shoulders back.
- Flare the outer two toes.
- Press the back foot and hands into each other.
- Pull the foot into the head and reach the head into the foot.
- For a more accessible entry to clasping the foot behind the head, see *eka pada rajakapotasana 2*.

refinement

This pose is either potent medicine or poison for the psoas, low back, and shoulders. It is more likely to be medicinal if you spend a few years refining *virabhadrasana 1, anjaneyasana, dhanurasana, ustrasana,* and *urdhva dhanurasana 1.* A few years? Yoga yep—patience is paramount to practice! A student told me that he didn't realize until recently that this pose is a backbend. He always thought of it as a shoulder stretch. That is because he was barely backbending when attempting *eka pada rajakapotasana 1,* which over-stretched and strained his shoulders. When he finally learned to bend deeply in his back, his shoulders were no longer an obstacle or even an issue.

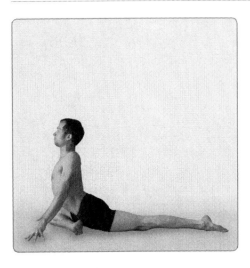

eka pada rajakapotasana 1 prep
one leg king pigeon pose 1

torso lifted

shape
(from *adho mukha svanasana*)

1. Inhale fully. Exhale, bend the right knee and place the knee to the right of and just behind the right wrist. Lower the hips and the outer right leg to the floor with the right heel touching the front of the left hip.
2. Slide the hips back slightly so the front of the back thigh touches the floor.
3. Bring the back leg parallel to the long edge of the mat. Point the back foot and squeeze the heel in.
4. Place the fingertips on the floor slightly wider than shoulder-distance apart in front of the top shin.
5. Inhale, lift the torso upright and look straight ahead. Hold the pose and breathe.
6. To come out, place the hands flat on the floor and curl the back toes under. Exhale, push the hands down and forward to lift the hips up and back. Step the front leg back.

Repeat on the second side.

safety
- Move the left hip forward and the right hip back to square the hips to the front of the mat.
- Center the weight in the hips and pelvis. The weight tends to lean into the hip of the bent leg.

- Press the outer edge/top of the front foot down.
- Clamp the front knee closed.
- Press the back foot down and straighten the leg.
- Isometrically squeeze the front knee and back leg toward each other.
- Rotate the inner thigh of the back leg up to point the kneecap straight down.
- Press the tailbone down and lift the low belly.
- Engage the glutes of the back leg.
- Press the hands down and back to stretch the spine and chest up.
- If there is pain or discomfort in the low back or to reduce the intensity of the stretch in the back quads, lift the hips slightly and/or place a blanket or block underneath the sit bone of the front leg.

refinement

Square your shoulders and torso to the top of the mat and turn your low belly and navel toward your front knee. Lift and widen your collarbones. Slide your ears back to center the crown of your head over your throat. Advanced practitioners can move the top foot forward to bring the shin parallel to the top of the mat.

Eka pada rajakapotasana 1 prep is a gateway pose into many of the asymmetrical backbends. For a more intense variation of this pose, place your palms together overhead and straighten your arms. When you can hold this variation for one minute, you are likely ready to attempt the full form of *eka pada rajakapotasana 1*.

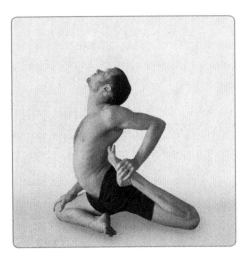

eka pada rajakapotasana 1 prep
one leg king pigeon pose 1

leg in frog

shape
(from *adho mukha svanasana*)

1. Inhale fully. Exhale, bend the right knee and place the knee to the right of and just behind the right wrist. Lower the hips and the outer right leg to the floor with the right heel touching the front of the left hip.
2. Slide the hips back slightly so the front of the back thigh touches the floor.
3. Place the right hand on the right thigh near the knee. Inhale, lift the torso upright and bend the back knee.
4. Hold the top of the back foot with the left hand.
5. Bend the knee even more and point the elbow back. Spin the hand to point the fingers forward, then bring the fingers to the outer edge of the foot and thumb around the arch.
6. Inhale fully. Exhale, press the inner edge of the back foot to the outer hip.
7. Square the shoulders and torso to the front of the mat. Lift the chin and look up. Hold the pose and breathe.
8. To come out, exhale, release the hands to the floor in front of the top shin, shoulder-width apart, and lower the back foot. Curl the toes under and press the hands down and forward to push the hips up and back. Step the front foot back.

Repeat on the second side.

safety
- Move the left hip forward and the right hip back to square the hips to the top of the mat.
- Center the weight in the hips and pelvis. The weight tends to lean into the hip of the bent leg, which will cause the back knee to widen.
- Press the outer edge/top of the front foot down.
- Clamp the front knee closed.
- Tone the back leg and rotate the inner thigh up.
- Push the hand into the back foot and push the back foot into the hand. Spread the toes.
- Press the tailbone down and lift the low belly.
- Engage the glutes of back leg.
- Lift the shoulders up and back.

- Isometrically squeeze the knees toward each other.
- Stretch the spine up.
- If there is pain or discomfort in the low back or to reduce the intensity of the stretch in the back quads, lift the hips slightly and/or place a blanket or block underneath the sit bone of the front leg.

refinement

Advanced practitioners can lower the hips to the floor. Although this pose is among the best preparatory poses for all backbends, it is also an excellent backbend in its own right. I used to regard the function of this pose as simply a preparatory pose. I no longer believe the primary purpose of any pose is to prepare a practitioner for another pose. Yoga yes, one pose does lead to another. Even so, each pose has something significant and unique to offer in its own right. Again and again, I find never-ending value in the seemingly simple and benign poses.

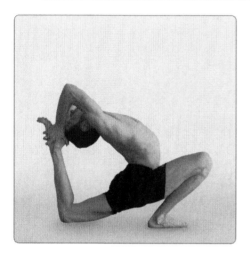

eka pada rajakapotasana 2
one leg king pigeon pose 2

shape
(from *adho mukha svanasana*)

1. Inhale fully. Exhale, step the right foot forward just inside the right hand.
2. Bend and close the front knee to bring the right hip as close to the front heel as possible.
3. Lower the back knee to the floor and lift the shin vertical.
4. Flex the back foot and turn the foot out. Turn the torso to the left and shorten the left side of the torso. With the palm facing up, hold the inner edge of the big toe mound with the fingers.
5. Curl the head and torso back and rotate the left arm so the elbow points up.
6. Inhale, lift the right arm vertical. Keep the chest full, and exhale, bend the right elbow. Clasp the left forearm with the right hand and walk the hand down the forearm to hold the foot.
7. Inhale fully. Exhale, bring the top of the head to the back heel. Look back. Hold the pose and breathe.
8. To come out, release the clasp. Keep the chest full and inhale, lift the torso and head. Release the hands to the floor in front of the hips. Exhale, lower the back foot to the floor. Curl the back toes under and press the hands down and forward to push the hips up and back.

Repeat on the second side.

safety

- If the hands cannot reach the foot behind the head, wrap a strap around the top foot and use the strap to bring the foot toward the head. Walk the hands down the strap to clasp the foot.
- Move the left hip forward and the right hip back to square the hips.
- Isometrically squeeze the back knee and front foot toward each other.
- Press the tailbone down, engage the back glutes, and lift the low belly.
- Move the base of the sternum back and stretch the spine and chest up while simultaneously moving the shoulders back.
- Pull the foot into the head and reach the head into the foot.

refinement

For a more challenging entry to clasp the foot behind the head, see *eka pada rajakapotasana 1*.

When was the last time you attempted this pose? In order to evolve in a given pose, you must create and then stay in relationship with it. If not daily, then weekly. If not weekly, then monthly. If not monthly, then yearly. If not yearly, then future forget about it!

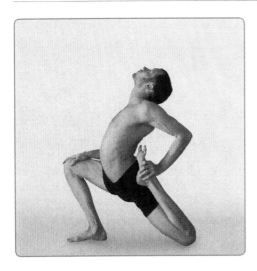

eka pada rajakapotasana 2 prep

one leg king pigeon pose 2

shape
(from *lunge pose*)

1. With the right leg forward, lower the back knee to the floor. Lift the back foot and bend the knee to capacity.
2. Place the right hand on the right thigh. Inhale, lift the torso upright and clasp the top of the back foot with the left hand. Wrap the fingers around the outer edge of the foot and the thumb around the arch of the foot. Bend the left elbow.
3. Inhale fully. Exhale, bring the inner edge of the back foot to the outer left hip.
4. Inhale, tone the low belly. Exhale, lower the hips down and forward. Allow the front knee to move forward, toward the toes.
5. Lift the chest and curl the head back. Look up. Hold the pose and breathe.

6. To come out, release the back hand and lower the foot. Exhale, lower the torso and place the hands directly below the shoulders. Curl the back toes under and lift the knee.

Repeat on the second side.

safety

- Move the left hip forward and the right hip back to square the hips.
- Press the back foot into the outer hip so there is no space between the hip and foot.
- Press the inner edge of the front foot down.
- Isometrically squeeze the back knee and front foot toward each other.
- Tone the back leg and spin the inner thigh back.
- Press the tailbone down and lift the low belly.
- Engage the glutes of the back leg.
- Press the front hand into the thigh and lift the shoulders up and back.
- Stretch the spine and chest up.
- If the back hand cannot reach the back foot, use a strap around the foot.
- If there is pain in the front knee, bring the front heel directly below the knee and tone the quads.
- If there is discomfort in the back knee, place a folded blanket underneath the knee for additional padding and/or reduce the bend in the knee. The top of the thigh, not the kneecap, should bear the weight of the body.

refinement

Eka pada rajakapotasana 2 prep provides a strong stretch for the back quad and hip flexor. Moving your front knee beyond your heel and dropping your hips down and forward will intensify this stretch. In order to approach your fullest expression of the pose, it is likely you will need to stay in this pose for more than just a couple of breaths. In addition, using long, full exhalations can help you release deeper into the pose. For a slightly less intense variation, hold the outer edge of your foot with your hand and/or lift your hips slightly.

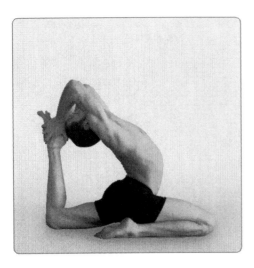

eka pada rajakapotasana 3
one leg king pigeon pose 3

shape
(from *adho mukha svanasana*)

1. Inhale fully. Exhale, place the right knee on the floor just inside the right hand.
2. Bring the right shin and the top of the foot to the floor parallel to the long edge of the mat.
3. Lower the hips as close to the floor as possible with the outer right hip and inner right heel touching.
4. Lift the back shin vertical.
5. Flex the back foot and turn the foot out. Turn the torso to the left and shorten the left side of the torso. With the palm facing up, hold the inner edge of the big toe mound with the fingers.
6. Curl the head and torso back and rotate the left arm so that the elbow points up.
7. Inhale, lift the right arm vertical. Keep the chest full, and exhale, bend the right elbow. Clasp the left forearm with the right hand and walk the hand down the forearm to hold the foot.
8. Inhale fully. Exhale, bring the top of the head to the back heel. Look back. Hold the pose and breathe.
9. To come out, keep the chest full and inhale, lift the torso and head. Release the hands to the floor in front of the hips. Exhale, lower the back foot to the floor. Curl the back toes under and press the hands down and forward to push the hips up and back.

Repeat on the second side.

safety

*   If the hands cannot reach the foot behind the head, wrap a strap around the top foot and use the strap to bring the foot toward the head. Walk the hands down the strap to clasp the foot.
*   Point the right toes back and squeeze the outer ankle in.
*   Move the left hip forward and the right hip back to square the hips.
*   Lift the back inner thigh up.
*   Press the tailbone down, engage the glutes, and lift the low belly.
*   Move the base of the sternum back and stretch the spine and chest up while simultaneously moving the shoulders back.
*   Pull the foot into the head and reach the head into the foot.

- To reduce the difficulty of the balance as the hands reach back for the foot, isometrically squeeze the legs toward each other and keep the hips slightly buoyant.

refinement

Eka pada rajakapotasana 3 is another pose that is rarely, if ever, taught in public classes. *Eka pada rajakapotasana 1,* however, is taught again and again and again. Clearly, these two poses are very similar. Contemplation: What makes one pose popular and another peripheral? I think it all too often comes down to personal preference and trends. So, why not start a new trend and practice *eka pada rajakapotasana 3,* instead of *eka pada rajakapotasana 1,* for the next few years? While we are at it, let's throw *eka pada rajakapotasana 2* into the mix!

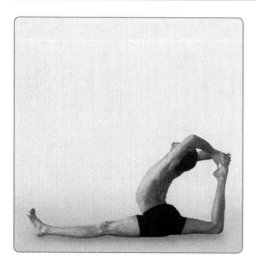

eka pada rajakapotasana 4
one leg king pigeon pose 4

shape
(from *hanumanasana*)

1. With the left leg forward and the right leg back, lift the back shin vertical.
2. Flex the back foot and turn the foot out. Turn the torso to the right and shorten the right side of the torso. With the palm facing up, hold the inner edge of the big toe mound with the fingers.
3. Curl the head and torso back and rotate the right arm so that the elbow points up.
4. Inhale, lift the left arm vertical. Keep the chest full, and exhale, bend the left elbow. Clasp the right forearm with the left hand and walk the hand down the forearm to hold the foot.
5. Inhale fully. Exhale, bring the top of the head to the back heel. Look back. Hold the pose and breathe.
6. To come out, keep the chest full and inhale, lift the torso and head. Release the hands to the floor next to the hips. Exhale, lower the back foot to the floor. Curl the back toes under, step the front foot back, and press the hands down and forward to push the hips up and back.

Repeat on the second side.

safety

- Tighten the front knee and press the back of the leg down.
- Move the right hip forward and the left hip back to square the hips as much as possible.
- Tone and lift the back inner thigh.
- Press the tailbone down, engage the glutes, and lift the low belly.
- Move the base of the sternum back and stretch the spine and chest up while simultaneously moving the shoulders back.
- Press the back foot and hands into each other.
- For a more accessible entry, wrap a strap around the back foot and inhale, lift the arms vertically. Exhale, walk the hands down the strap toward the foot.

refinement

Finding the balance is more challenging than the hamstring stretch and backbend in this pose. Although this is a pigeon pose, my sadhana-sister, who I call *Heather-Hero-of-Hilo,* considers it a form of *hanumanasana.* For many years her studio was called Balancing Monkey. She considered this pose the mascot of Balancing Monkey because as she said, "To attain the balance of Monkey Hanuman is nothing less than hatha-heroic."

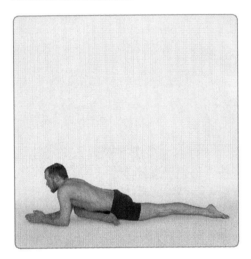

eka pada rajakapotasana prep
one leg king pigeon pose

forward fold

shape
(from *adho mukha svanasana*)

1. Inhale fully. Exhale, bring the right knee to the floor to the right of and just behind the right hand—knee slightly wider than the right hip.
2. Lower the right sit bone and leg to the floor.
3. Point the right foot and press the right heel to the front of the left hip.
4. Move the left hip forward and the right hip back to square the hips to the front of the mat.
5. Bring the back leg parallel to the long edge of the mat.
6. Inhale fully. Exhale, fold the torso forward over the front leg. Bring the forearms to the floor in front of the shin—elbows shoulder-width apart directly below the shoulders.

Press the palms together.

7. Point the back toes straight back with the heel straight up. Look forward or down. Hold the pose and breathe.

8. To come out, walk the hands back directly below the shoulders. Curl the back toes under and use the arms to push the hips up and back. Separate the feet hip-width apart.

Repeat on the second side.

safety

- If the weight of the body falls to the right, elevate the hips by placing one or several folded blankets underneath the right sit bone.
- To protect the front knee, press the top of the front foot down. Lift the outer ankle away from the floor.
- Strengthen the back leg and push the foot into the floor.
- Squeeze the front knee and back leg toward each other to lift and square the hips.

refinement

To deepen the stretch, move your front foot forward until your shin is parallel to the front edge of the mat—ankle in line with knee. In this variation, it is crucial to strongly flex your front foot and isometrically squeeze the front knee. This position will bring your back quad onto the floor. Lift the sit bone of your bent leg up away from the floor. Stretch your arms forward or overlap your hands to place the forehead down.

Rest is among the most important aspects of this practice. Most practices end with *savasana*. *Savasana* is practiced for 5 to 15 minutes. It is therefore usually held longer than any other pose in a given practice. If you have any kind of injury, give your body a chance to heal by resting. Many athletes have a short life span in their given sport (at least compared to the span of their life). They often play hard for maybe a decade or so and achieve their peak performance early on in life. Then, once retired, they may leave their sport with a plethora of physical issues and injuries. In yoga there is no off season. So, you must make rest a priority in your practice. As Swami Rudrananda says, "Longevity is everything." He also says that the one thing a spiritual practitioner must never give up is 8 to 10 hours of sleep per night![1] Be radical: rest! If you don't rest willingly it's likely your body will force you to rest due to injury.

---

[1]   John Mann, *Rudi: 14 Years with my Teacher* (Portland, Oregon: Rudra, 2001 p. 238).

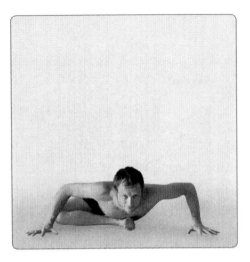

eka pada rajakapotasana prep
one leg king pigeon pose

foot to sternum

shape
(from *adho mukha svanasana*)

1. Step the right foot forward between the hands—knee over heel.
2. Move the back foot to the right in line with the front foot. Widen the hands beyond shoulder-width.
3. Drop the front knee out to the right and come onto the outer edge of the foot. Flex the foot.
4. Inhale fully. Exhale, slide the back foot back, and lower the body and front leg to the floor.
5. Lower the front knee out to the side—shin parallel to the top of the mat.
6. Inhale fully. Exhale, bring the center of the sternum to the inner edge of the front foot. Widen the hands until the wrists are directly below the elbows.
7. Bring the top of the back foot to the floor and point the foot back. Look forward or down. Hold the pose and breathe.
8. To come out, curl the back toes under and bring the hands shoulder-width apart. Inhale, lift the torso, hips and back knee. Step the front foot back. Lift the hips up and back.

Repeat on the second side.

safety
- Flex the front foot and squeeze the front knee.
- Press the outer edge of the front foot down. Lift the outer ankle up.
- Straighten the back leg. Lock the back knee into a straight position.
- Point the back kneecap down.
- Isometrically squeeze the legs toward each other.
- Engage the left glutes.
- To reduce the intensity in the outer hip, lower the back knee to the floor and lean onto the right hip. Press the left hand into the sole of the front foot. Press the right hand down and to the right. Inhale, shift the torso to the left and line up the sternum with the foot. If this is still too intense, fold the torso over the right shin or knee.

refinement

Engage your legs as you reach the front of your left quads down, and tilt your right sit bone up. Balance your weight evenly between the right and left sides of the body to emphasize the hip stretch. Extend out through your back foot and lift your knee off the floor to open the front of your thigh. To deepen the pose, inhale, lift your chest and lengthen your spine. Exhale, lower your forehead or chin to the floor. Hold the pose and breathe.

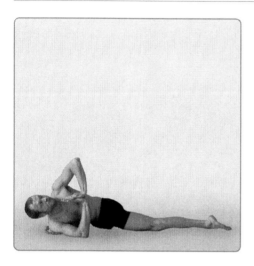

eka pada rajakapotasana prep
one leg king pigeon pose

shoulder to arch of foot

shape
(from *eka pada rajakopotasana*, foot to sternum)

1. Press the heel of the left palm into the toe mounds of the right foot.
2. Inhale, lift the torso. Exhale, weave the right arm between the space of left arm and right foot.
3. Place the right shoulder into the sole or arch of the right foot.
4. Inhale fully. Exhale, rotate the left shoulder over the right shoulder. Straighten the lower arm and point the palm up. Pause here and breathe.
5. Bend the right elbow and bring the hands together in *anjali mudra*.
6. Look up. Hold the pose and breathe.
7. To come out, exhale, look down. Release the hands and bring the hands to either side of the front shin. Inhale, lift the torso upright, curl the back toes under, and come to the outer edge of the right foot to lift the right knee slightly. Reach the right foot back next to the left foot— hip distance apart. Lift the hips up and back.

Repeat on the second side.

safety

- If the shoulder cannot come to the sole of the foot, place the elbow into the foot instead. Join the palms together and twist the chest open.
- Engage the front foot and press the foot into the shoulder. Squeeze the front knee.
- Push the shoulder into the foot to empower the twist.
- Straighten the back leg so there is little to no weight on the back knee.
- Point the back kneecap down, lower the left hip and lift the right hip slightly to level the hips.
- Point the back foot straight back. Squeeze the back heel in so the heel is vertical.
- If looking up is too intense for the neck or jaw, look down.
- To stay in the pose for an extended period of time, rest the face or back of the head on a block.

refinement

To deepen the pose, release your hands from *anjali mudra* and prop your left shoulder up with your right hand. Reach your left hand behind your back and hold the outer right thigh. Press your right hand into the your left shoulder/upper chest to facilitate the twist. Even walk the hand down toward the center of the chest. *Eka pada rajakapotasana*, shoulder to arch of foot, is a great preparatory pose for *yogadandasana*. It opens the hip via force more than flexibility. "*Hatha*" can translate to mean "forceful." If practiced properly, every pose has the potential to force weakness, tightness, stress, and anxiety out of the body.

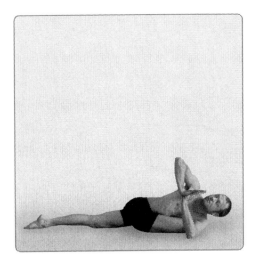

eka pada rajakapotasana prep
one leg king pigeon pose

shoulder to knee

shape
(from *eka pada rajakapotasana*, forward fold)

1. Place the hands shoulder-width apart in front of the top shin. Straighten the arms.
2. Lean onto the left hip.
3. Place the left shoulder on the floor in front of the front knee. Place the right fingertips on the floor in front of the face.
4. Inhale fully. Exhale, twist the torso to the right.

5. Lean the hips and torso to the right so that the hips return to center.
6. Bring the hands together in *anjali mudra*. Rotate the top shoulder over the bottom shoulder.
7. Look up. Hold the pose and breathe.
8. To come out, exhale, look down. Release the hands and bring the hands to either side of the front shin. Inhale, lift the torso upright and curl the back toes under. Step the right foot back next to the left foot. Lift the hips up and back.

Repeat on the second side.

safety

- Engage the front foot and press the front heel into the hip.
- Strengthen the back leg.
- Engage the left glutes.
- Press the bottom elbow into the floor.
- Press the palms into each other to empower the twist.
- Move the shoulders and head back.
- If looking up is too intense for the neck or jaw, place the head on a block or look down. If the hips fall to one side, place a blanket below the lower hip.

refinement

This is a good preparatory pose for *parivrtta parsvakonasana*. To deepen the stretch in your hip, bring your shin parallel to the top of the mat. The hip joint is the largest joint in the body and is protected by the gluteal muscles, some of the strongest muscles in the body. Because of the sheer size and strength of the hips in relation to other parts of the body, they can be an area of deeply stored trauma, stress, and anxiety. This stored stress however, is not indelible. Through proper yoga practice, it can be reduced, and even erased, to bring vitality, longevity, and health.

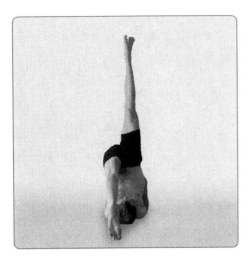

eka pada sarvangasana
one leg shoulderstand pose

shape
(from *sarvangasana 1*)

1. Inhale fully. Exhale, lower the left foot to the floor behind the head.
2. Keep the torso and top leg vertical.
3. Look past the tip of the nose. Hold the pose and breathe for 30 to 60 seconds.
4. To come out, inhale, lift the bottom leg vertical.

Repeat on the second side.

safety

- Press the shoulders down, in toward each other, and forward toward the head.
- Center the head. Bring the chin vertical—do not allow the chin to drop toward the chest.
- Press the head, shoulders, upper arms, and elbows down.
- Press the hands into the torso.
- Extend the inner edge of the top leg back so that the kneecap points straight ahead.
- Extend the outer edge of the bottom leg up. Lift the hip up and toward the top leg.
- Engage the glutes and move the hips and tailbone forward.
- Stretch the spine and top leg up. Spread the toes and center the foot over the hips.
- Relax the jaw, eyes, and face. Breathe evenly.
- If the bottom foot cannot reach the floor, bring the leg parallel to the floor instead.

refinement

If you practice *utthita hasta padangusthasana 1, virabhadrasana 3, hanumanasana,* and *supta padangusthasana 1,* you will be well-prepared for *eka pada sarvangasana.* Notice the tendency to become more goal-oriented in your bottom foot than your top foot. The bottom foot has the tangible goal of the floor to reach for. The top foot, on the other hand, is in the air, which often equals, "I don't really care." Give equal emphasis to the position of each foot. Yoga invites us to establish both concrete and subtle aims. Too much emphasis on one or the other can lead to imbalance.

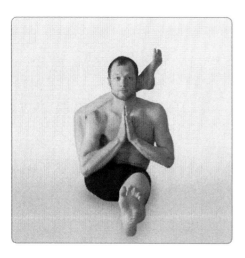

eka pada sirsasana
one leg behind the head pose

shape
(from *dandasana*)

1. Bend the right knee out to the side to hold the right heel with the left hand. Lift the heel as high as the head.
2. Bring the right arm to the inside of the right leg and hold the calf.
3. Round the back and turn the head to the left.
4. Inhale, lift the right shin up and over the head.
5. Exhale, place the shin on the back of the neck.
6. Move the head back and bring the torso upright.
7. Place the palms together in front of the chest. Look forward. Hold the pose and breathe.
8. To come out, release the hands, lean forward, and use the hands to release the top leg. Lower and straighten the leg.

Repeat on the second side.

safety

- If the shin does not reach the back of the head, bring the leg over the shoulder or upper arm instead.
- Engage both feet. Point the toes of the front leg up and push the heel down.
- Isometrically bend the top knee to engage the hamstrings. Push the shin into the upper back and the back of the head, and push the head into the leg.
- Press the shoulder into the knee.
- Straighten and strengthen the extended leg. Press the back of the knee down.
- Lift the pelvic floor and tone the low belly.

refinement

If your torso is long in proportion to your legs, you may have a more difficult time getting your leg over your head or sitting upright. There are certain body types that have an easier time getting into certain poses. In many forward folds, the legs are on the floor and the torso starts upright. Then the torso folds over the legs to stretch the spine. In *eka pada sirsasana* the torso starts and stays vertical, and it is the leg that is brought into position to bring the body into a forward fold. To do this, the torso has to resist the immense forward pressure of the back leg, which deeply stretches and strengthens the back.

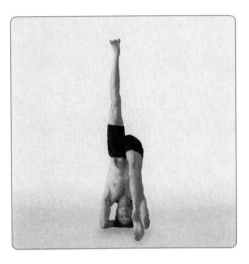

eka pada sirsasana
one leg headstand pose

shape
(from *sirsasana 1*)

1. Inhale fully. Exhale, touch the right foot to the floor in front of the face.
2. Keep the hips and top foot directly above the head. Look forward. Hold the pose and breathe.
3. To come out, lift the right leg vertical.

Repeat on the second side.

safety

*   Press the forearms and wrists down. Lift the shoulders up.
*   Extend down through the head. Stretch the top leg up.
*   Engage the left glutes.
*   Engage the abdomen.
*   Do not allow the upper back to round.
*   Move the inner edge of the top leg back so that the knee points straight ahead. Press the tailbone forward.
*   Keep the breath even and the eyes soft, yet determined.
*   If the balance is difficult, practice against or near a wall.

refinement

To reduce the intensity of the pose and enhance alignment, bring your bottom leg parallel to the floor. From here, lower your foot to the floor. As you lower your foot to the floor, you will likely lose some of the alignment of the first position.

The function of alignment is to promote health and safety. The function of alignment in asana is not the same as the function of form in diving and gymnastics, which is judged on its aesthetic beauty. If you compromise alignment simply to get into the aesthetic form, you may miss the benefits of the pose because you are too eager to advance or go to the next level, which can originate from a place of pride rather than a place of patience and modesty.

One of the physical benefits of *eka pada sirsasana* is to increase flexibility in the hamstrings of the bottom leg and the quads of the top leg while in an inverted position. By distorting the back, hips, and legs to achieve an expectation of what the pose should look like (rounding the back and dropping the top leg to lower the bottom leg to the floor) would, in fact, reduce the stability of the pose. At the same time, severe adherence to alignment can promote safety but create mental rigidity, which will block the very benefits you seek. If you were to always keep the bottom leg parallel to the floor in order to maintain so-called "perfect" alignment, you may never get any stretch at all.

Perfect alignment is not necessarily ideal in the context of practice. Practice, in my opinion, is not about avoiding poison at all costs. A little bit of poison can actually lead to purification. As Rumi says, "Good and bad are mixed. If you don't have both you don't belong with us."[1]

---

[1] Jalal al-Din Rumi, Coleman Barks (translator), *The Essential Rumi* (San Francisco: Harper Collins, 1995).

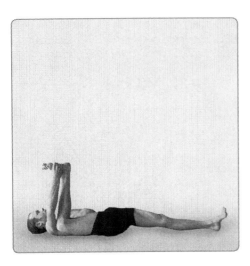

eka pada sukha balasana
one leg happy baby pose

shape
(from *supta tadasana*)

1. Bend the right knee and bring the thigh to the outer right torso. Stack the heel directly over the knee and hold the foot with both hands.
2. Inhale fully. Exhale, pull the right knee toward/to the floor. Look up. Hold the pose and breathe.
3. To come out, release the hands, and lower and straighten the leg.

Repeat on the second side.

safety

- Squeeze the knee of the extended leg straight and reach the underside of the thigh toward the floor. Point the toes up.
- Push the foot into the hands and pull the foot with the hands.
- Isometrically kick the heel of the bent leg down toward the sit bone.
- Relax the shoulders, throat, and jaw.

refinement

Eka pada sukha balasana is a good preparatory pose for *akarna dhanurasana 2* and *eka pada sirsasana*, although the word "preparatory" could be misleading. Every pose in a given sequence is in some way a preparatory pose. After all, one pose does lead to another. However, to practice one pose solely to prepare for another pose would be to miss much of the pose itself. Ideally every pose is a pivotal part of practice.

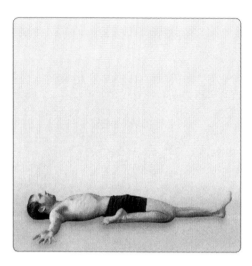

eka pada supta virasana
one leg reclined hero pose

shape
(from *virasana*)

1. Place the hands behind the hips.
2. Lift the hips, lean back, and extend the left leg straight ahead.
3. Lean back onto the elbows—upper arms vertical, forearms parallel.
4. Momentarily lift the hips and round the low back.
5. Lie down on the back. Extend the arms out to the sides—palms facing up. Look up. Hold the pose and breathe.
6. To come out, lift the chest, bend the elbows, and use the hands to push the torso to vertical. Lean to the side to release and straighten the bent leg.

Repeat on the second side.

safety

- Point the right toes straight back and flare the outer two toes.
- Press the inner right heel against the outer hip. Press the top of the foot down.
- To reduce the pressure on the low back or bent knee, place a bolster or 3 to 5 blankets underneath the torso. This will elevate the torso. The edge of the bolster or blankets must be above the top of the sacrum.
- If there is any pain in the knee, discontinue the pose immediately. It is also advisable to consult your doctor and/or seek guidance from a skilled yoga instructor if there is persistent pain in the knees.

refinement
The quads tend to be a storehouse for stress. This pose stretches away that stress.

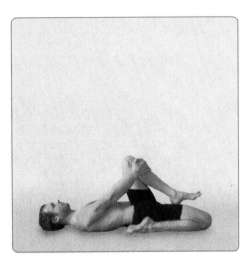

eka pada supta virasana
one leg reclined hero pose

knee bent toward chest

shape
(from *eka pada supta virasana*)

1. With the right leg in *virasana*, bend the knee of the extended leg and lift the foot off the floor. Interlace the fingers around the shin.
2. Look up. Hold the pose and breathe.
3. To come out, release the hands and straighten the top leg.

Repeat on the second side.

safety
- Point the right toes straight back and flare the outer two toes.
- Press the inner right heel against the outer hip. Press the top of the foot down.
- Engage the top foot.
- To reduce pressure on the bottom knee, widen the thigh slightly.
- If the head lifts away from the floor, place folded blankets underneath the head.

refinement
Resist the tendency to press your chin into your throat, which is often a sign of excessive effort. For a more intense variation, bend your elbows to pull your top knee toward your chest.

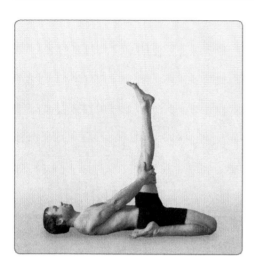

eka pada supta virasana
one leg reclined hero pose

straight leg lifted

shape
(from *eka pada supta virasana*)

1. With the right leg in *virasana*, lift the extended leg vertical and interlace the fingers behind the thigh just below the knee.
2. Look up. Hold the pose and breathe.
3. To come out, release the hands and lower the leg.

Repeat on the second side.

safety

- Point the right toes straight back and flare the outer two toes.
- Press the inner right heel against the outer hip. Press the top of the foot down.
- To reduce pressure on the bottom knee, widen the thigh slightly.
- Straighten and strengthen the extended leg.
- Bring the top foot into a position halfway between pointed and flexed. Spread the toes.
- Press the tailbone down and tone the low belly.
- Move the shoulders back and down.
- Keep the chin vertical.
- If lifting the leg directly above the hip is too intense on the hamstring or front of the opposite quads, use a strap around the top foot and lower the leg, or keep the knee slightly bent.

refinement

For a more intense variation, walk your hands up your extended leg toward your foot. If appropriate, interlace your fingers around your top foot and straighten your leg. It is fine if your right knee lifts off the floor as long as you do not experience any pain in the knee or low back.

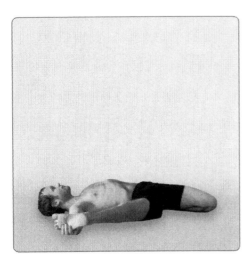

eka pada supta virasana
one leg reclined hero pose

leg to side

shape
(from *eka pada supta virasana*)

1. With the left leg in *virasana*, bend the right knee and lift the foot off the floor.
2. Bring the right arm to the inside of the leg and hold the outside of the foot. Straighten the arm and leg.
3. Inhale fully. Exhale, lower the right leg out to the side. Bring the outer edge of the foot toward/to the floor.
4. Look up. Hold the pose and breathe.
5. To come out, inhale, lift the leg vertical. Exhale, lower the leg.

Repeat on the second side.

safety
- Point the left toes straight back and flare the outer two toes.
- Press the inner left heel against the outer hip. Press the top of the foot down.
- To reduce pressure on the bottom knee, widen the thigh slightly.
- Straighten and strengthen the extended leg.
- Bring the top foot into a position halfway between pointed and flexed. Spread the toes.
- Press the tailbone down and tone the low belly.
- Move the shoulders back and down.
- Keep the chin vertical.
- If the hand cannot clasp the top foot, especially as the leg lowers to the side, use a strap.
- To reduce the intensity of the quad stretch for the leg in *virasana*, place a block or bolster under the outer edge of the left hip to keep the leg elevated. Or place the lifted foot against a wall.

refinement
It is likely that your left knee will lift up off the floor in this pose, which is fine as long as there is no pain in your knee or low back. Consider placing yoga sandbags or weights on the top of your thigh to prevent your leg from lifting. As your quads become more pliable, your knee will

not lift away from the floor. Personally, the stress I store in my quads has the potential to keep me awake at night. Every night before going to sleep I do *eka pada supta virasana,* leg to side variation, because it effectively and quickly removes the stress in my quads. I don't stretch to get flexible. And yet a certain amount of flexibility is required to access what these poses have to offer. I seek flexibility not for the sake of flexibility, but for the sake of accessibility.

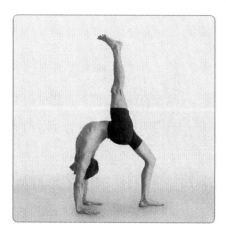

eka pada urdhva dhanurasana
one foot upward-facing bow pose

shape
(from *urdhva dhanurasana 1*)

1. Turn the left heel in slightly. Inhale, lift the right foot up, completely bend the knee, and bring the thigh to a vertical position.
2. Straighten the right leg until the foot is directly over the hips. Flex the foot.
3. Look at the tip of the nose. Hold the pose and breathe.
4. To come out, exhale, bend the right knee in toward the chest and lower the foot to the floor.

Repeat on the second side.

safety

- Press the fingertips and the perimeter of the palms down with equal pressure.
- Dig the thumbs into the floor.
- Lock the elbows into a straight position.
- Extend the shoulders back and chest forward.
- Flare the outer two toes and squeeze the shins in.
- Extend the inner edge of the bottom foot down. Rotate the inner thigh of the bottom leg down.
- Engage the glutes and abdomen and lift the tailbone.
- Point the knee of the top leg straight ahead. Strengthen the entire leg.
- Move the base of the sternum back and stretch the entire spine.
- Hold the pose without holding the breath.

refinement

Eka pada urdhva dhanurasana requires, and therefore develops, tremendous strength in the top leg. It also requires strength in the abdomen. This is a good preparatory pose for *eka pada viparita dandasana 1.*

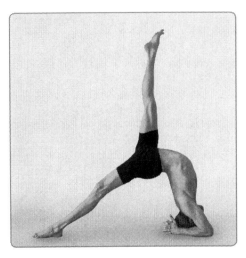
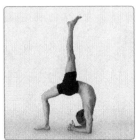

eka pada viparita dandasana 1
one leg inverted staff pose 1

shape
(from *dwi pada viparita dandasana*)

1. Press the left foot down. Inhale, lift the right leg vertical.
2. Look straight back. Hold the pose and breathe.
3. To come out, exhale, lower the lifted foot to the floor. Straighten the leg.

Repeat on the second side.

safety

- For a more accessible variation, begin in *dwi pada viparita dandasana* and bend both knees so that the shins are vertical. Lift the head off the floor and lift the right leg vertical.
- Press the wrists and forearms down.
- Move the shoulders back and extend the chest forward, beyond the shoulders.
- Strengthen the legs and lock them into a straight position.
- Move the inner edge of the bottom foot down. Rotate the inner thigh of the bottom leg down.
- Engage the glutes of the lifted leg and lift the tailbone. Tone the low belly.
- Spin the thigh of the top leg out so the kneecap points straight ahead.
- If the top thigh is not vertical to the floor, keep the leg straight and lower the leg, or bend the knee as much as is necessary.
- Move the base of the sternum back and stretch the entire spine.
- Breathe evenly and keep the eyes relaxed.

refinement

When Milo and I first released the *From Tadasana to Savasana* poster, we offered the manager of YogaOasis studios a framed photo of any pose in the poster. She chose the above photo. Surprised, I asked, "Why that one?" She said, "Because it is beautiful and it will give me something to aspire to. With steady practice one day I might just be able to do it." That made me hatha-happy. One of my aims for this eBook is that these photos and instructions inform and inspire people to practice, please practice.

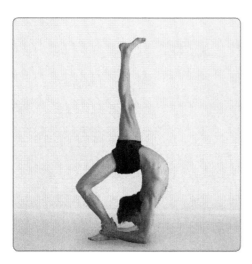

eka pada viparita dandasana 2
one leg inverted staff pose 2

shape
(from *urdhva dhanurasana 1*)

1. Bend the elbows and place the top of the head on the floor.
2. Lower the elbows to the floor shoulder-width apart. Interlace the fingers behind the head—thumbs pointing up.
3. Press the forearms down and lift the head. Reach the shoulders back and the chest forward until the upper arms are vertical. Look back at the heels.
4. Step the left foot back just in front of the hands—heel lifted.
5. Lower the heel to the floor and interlace the fingers around the left ankle.
6. Keeping the knee bent, lift the right leg up until the thigh is vertical.
7. Straighten the right leg to vertical and flex the foot.
8. Curl the head back and look past the bottom foot. Hold the pose and breathe.
9. To come out, keep the chest full, and inhale, release the clasp of the ankle. Exhale, lower the lifted foot to the floor. Step the left foot out. Place the hands near the head and straighten the arms.

Repeat on the second side.

safety

- Press the wrists and forearms down.
- Move the shoulders back and extend the chest forward.
- Press the inner edge of the bottom foot down. Rotate the inner thigh of the bottom leg down.
- Engage the glutes of the bottom leg and lift the tailbone. Tone the low belly.
- Tighten the lifted knee and lock the leg into a straight position.
- Spin the thigh of the top leg out so that the kneecap points straight ahead.
- If the top thigh is not vertical to the floor, keep the leg straight and lower the leg, or bend the knee as much as is necessary.
- Move the base of the sternum back and stretch the entire spine.
- Breathe evenly and keep the eyes relaxed.

refinement

The two most difficult aspects of this pose are interlacing the fingers around the ankle (as opposed to just touching the heel), and bringing the hips directly above the head. Making good choices under high stress is difficult to do. Some of the best advice my dad ever gave me was, "Never make a crucial decision in a negative state." I have pretty much done just that. So, when I need to make a big decision and my state is negative, the remedy for me is usually to practice. Every time I take the form of these poses my state shifts and I get some perspective on whatever problem I am dealing with. As I go from a negative to a positive state, I see how my negativity would have influenced me to make poor and problematic choices. Doing one thing (practicing) instead of another (making poor choices) is a difference that makes all the difference!

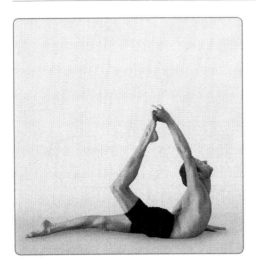

eka padangustha dhanurasana
one hand to big toe bow pose

shape

1. Bring the front body to the floor. Place the hands on the floor beside the chest—hands shoulder-width apart.
2. Bend the right knee to lift the shin vertical. Flex the back foot and turn the foot out. Turn the torso to the right and shorten the right side of the torso. With the palm facing up, hold the inner edge of the big toe mound with the fingers.
3. Momentarily press the left hand down to lift the chest and torso. Curl the head and torso back and rotate the right arm so that the elbow points up.
4. Hold the big toe with the first two fingers and thumb of the right hand.
5. Straighten the right arm. Lift the top hand and foot to capacity.
6. Lift the chin. Look back. Hold the pose and breathe.
7. To come out, exhale, lower the lifted leg and arm to the floor.

Repeat on the second side.

safety

- Pull the top foot forward with the hand, while simultaneously kicking the foot up and back into the hand.
- Tone and lift the inner thigh of the lifted leg.

- Press the tailbone down, engage the glutes, and tone the low belly.
- Squeeze the extended leg in toward the midline.
- Lock the top elbow into a straight position.
- Stretch the top arm up and back.
- Extend the spine and the top leg in opposite directions—away from the hips.
- For a more accessible entry, wrap a strap around the back foot and inhale, lift the arms. Simultaneously kick the back foot up and walk the hands down the strap toward the foot.

refinement

The most difficult aspect of so many backbends is the flexibility required in the shoulders. For example, *eka padangustha dhanurasana* is not any deeper of a backbend than *dhanurasana*. And yet it requires much more strength and stretch in the shoulders. My practitioner-point is that backbends require the full participation of the body, mind, and spirit.

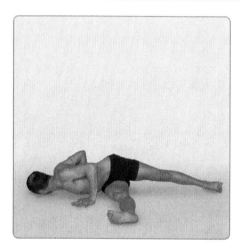

fallen sage

shape
(from *adho mukha svanasana*)

1. Step the right foot halfway between the left hand and left foot. Flex the foot and come onto the outer edge of the right foot.
2. Inhale, lift the hips and straighten the leg.
3. Exhale, slide the right foot out to the left and lower the outer right hip and leg to the floor. Line up both feet with the outer right hip—right leg parallel to the top of the mat and left leg parallel to the long edge of the mat. Spin your left heel down and turn the toes to the left.
4. Inhale, lift the torso. Exhale, lower the chest and head to the floor.
5. Turn the head to the right and look past the right fingertips. Hold the pose and breathe.
6. To come out, inhale, lift the head and torso. Straighten the arms, lift the hips and place the right foot back, next to the left foot—feet hip-width apart. Lift the hips up and back.

Repeat on the second side.

safety

- If the outer hip does not reach the floor, slide the right foot back so the right leg is no longer perpendicular to the back leg. Keep the leg straight.
- If the chest does not lower to the floor, keep the torso lifted. This variation of the pose will require more upper body strength.
- With the outer hip on the floor, slide the torso forward a few inches to externally rotate the right hip.
- Straighten and strengthen the legs. Engage the thighs. Lock the knees into a straight position.
- Flex both feet and press the outer edge of the right foot down.
- Engage the left glutes.
- Turn the abdomen away from the extended leg.
- Press the right hand down and lift the right shoulder up.

refinement

A unique feature of this pose is that the twist is initiated from the hips rather than the torso and shoulders as in most other twists. This is a good preparatory pose for *eka pada koundinyasana 1*. To deepen the twist, weave your left arm underneath your right armpit and place your left shoulder on the floor in line with your back foot, hips, and head. Walk your right hand out to the right with your elbow bent over the wrist, and come up onto your fingertips. Press your right fingertips into the floor and twist. Place the back of your left shoulder on the floor to facilitate the twist. Reach your left hand away from your right foot. Place a block underneath your head to stay in the pose for an extended period of time.

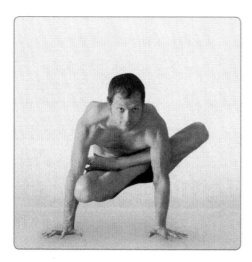

galavasana
Sage Galava's pose

shape
(from *padmasana*)

1. With the left shin on top in *padmasana*, lean back onto the hips and lift the knees vertical.
2. Hold the left shin with the right hand.
3. Pull the left shin toward the left armpit. Extend the left arm forward.
4. Place the left hand on the floor while squeezing the shin with the armpit. Straighten the left arm and move the shoulder back.
5. Place the right hand on the floor to the outside of the right thigh—hands shoulder-width apart. Spread the fingers and point the index fingers straight ahead.
6. Lean forward and transfer the weight of the body onto the hands. Inhale fully. Exhale, lift the hips off the floor.
7. Straighten both arms. Look straight ahead. Hold the pose and breathe.
8. To come out, exhale, lower the hips to the floor.

Repeat on the second side—switch the cross of the legs.

safety

- Press the fingertips and the perimeter of the palms— especially the mounds of the index fingers—into the floor with firm and equal pressure.
- Press the outer edges/tops of the feet into the upper thighs. Squeeze the heels toward the hips.
- Flare the toes.
- Engage the abdomen and lift the pelvic floor.

refinement

Advanced practitioners can enter this pose from *sirsasana 2*. Bring your right leg, then your left leg, into *padmasana*. Lower your knees toward the floor. Place your left shin on your left armpit. Lean back and transfer your weight from your head onto your hands. Lift your head and straighten your arms. Hold *galavasana* for five breaths. Lower your head to the floor and return to *sirsasana 2*. Recross your legs and repeat on the second side.

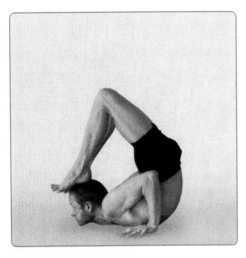 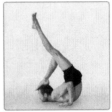 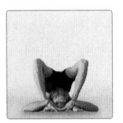

ganda bherundasana
formidable face pose

shape

1. Bring the front body to the floor. Curl the toes under and stretch the chin forward. Look straight ahead.
2. Place the hands by the chest—hands slightly wider than shoulder-distance apart.
3. Lift the shoulders as high as the elbows.
4. Inhale, kick one leg and then the other into a vertical position so the weight of the body comes into the hands, upper chest, and chin.
5. Exhale, bend the knees and lower the soles of the feet to the top of the head. Look forward. Hold the pose and breathe.
6. To come out, inhale, lift the legs. Exhale, lower the legs and feet to the floor.

safety

- Press the tips of the fingers and perimeter of the palms down with even pressure.
- Press the inner edges of the feet together and flare the outer two toes.
- Extend the inner thighs and inner edges of the feet down.
- Engage the glutes and press the tailbone in. Lift the low belly.
- Press the chest into the floor, move the base of the sternum back, and bend deeply and evenly in the spine.
- Extend the head and knees up.
- Do not hold your breath.

refinement

This is a good preparatory pose for *vrischikasana 1* and *2*. For a more advanced variation, practice *eka pada ganda bherundasana* by straightening one leg and lifting the foot above the head. Repeat on the second side. Advanced practitioners can also come into *paripurna ganda bherundasana* by lowering the feet to the floor in front of the head and placing the hands on the feet.

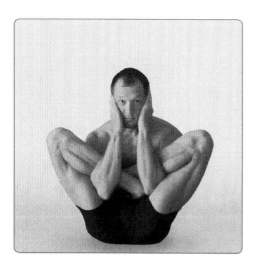

garbha pindasana
embryo in the womb pose

shape
(from *padmasana*)

1. Lean back, lift the knees, and balance on the hips.
2. Slide the right arm between the right calf and thigh. Slide the left arm between the left calf and thigh. Reach the elbows beyond the legs.
3. Bend the elbows and place the hands on the sides of the face. Look forward. Hold the pose and breathe.
4. To come out, release the hands and stretch the arms forward. One at a time, pull the arms out of the legs. Lower the knees.

Repeat on the other side—change the cross of the legs.

safety

- If the legs cannot fold into *padmasana*, perform the pose with the legs in *sukhasana*.
- Press the outer edges/tops of the feet into the thighs. Flare the toes.
- Squeeze the knees toward each other.
- Pull the legs toward the chest with the arms.
- Engage the abdomen and lift the pelvic floor.

refinement

Advanced practitioners can roll onto the back. Roll counter clockwise on the back 9 times, which represents the 9 months of gestation. Roll back and forth by engaging the abdomen and pelvic floor. Do not use the arms or head. Spin a complete 360-degree circle and on your ninth turn, roll up onto the hands and balance in *kukkutasana* for 5 breaths. This expression of *garbha pindasana* comes from Sri Pattabhi Jois' Ashtanga Yoga. Ashtanga Yoga is what really set me onto the path of hatha yoga. I practiced Ashtanga Vinyasa for 8 years in a roaring row. One of my favorite hatha yoga memories is doing the primary series of Ashtanga Yoga 40 days in a row.

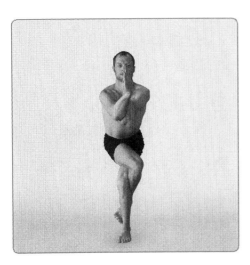

garudasana
eagle pose

shape
(from *tadasana*)

1. Inhale, lift the arms overhead.
2. Exhale, swing the right elbow under the left elbow, cross and wrap the left wrist around the right wrist. Press the palms together—thumbs toward the face.
3. Bend both knees slightly and press the knees together.
4. Cross the right thigh over the left thigh above the knee. Move the right knee to the left slightly.
5. Point the right foot and pull the foot back to hook the foot behind the left calf.
6. Center the elbows and knees.
7. Look straight ahead. Hold the pose and breathe.
8. To come out, unwind the legs, place the right foot on the floor, and straighten the legs. Unwrap the hands and arms and bring the arms by the sides.

Repeat on the second side.

safety

- If there is pain or discomfort in the knees, or if the leg position is not accessible, bring the feet and knees together and bend the knees slightly, or wrap the legs just once.
- If there is pain or discomfort in the shoulders or wrists, or if the hand position is not accessible, swing the elbow under the other elbow and press the backs of the hands and arms together.
- Engage the feet. Flare the outer two toes of the lifted foot.
- Squeeze the arms and legs together.
- Press the tailbone down and lift the low belly.

refinement

Garudasana is an unusual shoulder opener that also stretches the muscles of the upper back. It is good preparation for poses such as *mayurasana, parivrtta janu sirsasana, parivrtta paschimottanasana*, and *viparita salabhasana prep*.

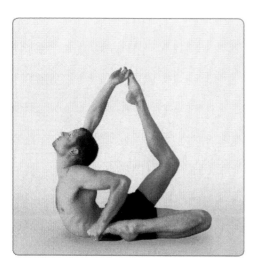

gherandasana 1
Sage Gheranda's pose 1

shape

1. Bring the front body to the floor—legs straight and feet outer hip-width apart.
2. Place the right forearm on the floor, parallel to the top of the mat, with the right elbow directly below the right shoulder.
3. Bend the left knee and hold the top of the left foot with the left hand. Inhale fully. Exhale, lower the inner left heel to the outer left hip.
4. Wrap the fingers around the tops of the toes and press the left heel down to the floor.
5. Bend the right knee to lift the shin vertical, flex the foot, and turn the foot out.
6. Turn the torso to the right and reach the right hand underneath the right foot—palm facing up. Hold the inner edge of the big toe mound with the fingers.
7. Inhale, curl the head and torso back. Exhale, rotate the right arm so that the elbow points up.
8. Hold the right big toe with the first two fingers and thumb of the right hand. Inhale, kick the right foot up and straighten the right arm.
9. Lift the chin and look up. Hold the pose and breath.
10. To come out, exhale, lower the top foot and hand. Release the hands and lower the leg to the floor.

Repeat on the second side.

safety

- Press the inner edge of the bottom foot into the outer hip.
- Tone and lift the inner thigh of the lifted leg. Engage the foot to avoid discomfort in the toe.
- Press the tailbone down, engage the glutes, and lift the low belly. Tone the pelvic floor.
- Lock the top elbow into a straight position.
- Stretch the right shoulder up and back.
- Move the base of the sternum back and stretch and strengthen the entire spine.

refinement

In my opinion, *gherandasana 1* and *2* are among the most exquisite forms in hatha yoga. Just looking at these forms *ananda*-alters my state. Which poses do you deem to be among the most exquisite?

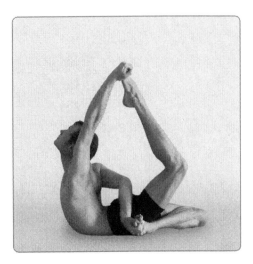

gherandasana 2
Sage Gheranda's pose 2

shape
(from *dandasana*)

1. Fold the right leg into *ardha padmasana*.
2. Bring the front body onto the floor.
3. Reach the right hand behind the back and clasp the big toe of the right foot with the first two fingers and thumb.
4. Bend the left knee to lift the shin vertical. Flex the foot and turn the foot out.
5. Reach the left hand underneath the left foot—palm facing up, and hold the inner edge of the big toe mound with the fingers.
6. Inhale, curl the head and torso back. Exhale, rotate the left arm to point the elbow forward.
7. Inhale fully. Exhale, straighten the left arm and hold the top of the foot with the hand.
   Lift the leg up and back to capacity.
8. Lift the chin. Look up. Hold the pose and breathe.
9. To come out, exhale, lower the left leg and arm to the floor. Release the right hand.
   Roll onto the left side of the body and straighten the right leg. Lift to sit.

Repeat on the second side.

safety
- Lift the outer edge of the right foot up.
- Tone and lift the inner thigh of the lifted leg.
- Press the tailbone down, engage the glutes, and lift the low belly. Tone the pelvic floor.
- Lock the top elbow into a straight position.
- Stretch the shoulder of the lifted arm up and back.
- Move the base of the sternum back and stretch and strengthen the entire spine.

refinement

Gherandasana 2 is twice as difficult as *gherandasana 1* due to the *ardha baddha padmasana* (half bound lotus) portion of the pose. One way to ease the difficulty is to use the foot in *ardha padmasana* to help lift the top leg.

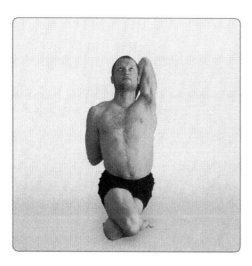

gomukhasana
cowface pose

shape
(from *bharmanasana*)

1. Inhale, lift the left leg up and back parallel to the floor.
2. Bend the left knee and place the shin and foot on the floor to the outside of the right calf and foot. Turn both sets of toes out slightly.
3. Exhale, lower the hips to sit on the feet. Bring the torso upright.
4. Bend the left elbow and place the back of the hand as far up the back as possible. Pull the left elbow in toward the spine with the right hand.
5. Inhale, lift the right arm vertical. Exhale, bend the elbow and bring the hand to the upper back. Clasp the hands behind the back.
6. Look between the eyebrows. Hold the pose and breathe.
7. To come out, exhale, release the clasp. Place the hands shoulder-width apart in front of the knees. Walk the hands forward and lift the hips. Lift the right leg and place the right knee hip distance away from the left leg.

Repeat on the second side.

safety

- To take pressure off the knees or calves, lift the hips.
- If the hands cannot clasp, use a strap to bind.
- Press the feet into the hips.
- Engage the abdomen.
- Move the base of the sternum back. Lift the chest.
- Press the tailbone down, move the low belly in, and lift the pelvic floor.

refinement

Sometimes the bulk of the calf muscle makes it difficult, painful, or uncomfortable to squeeze the legs together and support the weight of the body. Before lowering your hips, use your hands to move your calf muscles away from the backs of your knees to create space. (See *virasana*.) At first, this variation of *gomukhasana* is a challenging balancing pose. The balance becomes easier once you can fully rest your hips on your feet.

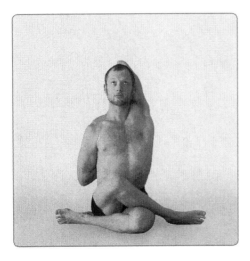
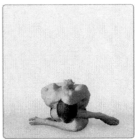

gomukhasana
cowface pose

feet separated

shape
(from *dandasana*)

1. Bend the right knee and place the heel on the floor against the outer left hip. Flex the foot and point the toes out to the left. Lower the knee.
2. Bend the left knee and place the heel on the floor against the outer right hip. Flex the foot and point the toes out to the right.
3. Stack the knees so the top knee is directly over the bottom knee.
4. Lift the right arm out to the side—arm parallel to the floor. Bend the right elbow and point the fingers toward the floor. Place the back of the hand as far up the back as possible. Pull the right elbow in toward the spine with the left hand.
5. Inhale, lift the left arm vertical. Exhale, bend the elbow and bring the hand to the upper back. Clasp the hands behind the back.
6. Lift the chin slightly and look up between the eyebrows. Hold the pose and breathe.
7. To come out, exhale, release the clasp. Place the hands next to the hips. Straighten both legs.

Repeat on the second side.

safety
- Squeeze the heels into the hips.
- Engage the feet and press the outer edges of the feet down. Spread the toes.
- Point the top elbow up and the bottom elbow down.
- Squeeze the shoulder blades together on the back.
- If the hands do not clasp, use a strap to bind.

refinement
It is easy to advance too quickly in this practice. For example, practitioners tend to clasp the hands just because they can despite pain in their shoulders. Discomfort comes with the territory of this practice. Yoga forces us to work our body and mind and breath in an unfamiliar manner, and for most of us, this brings discomfort. Pain, however, is always problematic. It is a sure sign that there is subtle or significant damage in the body. Discern between discomfort and pain and use discomfort to eliminate pain, current or future. Yoga motto: no pain, gain!

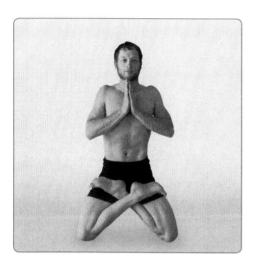

goraksasana
Sage Goraksa's pose

shape
(from *padmasana*)

1. Place the hands shoulder-width apart in front of the knees. Walk the hands forward and lift the hips to bring the weight forward into the hands.
2. Make the thighs as upright as possible. Walk the hands back toward the knees. Lift the torso upright.
3. Lift one hand, then the other. Use your arms, legs and low belly to achieve balance.
4. Place the palms together in front of the sternum. Hold the pose and breathe.
5. To come out, lean forward and lower the sit bones to the floor. Bring the hands next to the hips.

Repeat on the other side—change the cross of the legs.

safety

- If the legs cannot fold into *padmasana* or if there is pain or discomfort in the knees, do not attempt this pose.
- If necessary, place a blanket underneath the knees for padding. This will make the balance more difficult but the knees more comfortable.
- Be prepared to suddenly fall back to a sitting position. If necessary, place a blanket under the seat for padding. Lean forward to soften the fall.
- If the balance is difficult, place one hand on a wall, or release the top leg until the shin rests on the floor.
- Squeeze the outer edges/tops of the feet into the thighs and push the thighs into the feet.
- Press the tailbone down, tone the low belly, and lift the pelvic floor.

refinement

In *Light On Yoga*, B. K. S. Iyengar writes about *goraksasana*, "It is a difficult balancing pose and one feels elated even if one can only balance for a few seconds."[1]

---

[1]   B. K. S. Iyengar, *Light on Yoga* (New York: Schocken Books, 1977) p. 142.

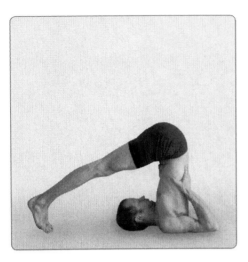

halasana
plow pose

shape

1. Lie down on the floor—arms along the sides of the body, palms facing down.
2. Roll back and bring the feet shoulder-width apart on the floor behind the head.
3. Elevate the hips above the shoulders until the spine is vertical.
4. Interlace the fingers and one at a time, walk the shoulders up toward the head and in toward the spine.
5. Place the hands as low on the back as possible to lift the hips.
6. Squeeze the elbows in until they are shoulder-width apart.
7. Bring the feet together and straighten the legs. Look past the tip of the nose. Hold the pose and breathe.
8. To come out, release the hands to the floor and straighten the arms. Roll the torso and legs to the floor.

safety

- Keep the seventh cervical (the bony protrusion at the base of the neck) off the floor. If your seventh cervical touches the floor in *halasana*, place folded blankets below the torso and shoulders as described in *sarvangasana 1*.
- If the feet do not reach the floor behind the head, place the feet on a wall or rest the legs on a chair. The feet should not hover in the air.
- Press the shoulders down, in toward each other, and forward toward the head.
- Center the head and press the head down. Bring the chin vertical—do not allow the chin to drop toward the chest.
- Press the hands into the torso and the elbows and forearms into the floor.
- Engage the glutes.
- Squeeze the inner knees, ankles, and feet together. Engage the legs and tone the thighs.
- Extend the hips and spine up. Attempt to curve the low back in.
- Relax the jaw, eyes, and face.
- Breathe evenly and deeply.

refinement

For better traction, place your hands directly on the skin as opposed to over your clothing. Discover the challenges and rewards of practicing different positions of the feet in *halasana*. Try coming onto the tips of your toes, the balls of your feet, as well as the tops of your feet. To stay in *halasana* for an extended period of time and use it as a restorative pose, place the tops of your thighs on the seat of a folding chair so your head is below the seat and your legs and feet stretch beyond the chair back and seat. Bring your arms next to your head and bend your elbows 90 degrees—fingers pointing in the same direction as the head. Stay for a minimum of five minutes to access the restorative benefits of the pose.

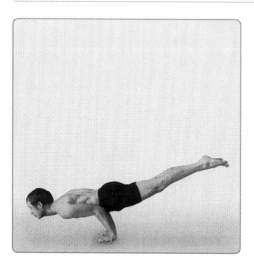

hamsasana

swan pose

shape

1. Come onto the hands and knees.
2. Place the tips of the thumbs together. Point the index fingers straight ahead.
3. Bend the elbows and squeeze the elbows together. Lean forward and place the elbows as close to the waistline as possible.
4. One at a time, straighten the legs and curl the toes under.
5. Lean forward even more until the elbows are forward of the wrists. This will put tremendous pressure on the hands and wrists.
6. Transfer all of the body weight onto the hands and lift the feet off the floor. Curl the head back to look forward. Hold the pose and breathe.
7. To come out, exhale, lower the feet and push the hands down to lift the hips.

safety

- Press the fingertips and the perimeter of the palms—especially the mounds of the index fingers—down into the floor with firm and equal pressure. Because of the flexed position of the wrists, it is important to root down through every part of the hand evenly. Do not attempt this pose if you have a wrist injury.
- Straighten and strengthen the legs. Extend out through the feet and flare the toes.
- Squeeze the inner edges of the feet and the legs together.
- Engage the glutes.

refinement

If you cannot yet perform this pose, try a hybrid of *mayurasana* and *hamsasana* by turning your hands out to the sides instead of backward or forward. *Viparita salabhasana prep* is a good pose to learn the necessary actions required in *hamsasana*.

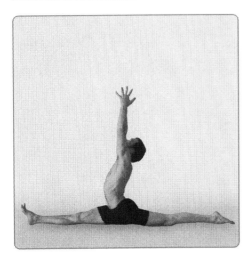

hanumanasana

monkey pose

shape
(from *bharmanasana*)

1. Step the right foot forward. Place the right heel on the floor—toes pointing up.
2. Straighten the right leg and slide the heel forward. Square the hips to the top of the mat.
3. Keeping the hips square, extend the front foot forward and back knee back. Lower the front leg, hips, and back leg to the floor.
4. Place the hands next to the hips and lift the torso upright. Pause here and breathe.
5. Inhale, lift the arms vertical. Place the palms together and straighten the arms.
6. Look up. Hold the pose and breathe.
7. To come out, look forward and release the hands next to the hips. Use the hands to lift the hips. Slide the front foot back, bend the knee, and place the knee on the floor next to the standing knee.

Repeat on the second side.

safety

- Press the back foot down and in, and press the front heel down. Engage the front foot and spread the toes.
- If the legs do not straighten to bring the hips to the floor, place the hands on one or more blocks to elevate the hips. Keep the front leg straight and lift the chest. This is more taxing on the arms and upper body, but is safest for those with tight hamstrings. Do not force the hips down.
- Straighten both legs and lock them into a straight position. Engage the hamstrings and quads of both legs.
- Press the back of the front knee and the front of the back thigh into the floor.

ingxout—

- Push the left hip forward and pull the right hip back.
- Press the tailbone down. Lift the pelvic floor and tone the low belly.
- Engage the abdomen, move the base of the sternum back, and lift the chest.
- Stretch the hands up. Squeeze the elbows in.

refinement

What makes *hanumanasana* so difficult is that it is simultaneously a forward fold and a backbend. The relationship of the front leg and pelvis shares a similar geometry to *dandasana* and other forward folds, while the relationship of the back leg and pelvis shares a similar geometry to *eka pada rajakapotasana 1* and other backbends. Explore entering *hanumanasana* by focusing on the different aspects of the pose. For the forward folding aspect, enter the pose by sliding your front heel forward (as described above). Keep the hips lifted and the front leg straight. Do not move the back knee. For the backbending aspect, enter the pose by sliding your back knee and foot back. Encourage your torso to be fully upright to equally experience the benefits of both categories of poses. Once in the pose, even discover a slight twist by rotating your navel toward your front leg.

Breath deeply and evenly in this pose. Mentally and emotionally allow the stretch to happen. With each inhalation, become fully present to the stress and tightness in the backs of the legs. With each exhalation, consciously release the stress.

Early on in my hatha yoga practice I asked my mom what it would take for me to be able to get into *hanumanasana*. She told me to practice it for one minute per day for 30 days in a row. I did just that, and it worked. Even so it still takes me seven sets of *hanumanasana* on each side to get into the full expression of the pose. And I like that because it helps me develop patience and perseverance.

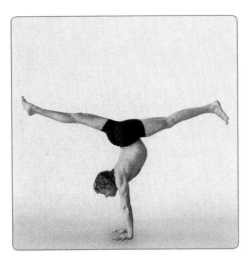

hanumanasana in adho mukha vrksasana
monkey in downward-facing tree pose

shape
(from *adho mukha vrksasana*)

1. Simultaneously extend the right leg back, the left leg forward, and move into a backbend.
2. Straighten the arms and legs. Hold the pose and breathe for five breaths. Bring the legs back to center.

Repeat on the second side.

safety

- To avoid falling over, place the back foot on a wall. Or if appropriate, learn to skillfully fall back into *urdhva dhanurasana 1*.
- Press the fingertips and the perimeter of the palms down into the floor with equal pressure.
- As the back leg extends back, move the inner edge of the leg down and press the tailbone in.
- As the front leg moves forward, move the outer edge of the leg up.
- Squeeze the elbows and knees straight.
- Engage the abdomen and legs.

refinement

This pose is a good way to learn the actions required to perform *vrischikasana 1 & 2*. While it is necessary to backbend in the low back for the *hanumanasana* leg position, continue to engage the core to protect the low back.

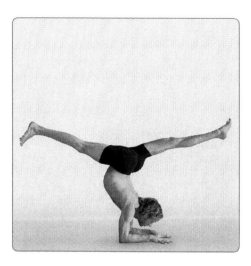

hanumanasana in pincha mayurasana
monkey in peacock feather pose

shape
(from *pincha mayurasana*)

1. Move into a backbend to simultaneously extend the left leg back and the right leg forward.
2. Straighten the legs. Hold the pose and breathe for five breaths. Bring the legs back to center.

Repeat on the second side.

safety

- To avoid falling over, place the back foot on a wall.
- Do not allow the hands to move in or the elbows to move out.
- Press the hands, forearms, and elbows down. Stretch the shoulders, spine, and legs away from the floor.
- As the back leg extends back, move the inner edge of the leg down and press the tailbone in.
- As the front leg moves forward, move the outer edge of the leg up.
- Squeeze the knees straight.
- Engage the abdomen and legs.
- If the wrists and hands slide in and/or the elbows and forearms slide out, use a block between the hands to keep the forearms parallel and in place.

refinement

While it is necessary to backbend in your low back for the *hanumanasana* leg position, continue to engage your core to protect your low back. Inverted backbends with the legs split can be a difficult place to know where your body is in space. Practicing in front of a mirror can be beneficial to see if your body is actually doing what you think it is doing in the pose. The tendency in this pose is to bring the front leg lower than the back leg. Lower your back foot faster than your front leg to resist this tendency.

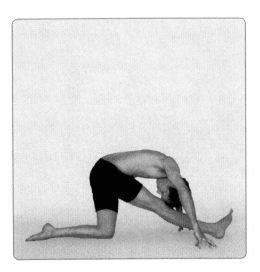

hanumanasana prep
monkey pose

shape
(from *bharmanasana*)

1. Step the right foot forward. Place the right heel on the floor—toes pointing up.
2. Straighten the right leg and slide the heel forward to square the hips to the top of the mat.
3. Inhale fully. Exhale, fold the torso over the leg and lower the forehead toward/to the knee.
4. Walk the hands forward and bend the elbows out to the sides. Look at the tip of the nose. Hold the pose and breathe.
5. To come out, walk the hands back directly below the shoulders. Inhale, look up. Exhale, bend the front knee and slide the foot back.

Repeat on the second side.

safety
*   To reduce the intensity of the hamstring stretch, place the hands on blocks.
    If there is pain or discomfort in the low back, keep the torso lifted and lengthen the spine.
*   Flex and engage the front foot.
*   Press the front heel down and back. Squeeze the front heel and back leg toward each other.
*   Engage the front thigh and squeeze the kneecap up.
*   Move the left hip forward and the right hip back.
*   Lift the pelvic floor and tone the low belly.

refinement
Press the top of your back foot down. Keep your back thigh perfectly vertical so your hip is directly over your knee. Turn your navel toward your extended leg. Round your back evenly to bring your forehead to your knee.

This pose is a good preparation for *dwi hasta padasana* and the torso lifted variation. Because the bottom knee is bent, *hanumanasana prep* offers a similar hamstring stretch but without the pressure on the low back. If you have low back pain or discomfort, that kind of pressure is often problematic. If you do not, poses like *dwi hasta padasana* will keep your back strong and pliable.

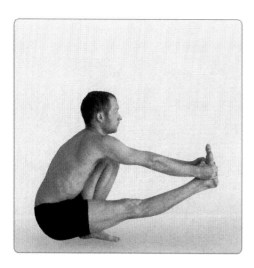

hasta padasana
hand to foot pose

squatting

shape
(from *tadasana*)

1. Lower into a squat position with the knees together.
2. Lean onto the left foot. Lift the right foot off the floor and hold the foot with both hands. Straighten the right leg. Hold the pose and breathe.
3. To come out, release the hands and place the right foot next to the left foot. Lift to stand.

Repeat on the second side.

safety

- To reduce the intensity of the hamstring stretch, use a strap around the sole of the front foot.
- Engage the extended leg—tighten the quads and flex the foot.
- Pull the foot with the hands and press the foot down and forward into the hands.
- Squeeze the bent knee.
- To reduce the intensity on the bent knee, lower the hips to the floor and practice *hasta padasana* seated.

refinement

Hasta padasana requires, and therefore develops, balance and agility. Advanced practitioners can go from *hasta padasana,* standing, into the squatting variation of this pose. From there, return to *hasta padasana* standing.

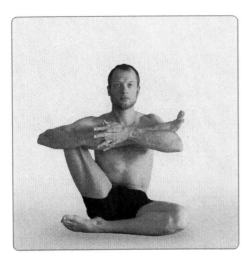

hindolasana
baby cradle pose

shape
(from *dandasana*)

1. Hold the right ankle with the right hand in front of the chest.
2. Bend the left knee and place the left heel to the right sit bone. Lower the leg to the floor.
3. Place the right foot into the crease of the left elbow.
4. Wrap the right elbow around the right knee.
5. Interlace the fingers around the outer shin.
6. Bring the shin parallel to the floor and the top of the mat.
7. Sit upright. Curve the low back in and up.
8. Press the inner shin against the chest. Look straight ahead. Hold the pose and breathe.
9. To come out, release the upper leg to the floor and straighten both legs. Place the hands
   next to the hips.

Repeat on the second side.

safety
- Press the outer edge of the right foot into the crease of the left elbow. Press the inner edge of
  the foot into the biceps.
- Flex the lifted foot, especially the outer two toes.
- Press the elbows into the knee and foot.
- Isometrically pull the right heel down.
- Bring the shoulders down the back.
- To reduce the intensity of the hip stretch, hold the right foot with the left hand. Place the right
  elbow against the inner right thigh and hold the outer right shin with the right hand.

refinement
Seated poses that mirror standing poses are usually more difficult to perform, at least in terms
of flexibility. In the case of *hindolasana*, however, the opposite is true. Therefore, if the standing
variation, *utthita hindolasana*, is too intense for the low back or hip, practice the seated variation
instead.

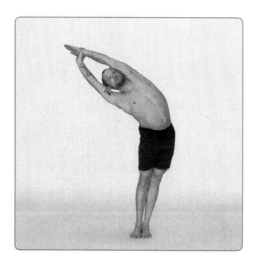

indudalasana
standing crescent pose

shape
(from *tadasana*)

1. Inhale, extend the arms overhead—elbows directly above shoulders.
2. Lock the left arm into straight position and hold the left wrist with the right hand.
3. Exhale, sway the hips to left, torso to the right.
4. Keep the head placed evenly between the arms.
5. Look straight ahead. Hold the pose and breathe.
6. To come out, inhale, lift the torso to center. Exhale, lower the arms.

Repeat on the second side.

safety

- Squeeze the feet and legs together.
- Tone the thighs, lift the kneecaps.
- Engage the glutes.
- Move the tailbone down and the low belly in.
- Move the base of the sternum back and lift the chest.
- Do not overstretch or compress either side of the torso—yoga is not about breaking, but creating and expanding boundaries.

refinement

Turn your hips and torso slightly to the left—move your left hip and shoulder back. Extend down through your left foot. Stretch your left hand away from your left foot and press the inner edge of your left foot down. Stretch your entire spine. With your right hand, lift and extend your left arm. Very few poses strengthen and stretch the obliques. I, therefore, do *indudalasana* almost every time I practice—it serves as a great warm up. It can be held for fifteen to thirty seconds, or you can move into and out of it with your breath. For example: exhale, *indudalasana* to the right. Inhale, come back to center. Exhale, *indudalasana* to the left and so on and so forth. Consider making *indudalasana* part of your regular *surya namaskar* (sun salutation) practice. You could do five sets on each side, moving with your breath, as described above, each time you cycle back to *tadasana*.

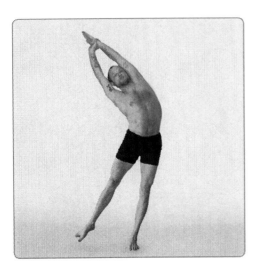

indudalasana
standing crescent pose

one leg lifted

shape
(from *tadasana*)

1. Inhale, extend the arms overhead—elbows directly above shoulders.
2. Lock the left arm into straight position and hold the left wrist with the right hand.
3. Exhale, sway the hips to left, torso to the right.
4. Keep the head placed evenly between the arms.
5. Lift the right leg out to the side. Hold the pose and breathe. Look straight ahead.
6. To come out, lower the foot. Inhale, lift the torso to center. Exhale, release the arms.

Repeat on the second side.

safety
- Squeeze the feet and legs together.
- Tone the thighs, lift the kneecaps.
- Engage the glutes.
- Move the tailbone down and the low belly in.
- Move the base of the sternum back and lift the chest.
- Do not overstretch or compress either side of the torso.

refinement
When you lift your right leg out to the side, extend your left hand and right foot away from your hips.

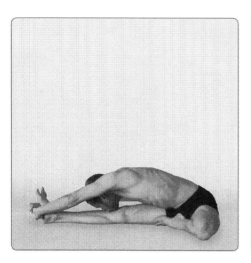
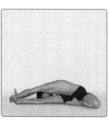
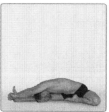
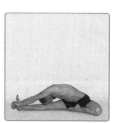

janu sirsasana
head to knee pose

shape
(from *dandasana*)

1. Bring the left palm to the inner left knee. Pull the knee as far back as possible, creating an obtuse angle with the legs.
2. Move the foot to the groin—heel to pubic bone. Lift the heel and point the left foot. Spin the top of the foot down to the floor. Point the heel up.
3. Lean to the right and place the right hand to the inner left thigh—fingers between the calf and thigh. As the hip lowers to the floor, spin the thigh down with the right hand and pull the left glutes back with the left hand. Repeat on the other side.
4. Place the hands shoulder-width apart on either side of the front leg.
5. Turn the torso to the right. Line up the navel and center of the sternum with the front kneecap.
6. Inhale, lift and lengthen the torso.
7. Exhale, fold the torso over the leg.
8. Reach the backs of the hands in front of the right foot. Hold the right wrist with the left hand.
9. Inhale, stretch the spine. Exhale, place the chin on the shin. Look down. Hold the pose and breathe.
10. To come out, release the clasp and bring the hands underneath the shoulders. Inhale, press the hands down to lift the torso upright. Bring the left hand to the outside of the left knee and lift the knee to a vertical position. Straighten the legs, square the hips, and place the hands next to the hips.

Repeat on the second side.

safety

- Before folding forward, tilt the pelvis forward and curve the low back in. If the low back rounds, sit up on one or more blankets.
- Squeeze the foot into the groin and press the top of the foot down.
- Clamp the bent knee closed.
- Pull the front calf out away from the midline.
- Engage the front leg—press the back of the front knee down.
- Reach the front foot forward into the hands and press the heel down into the floor. Point the toes straight up.

- Push the inner edge of the front foot forward. Pull the outer edge of the front foot back. Ground the sit bone of the bent leg and stretch the outer left waist.
- If holding the wrist is not possible, hold the outer edges of the feet, ankles, or calves, or use a strap around the foot. Straighten the arms and hold the strap as close as possible to the front foot (do not bend the elbows when using the strap).
- Tone the pelvic floor and lift the low belly.
- Breathe into and inflate the right waist and ribcage.
- Lift the shoulders up.

refinement

Janu sirsasana can benefit students of any level. This pose can challenge even the most flexible students. If it is easy to hold your wrist with your hand, walk your hand up the forearm of your opposite arm, and bend your elbows out to the sides. One variation is to place your forehead firmly on the floor on the inside of your front shin. Another variation is to place your forehead on the floor on the outside of your front shin. Both of these variations require an immense amount of strength, flexibility, and twist.

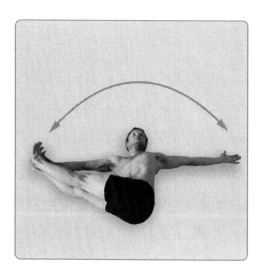

jathara parivartanasana
firmly rotated pose

shape
(from *supta tadasana*)

1. Extend the arms out to the sides—wrists in line with the shoulders, palms facing up.
2. Inhale, lift the legs vertical.
3. Exhale, turn the abdomen to the left and lower the feet toward/to the right hand.
4. Inhale, lift the legs vertical.
5. Exhale, turn the abdomen to the right and lower the feet toward/to the left hand.
6. Inhale, lift the legs vertical.

Repeat for several rounds and then lower the legs.

safety

- Engage the arms and legs—lock the elbows and knees into a straight position.
- Press the inner feet, ankles, and knees together.
- Press the backs of the shoulders, arms, and hands into the floor to aid slow, controlled movements.
- Keep the feet flush and both shoulders on the floor.
- Extend the top hip away from the head.
- Lift the pelvic floor and tone the low belly.

refinement

While this pose involves dynamic movements to heat the body and strengthen the core, it can also be used as a deep twisting pose by holding the pose for several breaths on each side. *Jathara parivartanasana* is a good preparatory pose for *dwi pada koundinyasana*.

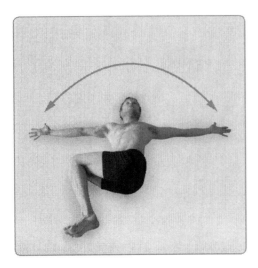

jathara parivartanasana
firmly rotated pose

knees bent

shape
(from *supta tadasana*)

1. Extend the arms out to the sides—wrists in line with the shoulders, palms facing up.
2. Inhale, lift the feet, and bend the knees. Stack the knees directly over the hips.
3. Exhale, turn the abdomen to the left and lower the legs to the right.
4. Inhale, lift the knees vertical.
5. Exhale, turn the abdomen to the right and lower the legs to the left.
6. Inhale, lift the knees vertical.

Repeat for several rounds and then lower the legs.

safety
- Engage the arms and legs. Lock the elbows into a straight position.
- Press the inner feet, ankles, and knees together.
- Press the backs of the shoulders, arms, and hands into the floor to aid slow, controlled movements.
- Keep the knees flush and both shoulders on the floor.
- Extend the top hip away from the head.
- Lift the pelvic floor and tone the low belly.
- To reduce the intensity of the pose, bring the heels toward the sit bones.

refinement
This is a good preparatory pose for *parsva bakasana*. For a more intense variation of *jathara parivartanasana*, knees bent, bend your knees completely and bring them to your elbow. Do not rest your knees on your arms. Hold the pose and then switch sides.

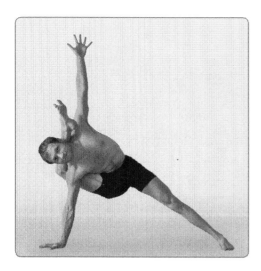

kala bhairavasana
death slayer pose

shape
(from *chakorasana*, right leg behind the head)

1. Swing the left leg back through the hands.
2. Place the left foot on the floor.
3. Straighten the right arm and left leg.
4. Lift the left arm vertical. Look forward. Hold the pose and breathe.
5. To come out, lower the top hand, bring the back foot forward and lower the hips to the floor.

Repeat on the second side.

safety
- Engage both feet, especially the top foot.
- Isometrically bend the top knee to engage the hamstrings.
- Straighten and strengthen the extended leg. Tighten the knee.
- Press the neck and back of the head into the leg.
- Push the hand down to lift the hips up.
- Lift the pelvic floor and tone the low belly.

refinement
Kala bhairavasana is Shiva in his ferocious and formidable form. He is the male aspect of Kali.
As my friend, Mira Shani once said: "This pose beats death to death."[1]

1   Mira Shani, personal communication, 2007.

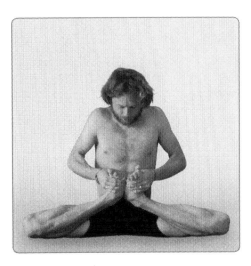

kandasana
central energy nexus pose

shape
(from *baddha konasana,* torso upright)

1. Hold the feet with the hands.
2. Lean back on the hips and lift the heels and knees slightly higher than the pubic bone.
3. Simultaneously pull the soles of the feet into the abdomen, rotate the inner thighs toward the floor, and lower the knees. Hold the pose and breathe.
4. To come out, release the hands and lower the feet.

safety
- If there is pain or discomfort in the knees, do not attempt this pose.
- If the arms are not strong enough to lift the feet and legs, place a block beneath the outer ankles and lean forward.

refinement
When I first started hatha yoga, my knees were six inches off the floor in *baddha konasana*. It was out of the question for me to even attempt this pose for many years. Although this pose does not come naturally or easily to me, I was dharma-determined to at least get in the neighborhood of *kandasana*. There were times where I spent 90 minutes alone working on just this pose. Although it didn't yield all that much compared to those that can do *kandasana* deeply, I progressed above and beyond what I thought my capacity. When you reach the limit of your capacity, if you are paying attention, you will know it. And anytime you achieve your capacity, that is an accomplishment in and of itself.

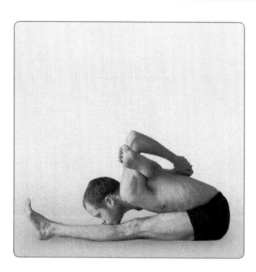

kapilasana
Sage Kapila's pose

shape
(from *buddhasana*)

1. Bend the right elbow and clasp the hands behind the back.
2. Inhale fully. Exhale, fold the torso over the extended leg and place the chin and tip of the nose on the shin. Look down. Hold the pose and breathe.
3. To come out, inhale, lift the torso vertical. Exhale, release the hands.

Repeat on the second side.

safety

- Engage both feet, especially the top foot.
- Isometrically bend the top knee to engage the hamstrings.
- Flare the outer two toes of the top foot.
- Press the shoulder and neck into the top ankle.
- Little by little, use deep exhalations to move the top foot down the back.
- Lift the pelvic floor and tone the low belly.
- If the hands cannot clasp behind the back, use a strap.

refinement

If you look at the photo of this pose you can see what an intense shoulder stretch it is.
To prepare for *kapilasana*, practice shoulder openers such as forward folds with hands bound and even *sarvangasana 1* with your hands as close to your upper back and head as possible.

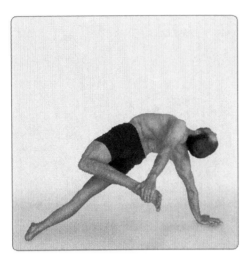

kapinjalasana prep
chathaka bird pose

shape
(from *vasisthasana*, legs together)

1. With the right hand and foot on the floor, look down at the floor.
2. Bring the left hand just behind the left hip—palm pointing down. Straighten the arm.
3. Bend the top knee and hold the top of the foot with the hand.
4. Lift the hips to lower the sole of the right foot to the floor.
5. Kick the left foot straight back and move the hips forward. Curl the chest and head back to come into a backbend.
6. Look back. Hold the pose and breathe.
7. To come out, release and lower the top leg.

Repeat on the second side.

safety
*   If the hand cannot reach the top foot, draw the top knee in toward the chest, point the foot and use the top hand to hold the foot. Then reach the knee back and kick the heel away from the hip.
*   Separate the fingers of the bottom hand. Point the index finger and biceps straight ahead.
*   Press the fingertips and the perimeter of the palm evenly into the floor.
*   Push the bottom hand down to lift the hips up.
*   Strengthen the bottom leg and arm—squeeze the knee and elbow straight.
*   Bring the top foot into a position halfway between pointed and flexed.
*   Engage the glutes and abdomen. Press the tailbone forward.
*   If the balance is difficult, look down.

refinement
Kapinjalasana prep is a challenging balancing pose. Hatha yoga requires that we become capable of focusing on many parts of the body at once. I like to call that "circumferential awareness." This pose is a good preparatory pose to *parsva dhanurasana*.

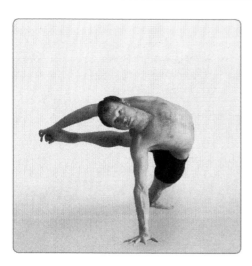

kapinjalasana
chathaka bird pose

shape
(from *kapinjalasana prep*)

1. With the right hand and foot on the floor, rotate the back of the left hand to the outer edge of the left foot. Point the thumb down. Pinch the outer edge of the foot with the thumb and index finger.
2. Point the top biceps up and turn them out to capacity.
3. Bend the top elbow and swing the elbow up and then forward. Extend the hips forward and the chest back to deepen the backbend.
4. Hold the big toe with the first two fingers and thumb.
5. Kick the foot back and straighten the top arm.
6. Look up and back slightly. Hold the pose and breathe.
7. To come out, bend and lift the top elbow, and move the arm closer to the hips. Release the hand and straighten the top leg.

Repeat on the second side.

safety

- To make this pose more accessible, place a strap on the sole of the top foot and hold it with the top arm. Bring the leg into *kapinjalasana* prep. Then bend the top elbow, point it up, and extend the arm toward straight just behind the torso and head.
- Separate the fingers of the bottom hand. Point the index finger and biceps straight ahead.
- Press the fingertips and the perimeter of the palm evenly into the floor.
- Strengthen the bottom leg and arm—squeeze the knee and elbow straight.
- Engage the top foot—press the big toe into the hand. Tone the glutes.
- Press the tailbone forward and tone the low belly.
- Before straightening the top arm, engage the biceps and shrug the shoulder. Then move the shoulder toward the back plane of the body.

refinement

I'm really not sure why, but *kapinjalasana* is much more doable than *natarajasana 1*. Perhaps it is because in *natarajasana* gravity is pulling the spine and shoulders down. It's also easier to balance in *kapinjalasana* because the hand and foot are on the floor. In *natarajasana 1* only one foot touches the floor. In B. K. S. Iyengar's *Light On Yoga*, he gives each pose a degree of difficulty from 1–60. He gives *kapinjalasana* a 43 and *natarajasana* a 58. That confirms that *natarajasana 1* is indeed more difficult, but what does not make sense to me is the difference in degree of difficulty. Take a look at some of the other advanced backbends, like *valakhilyasana*, *gherandasana*, *sirsa padasana*, and *ganda bherundasana*. Are they any less difficult than *natarajasana 1*? No way! My guess is that B. K. S. Iyengar is giving *natarajasana* a 58 because it is named after Shiva Himself. As he says, "This vigorous and beautiful pose is dedicated to Siva, Lord of the Dance, who is also the fountain and source of Yoga."[1]

---

[1]   B. K. S. Iyengar, *Light on Yoga* (New York: Schocken Books, 1977) p. 420.

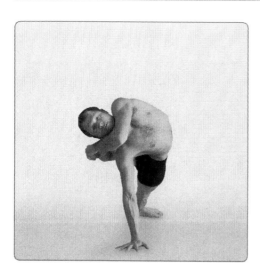

kapinjalasana
chathaka bird pose

arm across chin

shape
(from *kapinjalasana*)

1. With the right hand and foot on the floor, bend the left elbow.
2. Curl the head back to capacity.
3. Pull the left foot toward the head.
4. Bring the left elbow across the face and in front of the throat.
5. Look up and back. Hold the pose and breathe.
6. To come out, lift the left elbow, extend the arm and leg back.

Repeat on the second side.

safety
- To make this pose more accessible, hold a strap on the sole of the top foot with the hand while balancing in *kapinjalasana prep*. Move the top elbow forward and up, then bring it across the face and in front of the throat.
- Separate the fingers of the bottom hand. Point the index finger and biceps straight ahead.
- Press the fingertips and the perimeter of the palm evenly into the floor.
- Strengthen the bottom leg and arm—squeeze the knee and elbow straight.
- Engage the top foot and glutes.
- Press the tailbone forward and tone the low belly.

refinement
The most challenging aspect of this pose is balancing as you bring the elbow in front of the throat. This variation of *kapinjalasana* is a deeper backbend, yet less of a shoulder stretch.

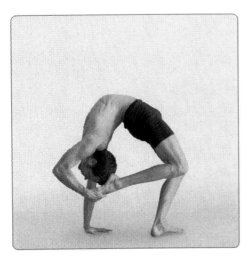

kapinjalasana in urdhva dhanurasana
chataka bird in upward-facing bow pose

Shape
(from *urdhva dhanurasana 1*)

1. Bring the inner edges of the feet together.
2. Keeping the heels together, turn the toes out.
3. Lift the chin and look up.
4. Lift the right leg and arm. Pause and breathe while establishing the balance.
5. Bend the right knee and clasp the outer edge of the right foot with the thumb and index finger—palm facing out.
6. Point the right elbow straight ahead and bring the right foot and head together. Wrap the right palm around the top of the foot.
7. Inhale fully. Exhale, curl the head back. Look at the tip of the nose. Hold the pose and breathe.
8. To come out, exhale, release the lifted hand and foot to the floor. Separate the feet outer hip-width apart.

Repeat on the second side.

Safety
- Press the fingertips and the perimeter of the bottom palm down with equal pressure. Dig the thumb into the floor and squeeze it isometrically toward the palm.
- Lock the left elbow into a straight position.
- Simultaneously move the left shoulder back and the chest forward.
- Move the right shoulder back and toward the spine.
- Extend the inner edge of the bottom foot down. Rotate the inner thigh of the bottom leg down.
- Flare the outer two toes. Squeeze the shins in.
- Engage the glutes and abdomen. Lift the tailbone.
- Press the head into the foot.
- Press the foot and hand into each other.
- Move the base of the sternum back and stretch the entire spine.

refinement

The backbending aspect of this pose is challenging, but the balancing aspect is even more challenging. A teaching I once heard from Lee Lozowick is, "Unless it can go either way, it is not the Work." The "Work" refers to spiritual evolution. This pose gives a glimpse into the precarious and precious balance of THAT. And THAT can always go either way!

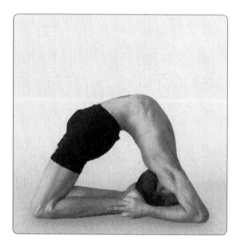
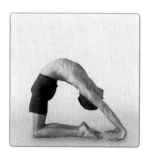

kapotasana

pigeon pose

shape

(from *supta virasana*)

1. Place the hands flat on the floor by the head—thumbs facing in. Point the elbows up.
2. Inhale, lift the hips and torso. Straighten the arms.
3. Walk the hands toward the feet until the thighs are vertical.
4. Place the inner edges of the feet together, bend the elbows, and lower the top of the head to the soles of the feet.
5. Lower the elbows to the floor and clasp the ankles with the hands.
6. Look at the tip of the nose. Hold the pose and breathe.
7. To come out, walk the hands away from the feet and place the hands on the floor next to the feet—thumbs facing in. Keep the chest full and inhale, lift the torso vertical. Once the torso is upright, lift the head.

safety

- Press the inner edges of the feet together and flare the outer two toes.
- Isometrically squeeze the knees in, and move the inner thighs back.
- Press the tailbone forward and engage the glutes.
- Lift the pelvic floor and tone the low belly.
- Press the tops of the feet down, move the hips forward, and stretch the entire spine.
- Press the head and feet into each other.
- Press the wrists down. Move the shoulders back while simultaneously moving the chest forward.
- To make this pose more accessible, place a block between the feet in *supta virasana* and place the top of the head on the block. Squeeze the feet and shins in toward the block to prevent the block from slipping.

refinement

Another way to get into *kapotasana* is from an upright kneeling position. Curl your head and torso back and place your hands on the backs of your knees. One at a time extend your arms overhead and place your hands flat on the floor. From there, walk your hands toward your feet and lower your head to the soles of the feet.

In the practice of hatha yoga, practitioners both shape shift and state shift. *Kapotasana* requires an immense amount of shape shifting that pays off by creating a significant shift in state. This pose is among the most deliciously calming asanas I've ever practiced.

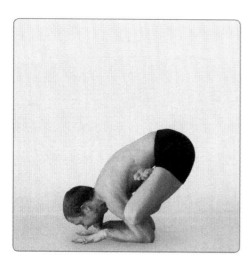

karandavasana

goose pose

shape

(from *padmasana* in *pincha mayurasana*)

1. Inhale, extend out through the knees. Exhale, lower the shins parallel to the floor. Pause and breathe.
2. Draw the navel toward the spine as much as possible.
3. Isometrically, pull the hands and forearms back to bring the shoulders forward toward the wrists. Simultaneously lower the shins onto the upper arms and round the back completely.
4. Look down. Hold the pose and breathe.
5. To come out, lift the knees.

Repeat on the second side—switch the cross of the legs.

safety

- Engage the abdomen.
- Press the outer edges/tops of the feet into the thighs.
- Squeeze the heels into the hips.
- Practice this pose with a skilled instructor if there is not enough strength in the arms, core, and/or back to lower slowly and with precision.

refinement

There are two key points to come into this pose from *pincha mayurasana*: 1. Come into a back-bend with your knees over your shoulders, but with the shoulders reaching forward—toward your hands—so the upper arms are no longer vertical. Once in this position, reach your hips back as you lower your knees. 2. Lift your navel and low belly in and up toward the spine to capacity. This upward lifting energy in the abdomen, sometimes referred to as *uddiyana bandha*, is essential in resisting gravity and preventing the tremendous weight of the hips and lower body from crashing down. Once in the pose, it is tempting to rest the knees and shins against the arms, but if there is any hope of lifting the legs to return to *pincha mayurasana*, you must keep the weight of the legs and hips off the arms. The most difficult part of this pose is the entry and exit rather than the pose itself. It is easier, for example, than *bakasana* with straight arms.

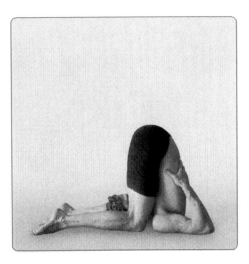

karnapidasana
ear pressure pose

shape
(from *halasana*)

1. Separate the feet shoulder-width apart.
2. Inhale fully. Exhale, bend the knees and walk the feet toward the head to bring the shins toward/to the floor. Point the feet and lower the tops of the feet to the floor.
3. Press the knees into the ears. Look past the tip of the nose. Hold the pose and breathe.
4. To come out, straighten the legs and walk the feet away from the head.

safety
- Keep the seventh cervical (the bony protrusion at the base of the neck) off the floor. If your seventh cervical touches the floor in *halasana*, place folded blankets below the torso and shoulders as described in *sarvangasana 1*.
- Press the shoulders down, in toward each other, and forward toward the head.
- Center the head and press the head and elbows down. Bring the chin vertical—do not allow the chin to drop toward the chest.
- Push the torso with the hands to move the hips forward and the knees down.
- Engage the biceps and press the hands into the torso.
- Extend the hips and spine up.
- Breathe evenly.

refinement
To get your knees to the floor in this pose, your spine will have to forward fold. Once you attain the full form of *karnapidasana*, straighten your legs to come into a deeper expression of *halasana.* Keep the feet pointed in this variation.

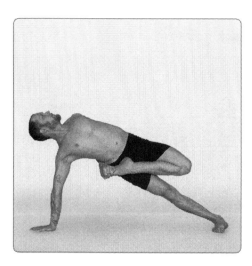

kasyapasana
Sage Kasyapa's pose

shape
(from *vasisthasana*, legs together)

1. Bend the left knee toward the chest and hold the top of the foot with the left hand.
2. Bring the left leg into *ardha padmasana* by placing the outer edge of the foot on the upper right thigh.
3. Inhale fully. Exhale, swing the left arm behind the back and catch the inner edge of the left foot with the hand. Hold the left big toe with the first two fingers and thumb.
4. Lower the top knee as much as possible.
5. Look up. Hold the pose and breathe.
6. To come out, release the hand and straighten the top leg.

Repeat on the second side.

safety

- To reduce the pressure on the lower wrist, move the hand a few inches forward—toward the top of the mat—so that the wrist is in front of the shoulder.
- Separate the fingers of the bottom hand. Point the index finger and biceps straight ahead.
- Press the fingertips and the perimeter of the palm evenly into the floor—press the mound of the index finger down and lift the outer wrist up.
- Push the lower hand down and lift the hips up and back.
- Press the outer edge/top of the *ardha padmasana* foot into the thigh and clamp the knee closed.
- Move the tailbone forward and tone the low belly. Press the base of the sternum back.
- If looking up is too intense for the neck or jaw, look down.

refinement

To make binding the top foot with the hand more accessible, try one of the following:
1. Bend your bottom knee, move your hips back, backbend slightly in your low back, and swing the left arm behind your back to catch your foot.
2. Once in *ardha padmasana*, come into a one-handed *adho mukha svanasana*. Lean onto your right foot and right hand. Wrap your left arm behind your back and bind the big toe. Inhale fully.

Exhale, come into *kasyapasana*.

3. Come into *ardha padmasana* in a seated position. Bind your left foot with your left hand. Balancing on your right hand and right foot, lift your hips into *kasyapasana*.

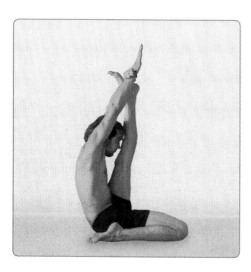

krounchasana
heron pose

shape
(from *dandasana*)

1. Bend the right knee and place the inner ankle against the right outer hip. Lower the leg to the floor and point the foot back.
2. Lean to the left and pull the right glutes back with the right hand. Repeat on the other side.
3. Place the left foot on the floor in front of the sit bone.
4. Flex the left foot—heel on the floor, toes lifted.
5. Clasp the right wrist with the left hand beneath the left foot.
6. Inhale fully. Exhale, lift and straighten the left leg.
7. Bend the elbows out to the sides and bring the forehead or chin toward/to the shin.
8. Look forward. Hold the pose and breathe.
9. To come out, bend the top knee and release the hands and leg—straighten the leg. Stretch the right leg forward and place the hands next to the hips.

Repeat on the second side.

safety

- If the low back rounds, sit on one or more folded blankets—foot off the blanket.
- To reduce the intensity of the hamstring stretch, hold the top foot with both hands or use a strap around the top foot. Walk the hands up the strap to straighten the arms.
- Tone the top thigh and tighten the knee.
- Press the hands into the foot and the foot into the hands.
- Lift the pelvic floor and tone the low belly.
- Lengthen the spine and lift the chest.

refinement

Sit toward the fronts of your sit bones rather than rolling toward the backs of your sit bones to prevent excessive rounding in your low back. Lift your ribcage away from your hips to lengthen the waist. On the lifted leg, reach the mound of your big toe forward and pull your outer foot back. Spread your toes and flare the outer two toes. Articulate the arch of your foot. *Krounchasana* has so much to offer it's worth the aspiration and perspiration it takes to attain it. Often what these poses offer is what they take away from us.

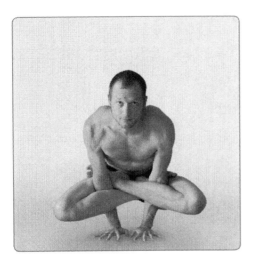

kukkutasana
rooster pose

shape
(from *padmasana*)

1. With the left shin on top in *padmasana*, place the hands behind the hips and lean back. Lift the knees away from the floor.
2. Hold the left shin with the left hand. Slide the right forearm between the right calf and thigh—in front of the left ankle. Bring the inner elbow to the back of the outer calf.
3. Slide the left forearm between the left calf and thigh—in front of the right ankle. Bring the inner elbow to the back of the outer calf.
4. Lean forward and place the hands on the floor with the tips of the thumbs touching.
5. Inhale fully. Exhale, lift the hips off the floor. Straighten the arms.
6. Look straight ahead. Hold the pose and breathe.
7. To come out, exhale, lower the hips to the floor. Release the arms one at a time and place the hands on the thighs.

Repeat on the second side.

safety
- If the legs cannot fold in *padmasana*, fold the legs into *sukhasana* instead.
- Press the fingertips and the perimeter of the palms into the floor with firm and equal pressure.
- Press the outer edges/tops of the feet into the upper thighs. Squeeze the heels toward the hips.
- Flare the toes.
- Engage the abdomen and lift the pelvic floor.

refinement
Before moving into *kukkutasana*, consider performing *garbha pindasana*. Roll counter clockwise on the back nine times, which represents the nine months of gestation, until you return to face your starting direction. Roll back and forth by engaging your abdomen and pelvic floor. In other words, don't use your arms or head to create the rolling movement. After rotating 360 degrees in nine movements, roll up onto your hands and balance in *kukkutasana* for five breaths. This expression of *garbha pindasana* comes from Sri Pattabhi Jois' Ashtanga Yoga.

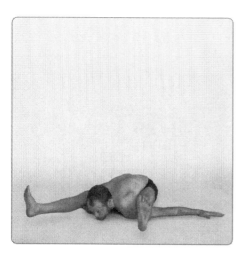

kurmasana
tortoise pose

shape
(from *dandasana,* facing long edge of mat)

1. Separate the legs wider than shoulder-width apart and bend the knees slightly.
2. Flex the feet so the heels are the only part of the legs touching the floor. Point the toes and knees up.
3. Inhale fully. Exhale, fold the torso forward between the knees.
4. One at a time, bring the hands, arms, and then shoulders underneath the knees. Stretch the arms out to the sides.
5. Straighten the arms. Place the palms on the floor and separate the fingers.
6. Squeeze the thighs into the torso and straighten the legs.
7. Lower the shoulders and chin toward/to the floor.
8. Lift the feet and hips off the floor so the shoulders, arms, and chin are the only parts of the body touching the floor. Hold the pose and breathe.
9. To come out, exhale, lower the feet and hips to the floor. Bend the knees enough to release the torso and shoulders from underneath the legs. Lift the torso upright and use the hands to bring the knees together and straighten the legs. Place the hands next to the hips.

safety
- To reduce the intensity of the hamstring stretch, keep the knees slightly bent and press the heels into the floor.
  If the shoulders do not rest below the knees, bring the backs of the upper arms under the knees and widen the legs slightly.
- Straighten and strengthen the arms and legs. Extend out through the hands and feet.
- Engage the triceps and quads.
- Lock the knees and elbows into a straight position.
- Lift the pelvic floor and tone the low belly.

refinement
Advanced practitioners can move from here into the following variation of *kurmasana*: Turn your palms up and bend your elbows to bring the backs of your hands to the outer waist or hips. Bind your hands and squeeze your arms into your legs and press your legs into your arms. Cross your

right ankle over your left ankle or vice versa. Rest your forehead on the ankles. Once you can perform this variation of *kurmasana*, you are ready to proceed into *tittibhasana*.

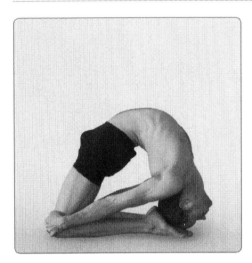

laghuvajrasana
graceful thunderbolt pose

shape
(from *supta virasana*)

1. Place the hands flat on the floor by the head—thumbs facing in. Point the elbows up.
2. Inhale, lift the hips and torso. Straighten the arms.
3. Walk the hands toward the feet until the thighs are vertical.
4. Place the inner edges of the feet together, bend the elbows, and lower the top of the head to the soles of the feet.
5. Slide the hands up the shins to clasp the knees with the hands.
6. Look at the tip of the nose. Hold the pose and breathe.
7. To come out, walk the hands back toward the feet and place the hands on the floor next to the feet—thumbs facing in. Keep the chest full and inhale, lift the torso vertical. Lift the head once the torso is upright.

safety
- Press the inner edges of the feet together and flare the outer two toes.
- Isometrically squeeze the ankles, shins, and forearms in.
- Squeeze the knees in and move the inner thighs back.
- Press the tailbone forward and engage the glutes.
- Lift the pelvic floor and tone the low belly.
- Press the tops of the feet down, move the hips forward, and stretch the entire spine.
- Press the head and feet into each other.
- To make this pose more accessible, place a block between the feet in *supta virasana* and enter into the pose with the top of the head on the block. Squeeze the feet and shins in toward the block to prevent the block from slipping.

refinement
Laguvajrasana is among the best preparatory poses for *vrischikasana 2* and *ganda bherundasana*.

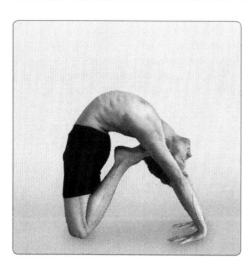

laghuvajrasana
graceful thunderbolt pose

feet to back of head

shape
(from *supta virasana*)

1. Place the hands flat on the floor by the head—thumbs facing in. Point the elbows up.
2. Inhale, lift the hips and torso. Straighten the arms.
3. Walk the hands toward the feet until the thighs are vertical.
4. Place the inner edges of the feet together, bend the elbows, and lower the top of the head to the soles of the feet.
5. Lower the elbows to the floor and clasp the ankles with the hands.
6. With the support of the hands, lift the feet one at a time to the back of the head—toes to the base of the skull.
7. Place the hands flat on the floor underneath the shoulders.
8. Straighten the arms.
9. Walk the hands toward the knees until the thighs are vertical. Curl the head back. Hold the pose and breathe.
10. To come out, bend the elbows and lower the head to the floor. Release the feet from the back of the head. Keep the chest full, inhale, and lift the torso vertical. Lift the head once the torso is upright.

safety

- Press the inner edges of the feet together and flare the outer two toes.
- Squeeze the knees in and move the inner thighs back.
- Press the tailbone forward and engage the glutes.
- Lift the pelvic floor and tone the low belly.
- Press the head and toes into each other.
- Press the hands down and forward while simultaneously moving the shoulders back. Stretch the entire spine.

refinement

The most difficult aspect of this pose is getting the feet on the head. The key is to not lose the depth of the backbend as you lift your feet onto the back of your head with your hands. How does one do that? Focus and will power. All of the advanced backbends require intense focus, willpower, discipline, and awareness. What they require is what they offer.

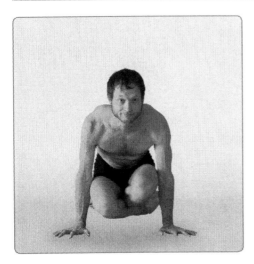

lolasana
tremulous pose

shape
(from *bharmanasana*)

1. Cross the left shin over the right shin.
2. Lower the hips and place the arch of the left foot directly under the right sit bone and the arch of the right foot directly under the left sit bone.
3. Place the hands on the floor beside the hips.
4. Separate the fingers and point the index fingers straight ahead.
5. Lean forward, push the hands down and straighten the arms to lift the hips and legs off the floor.
6. Kick the feet into the hips.
7. Swing the hips back and forth slowly—inhale as the knees move forward, exhale as the knees move backward. Repeat this five times. Look straight ahead.
8. To come out, exhale, lower the hips and legs to the floor. Uncross the legs.

Repeat on the second side.

safety
- Press the fingertips and the perimeter of the hands evenly into the floor—press the mounds of the index fingers down and lift the outer wrists up.
- Lift the pelvic floor and low belly. In other words, shorten the distance between the pelvic floor and the shoulders by lifting up, up, and up. It is this action, combined with the strength of the arms pressing down, that will make "floating" in this pose possible.
- If the hips and legs cannot lift off floor, place blocks underneath the hands.

refinement

To progress toward the full form of *lolasana*, follow steps 1–4 in the shape instructions. Then lean forward, taking your weight into your knees while kicking your heels into your hips. Lean back, taking your weight into your hips while lifting your knees into your chest. Repeat this sequence several times and then recross your legs and repeat. This will help you feel the actions that *lolasana* requires of you.

I know a practitioner from Prescott, Arizona who attempted *lolasana* several times a week for about two years without being able to lift her hips and feet off the floor. After two years of such dedication, one day she suddenly lifted into *lolasana*. What a tenacious practitioner! Often we cannot see or feel our progress. Please rest assured that if you are practicing, you are progressing. In the Twelve-Step Program there is a saying, "Progress not perfection." A good hatha yoga saying might be, "Practice *is* progress."

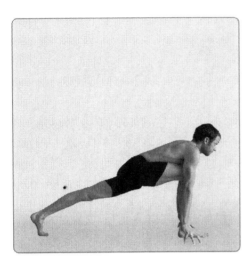

lunge pose

shape
(from *adho mukha svanasana*)

1. Step the right foot forward to the inside of the right hand—feet outer hip-width apart. Point the front foot straight ahead.
2. Bring the front knee above the front heel. If the right hip is higher than the knee, take a longer stance via the back foot until the front thigh is parallel to the floor.
3. Bring the fingertips to the floor directly below the shoulders and straighten the arms.
4. Straighten the back leg.
5. To square the hips to the front of the mat, move the left hip forward, right hip back.
6. Look straight ahead. Hold the pose and breathe.
7. To come out, exhale, step the right foot back to *adho mukha svanasana*.

Repeat on the second side.

safety
- Do not allow the front knee to move beyond the heel.
- Move the front knee out to the side until the thigh is in line with the long edge of the mat.
- Without moving the front knee, move the back heel forward until it is vertical.
- Isometrcially squeeze the feet toward each other.
- Keep the hips slightly lifted and the abdominal muscles toned. The hips tend to drop, which can cause the back thigh to collapse and the low back to compress.
- Move the tailbone down and lift the low belly.
- Press the fingertips down.

refinement
Extend your back foot and sternum away from each other, but keep both your back heel and front shin vertical. Lunge pose is one of the few standing poses where the back heel is vertical rather than on the floor. A common practice is moving from lunge into a modified *virabhadrasana 1* (with the back heel up). This foot position is one of the few poses that stretches the toes and the sole of the foot.

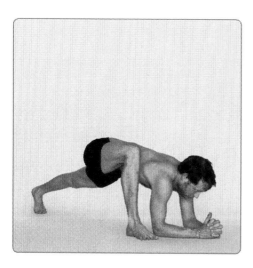

lunge pose

forearms to floor

shape

1. Begin in lunge pose, and bring both arms to the inside of the right foot. Place the forearms on the floor—right elbow next to right foot.
2. Separate the elbows shoulder-width apart.
3. Interlace the fingers and press the palms together.
4. Look straight down. Hold the pose and breathe.
5. To come out, lift onto the hands. Bring the hands to either side of the foot.

Repeat on the second side.

safety

- Press the front big toe down; flare the outer two toes of both feet.
- Press the back foot down and back. Lift the back thigh up.
- Without moving the front knee, bring the back heel vertical and lift the hips slightly.
- Move the tailbone down and the low belly in.
- Engage the left glutes.
- If the forearms do not reach the floor, place blocks under the forearms.

refinement

Press your forearms down and forward. Isometrically extend your front knee and back heel away from your hips.

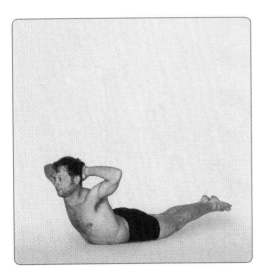

makarasana
crocodile pose

shape

1. Bring the front body and forehead to the floor.
2. Interlace the fingers behind the head and lift the elbows so the arms are parallel to the floor.
3. Straighten the legs and bring the inner edges of the legs and feet together. Point the feet.
4. Inhale, lift the chin, torso, and legs. Look straight ahead. Hold the pose and breathe.
5. To come out, exhale, lower the head, torso, and legs to the floor. Release the hands.

safety

- If there is pain or discomfort in the low back, separate the feet outer hip-width apart.
- Lock the legs into a straight position.
- Point the kneecaps straight down.
- Point the toes straight back and squeeze the inner feet together.
- Press the tailbone down, engage the glutes, and lift the low belly.
- Press the head into the hands and lift the back of the head with the hands.
- Stretch the spine forward and up.

refinement

The prevalence of low back pain is preventable. Often low back pain comes from, or is aggravated by, our lifestyles. Sitting at a desk for hours at a time for example, especially with poor posture and lack of awareness, can weaken the abdomen and overstretch the low back. Over time the body responds to this misuse and abuse with discomfort or pain. Regular practice of *makarasana* and variations is a great way to keep your low back both strong and supple. The practice of hatha yoga is as much about strength as it is about stretch.

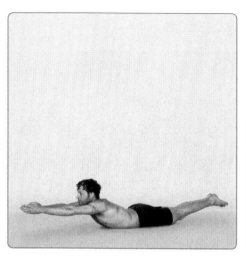
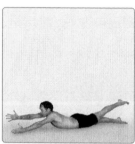

makarasana
crocodile pose

arms extended

shape

1. Bring the front body to the floor.
2. Straighten the legs and bring the inner edges of the legs and feet together. Point the feet.
3. Lift the chin and place the chin on the floor.
4. Extend the arms forward and place the outer edges of the hands on the floor—thumbs pointing up. Straighten the arms.
5. Press the hands down and lift the shoulders up and back to capacity. This will cause the hands to slide back slightly.
6. Inhale, lift the arms, legs, and torso. Bring the arms parallel to the floor and press the palms together.
7. Look forward past the thumbs. Hold the pose and breathe.
8. To come out, exhale, lower the arms and legs to the floor.

safety

- If there is pain or discomfort in the low back, separate the feet outer hip-width apart.
- If there is pain or discomfort in the shoulders, separate the arms outer shoulder-width apart.
- Lock the arms and legs into a straight position.
- Point the kneecaps straight down.
- Point the toes straight back and squeeze the inner feet together.
- Press the tailbone down, engage the glutes, and lift the low belly.
- Stretch the spine forward and up.

refinement

This pose can also be done with the heels firmly pressed together. I call this pose "superhero pose" when teaching it in class because it comes to the rescue of weakness in the low back.

The arms extended variation of *makrasana* can be practiced asymmetrically with just one arm and the opposite leg lifted. This is the most doable variation of *makarasana* and yet it is still a great warm up for the legs, arms, and back. This asymmetrical version is an important exercise for those with scoliosis because it engages the muscles along one side of the spine as it releases the muscles on the other side. In doing so, this pose can strengthen the weak side as it releases the strong side, which can reduce back pain for those with scoliosis.

I once had a 40-degree scoliosis C-curve and was in pain on a daily basis. Yoga has significantly reduced my C-curve and completely taken away my back pain. If you have scoliosis, you will need to learn to practice accordingly in order to really shift your curve. For example, the way I twist to the right is completely different than how I twist to the left. My spine will never be perfectly straight or so-called "normal"—the back of my left ribcage is flat, my right ribcage overly rounded; the muscles along the right side of my spine are overly developed, the left side underdeveloped. Even so, my back is hatha happy and healthy. I used to be embarrassed about my scoliosis, but yoga has helped me to love my body as it is.

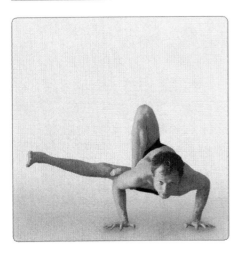

maksikanagasana 1
dragonfly pose 1

shape

1. Come to sit on the floor.
2. Bend both knees and bring the heels about a foot in front of the sit bones.
3. Place the hands behind the hips, lean back and place the right outer ankle on top of the left thigh.
4. Inhale, lift the right arm vertical.
5. Exhale, twist the torso to the left and bring the outer right shoulder to the arch of the right foot.
6. Place the right hand on the floor. Separate the hands outer shoulder-distance apart.
7. Lift the hips off the floor and lean forward into the hands. Bend the elbows 90 degrees.
8. Straighten the lower leg out to the side. Look forward. Hold the pose and breathe.
9. To come out, exhale, bend the bottom knee, lower the hips and straighten the legs.

Repeat on the second side.

safety

- Press the fingertips and the perimeter of the left hand down onto the floor with firm and equal pressure.
- Lift the shoulders up.
- Straighten and strengthen the extended leg. Flex the foot and flare the toes.

refinement

Another entry point is to start from a standing position. Bend your knees slightly and place your right ankle on top of your left thigh above the knee. Twist to the lift and place your hands outer shoulder-distance apart, with your right foot against your right upper armpit. Lean forward and bend your elbows 90 degrees. Lift your bottom foot and straighten your leg out to the side.

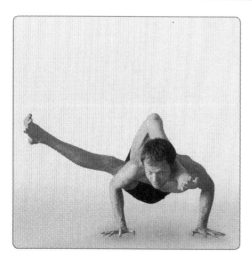

maksikanagasana 2
dragonfly pose 2

shape
(from *eka pada sirsasana*)

1. With the right leg behind the head, bend the left knee and place the sole of the foot directly in front of the right sit bone.
2. Place the left hand on the floor to the outside of the left hip. Point the fingers away from the hips.
3. Move the left knee to the right and twist the torso to the left. Bring the shoulder to the outside of the knee and place the hands outer shoulder-width apart.
4. Press the hands and left foot down. Lift the hips up and to the right and bring the left thigh to the right elbow.
5. Lean onto the hands and lift the left foot off the floor. Straighten the left leg.
6. Bend the elbows 90 degrees so the forearms are vertical.
7. Lift the chin and look straight ahead. Hold the pose and breathe.
8. To come out, bend the extended leg and place the foot underneath the hips. Lower the hips and stretch the leg forward.

safety

- Flex the feet and flare the toes.
- Isometrically bend the top knee to engage the hamstrings.
- Straighten and strengthen the extended leg.
- Tone the pelvic floor and low belly.

refinement

This pose is as difficult as it looks. In order to get into this pose you must curl your head back with all your strength, otherwise the leg is likely to slip from behind the head. Another entry point: start from *eka pada sirsasana*, and come into a standing forward fold. Bend your left knee and bring your right elbow to the outside of your left knee and place your hands outer shoulder-width apart—fingers facing forward. Lean onto your elbow, lift your left foot and straighten your leg.

maksikanagasana 2
dragonfly pose 2

hand to chin

shape
(from *eka pada sirsasana*)

1. With the right leg behind the head, bend the left knee and place the sole of the foot directly in front of the right sit bone.
2. Lean to the left and lower the left forearm and hand to the floor.
3. Place the right hand in front of the left knee—in line with the left elbow—hands outer shoulder-width apart.
4. Bring the right elbow to the outside of the left thigh just above the knee.
5. Lean forward and lift the hips up and to the left.
6. Lift the left foot off the floor and straighten the leg.
7. Lift the left hand to hold the left side of the face. Look forward. Hold the pose and breathe.
8. To come out, lower the lifted hand and hips to the floor. Release and straighten the top leg.

Repeat on the second side.

safety
- Flex the feet and flare the toes.
- Isometrically bend the top knee to engage the hamstrings.
- Straighten and strengthen the extended leg. Flare the toes.
- Tone the pelvic floor and low belly.

refinement
The point of taking the hand to the chin in a pose like this is to invoke playfulness. Play must always remain part and parcel of this path. Otherwise seriousness will stifle instead of stoke your *sadhana*.

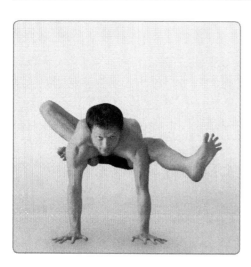

maksikanagasana 3
dragonfly pose 3

shape
(from *yogadandasana*)

1. With the right foot in the right armpit, place the right hand on the floor.
2. Place the left hand on the floor behind the hips. Lift the hips off the floor and stand on the left foot.
3. Bring the left arm inside and under the left leg. Place the left hand on the floor outside of the left foot.
4. Lean back, lift the left foot, and extend the leg forward.
5. Straighten the arms and look straight ahead. Hold the pose and breathe.
6. To come out, bend the front knee and lower the foot to the floor. Lower the hips and release the top leg.

Repeat on the second side.

safety

- Press the fingertips and the perimeter of the left hand down onto the floor with firm and equal pressure.
- Press the right shoulder into the right foot and the left shoulder into the left knee.
- Straighten and strengthen the front leg. Extend the inner edge of the front leg down. Squeeze the extended leg into the arm.
- Round the back and press the tailbone forward.
- Lift the pelvic floor and tone the low belly.

refinement

The tightness in the hip of the bent knee makes this arm balance feel effortless in the arms. The hips and legs will feel like they are weightless.

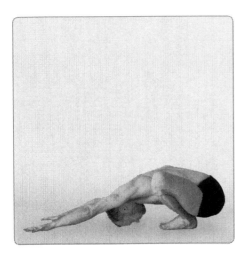
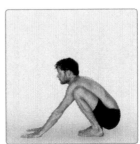

malasana prep
garland pose

shape
(from *tadasana*)

1. Lower into a squat position.
2. Squeeze the feet together and separate the knees as wide as possible.
3. Place the palms flat on the floor shoulder-width apart. Stretch the hands forward.
4. Inhale fully. Exhale, fold the torso forward between the legs. Walk the hands forward to capacity.
5. Rest the forehead on the floor. Hold the pose and breathe.
6. To come out, inhale, lift the head. Walk the hands back until they are directly below the shoulders. Lift to stand.

safety

- If the heels do not reach the floor, place a rolled-up mat or folded blanket underneath the heels. Do not allow the heels to lift and the weight to come forward toward the toes. *Malasana* is meant to stretch the Achilles tendon and low back. If the heels are lifted, the Achilles tendon will not fully stretch.
- If the inner edges of the feet lift away from the floor, keep the heels together and open the feet 60 degrees.
- Press the inner edges of the feet down and squeeze the torso with the thighs.
- Press the tips of the toes into the floor. Press the hands down.
- Lift the pelvic floor and tone the low belly.

refinement

Stretch your arms away from your hips to gain length in your waist and torso. Keep your head low but lift your hips slightly. Stretch your arms forward, drop your sit bones toward the floor, and fold your torso down and forward between your legs. Use your abdomen to draw your body into a tight, closed position. If your head remains lifted due to restrictions of the body or mental agitation or excitement, it is difficult to receive the full benefits of the forward fold. If your forehead does not reach the floor, place it on the edge of a block. Allowing your head to come into contact and rest on a solid surface is both grounding and pacifying. Stay in the pose for an extended period of time and release into the pose. Use forward folds to learn to soften in your practice and in your body, and to draw your attention and energy inward.

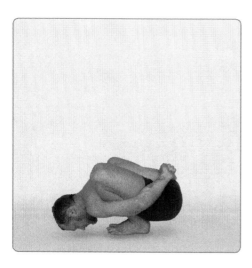

malasana 1
garland pose 1

shape
(from *malasana prep*)

1. Lift the hips slightly, bend the elbows and bring the backs of the upper arms to the shins. Point the elbows back and lower the hips.
2. Walk the outer shoulders down the shins one at a time. Bring the shoulders as low as possible until the head is near the floor.
3. Straighten the arms out to the sides, then turn the palms up and reach the arms back. Pause and breathe.
4. Bend the right arm and place the back of the hand on the outer right hip. Squeeze the right thigh into the torso with the right arm. Repeat on the other side.
5. Little by little move the hands together. Turn the right hand so the thumb points down. Clasp the fingers or hands.
6. Rest the forehead on the floor. Hold the pose and breathe.
7. To come out, release the clasp of the hands. Inhale, look up and stretch the arms forward.

safety
- If the heels do not reach the floor, place a rolled-up mat or folded blanket underneath the heels.
- If the inner edges of the feet lift away from the floor, keep the heels together and open the feet 60 degrees.
- Press the inner edges of the feet down and squeeze the shins in.
- Keeping the hands clasped, pull the hands in opposite directions.
- Squeeze the elbows in.
- Tone the low belly and lift the pelvic floor.
- If the hands do not clasp, use a strap to bind.
- If the head does not reach the floor, place the forehead on the edge of a block.
- To reduce the intensity of the pose, sit on a block.

refinement
This is among the most difficult poses to clasp the hands in. The creativity and tenacity it requires makes it a good preparatory pose for *pasasana*. *Malasana 1* is also excellent preparation

for *bakasana*. They are similar in shape in that the back is rounded and the knees hug the outer, upper arms. Both poses also require flexibility in the hips. Understanding the shape of the pose on the ground can provide the basic framework for taking the pose into flight in *bakasana*.

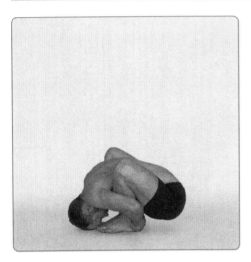

malasana 2
garland pose 2

shape
(from *tadasana*)

1. Bend the knees slightly.
2. Inhale fully. Exhale, fold the torso forward and hold the backs of the heels with the hands.
3. Lower into a squat position—inner knees to outer shoulders.
4. Lean back and move the hips down toward the floor.
5. Inhale, keep the torso low and lift the hips slightly. Exhale, fold the torso between the legs.
6. Place the forehead on the floor. If possible, touch the toes with the forehead. Hold the pose and breathe.
7. To come out, inhale, look forward. Exhale, release the hands and lift the torso to stand.

safety
*   Press the inner edges of the feet down.
*   If the inner edges of the feet lift away from the floor, keep the heels together and open the feet 60 degrees.
*   Squeeze the torso with the thighs.
*   Squeeze the elbows into the shins.
*   Tone the low belly and lift the pelvic floor.
*   If the forehead does not reach the floor, place the forehead on the edge of a block.
*   To reduce the intensity of the pose, sit on a block.

refinement
Pull up on your heels with your hands and press your shoulders into your shins to help get your forehead to the floor. Engage your arms and abdomen to bring your forehead and toes together. *Malasana 1* is more difficult than *malasana 2*. And yet, *malasana 2* requires vigor, which makes it an optimal warm up pose.

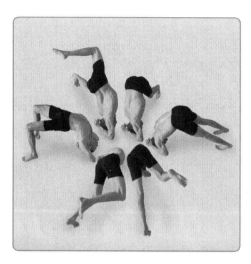

mandalasana
orbit pose

shape
(from *dwi pada viparita dandasana,* knees bent)

1. Press the head and forearms down and walk the feet to the right.
2. Once the feet are in line with the right ear, lift the left leg up and over the right leg.
3. Pivot on the right foot and turn the hips and torso to the right to place the left foot on the floor on the other side of the right foot. The toes now point in toward the head, and the torso faces the floor.
4. Walk the feet to the left until they are in line with the left ear. Then lift the right leg up and over the left leg.
5. Pivot on the left foot and turn the hips and torso to the left to place the right foot on the other side of the left foot. The toes now point away from the head, and the torso faces upward.
6. Walk the feet back into *dwi pada viparita dandasana,* knees bent.
7. Circumambulate the head again moving in the opposite direction.

Do one to ten sets.

safety
- Press the wrists down and move the shoulders back.
- Engage the abdomen and move the base of the sternum back.
- Do not move the wrists or elbows. Keep the head in the same place on the floor from start to finish.
- Keep the top leg as close to the floor as possible when crossing over the bottom leg.
- Keep the feet equidistant from the head from start to finish.

refinement
Once you become familiar with *mandalasana,* it is easier to perform when moving quickly. Advanced practitioners can drop over into *dwi pada viparita dandasana* from *sirsasana,* and then perform *mandalasana.* Once *mandalasana* is completed, return to *sirsasana* in one fluid movement.

This pose requires a unique kind of mobility in the low back. In a way, your spine must move like liquid. Good preparatory poses for *mandalasana* are *indudalasana, parighasana, parivrtta supta padangusthasana, parsva halasana, parsva sarvangasana, camatkarasana,* and *parivrtta pada visama pincha mayurasana.* If your shoulders and/or back are not open enough to perform this pose, you will likely fall over onto your side.

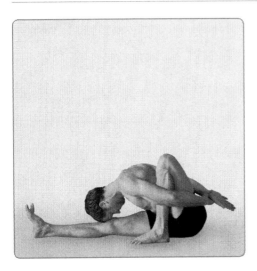

marichyasana 1
Sage Marichi's pose 1

shape
(from *dandasana*)

1. Bend the left knee. Place the heel in front of the left sit bone. Point the knee up.
2. Press the hands down. Lift the hips up and forward. Bring the left sit bone against the left heel. Lower the hips to the floor.
3. Curve the low back in and up.
4. Inhale, lift the left arm vertical. Exhale, fold the torso forward and hold the inner edge of the right foot with the left hand.
5. Inhale, lift and lengthen the spine. Exhale, lean forward and wrap the left arm around the left leg. Place the back of the left hand on the outer left hip.
6. Swing the right arm behind the back and hold the right wrist with the left hand.
7. Straighten the back arm. Turn the abdomen to the right and lower the forehead to the knee. Hold the pose and breathe.
8. To come out, inhale, look forward and lift the head and torso. Exhale, release the hands next to the hips. Straighten the bent leg.

Repeat on the second side.

safety
- If the low back rounds, sit on one or more blankets and/or step the foot of the bent leg forward.
- If the hand does not clasp the wrist behind the back, hold the hand or fingers, or use a strap.
- Engage the extended leg. Press the back of the knee into the floor.
- Press the back foot down into the floor and squeeze the knee.
- Allow the sit bone of the bent leg to lift away from the floor.

- Lift the right shoulder up.
- Squeeze the elbows in.
- Lift the pelvic floor and tone the low belly.
- If the head does not reach the knee, stack one or more blankets on top of the leg and rest the forehead on the edge of the blankets.

refinement

Marichyasana 1 is a unique forward fold in that the hands do not hold the foot of the extended leg. To get your forehead to your front knee will require core engagement. In *Light On Yoga,* B. K. S. Iyengar says that *janu sirsasana, ardha baddha padma paschimottanasana, triang mukhaikapada paschmiottanasa,* and *marichyasana 1* are the four key poses that prepare practitioners for *paschimottanasana.*[1] As you practice one pose, you are also preparing for another. None of the poses are meant to be practiced in isolation.

[1]   B. K. S. Iyengar, *Light on Yoga* (New York: Schocken Books, 1977) p. 161.

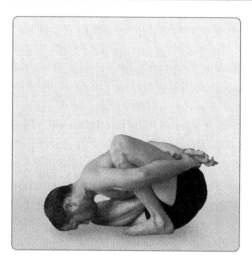

marichyasana 2
Sage Marichi's pose 2

shape
(from *dandasana*)

1. Bring the right palm to the inner right knee.
2. Pull the knee as far right and back as possible so that the legs come into an obtuse angle—outer leg and knee to floor.
3. With the hands, lift the right foot and place the outer right foot on the upper inner left thigh at the crease of the groin. Point the right knee forward and lower the leg.
4. Lean to the left and place the left hand to the inner right thigh—fingers between the calf and thigh. As the hip lowers to the floor, spin the thigh down with the left hand and pull the right glutes back with the right hand.
5. Keep the right knee on the floor and place the left heel just in front of the left sit bone—knee pointing up.
6. Inhale fully. Exhale, fold the torso to the inside of the left leg—outer shoulder to inner knee.
7. Wrap the left arm around the leg. Place the back of the hand on the outer left hip.

8. Swing the right arm behind the back. Clasp the right wrist with the left hand.
9. Inhale, lengthen the spine. Exhale, fold the torso forward and lower the forehead toward/to the floor to the inside of the bottom knee. Look down. Hold the pose and breathe.
10. To come out, inhale, look up and lift the torso. Exhale, release the hands and straighten both legs. Place the hands next to the hips.

Repeat on the second side.

safety

- If *ardha padmasana* is not possible, bring the lower leg and foot to the floor in front of the pubic bone (as in *baddha konasana*). Or, practice *marichyasana 1* instead.
- Allow the sit bone of the upright knee to lift away from the floor, especially to come into the forward fold. Keep the thigh of the *ardha padmasana* leg on the floor.
- Flex the foot in *ardha padmasana* and press the top of the foot into the thigh. Press the heel into the belly. Spread the toes.
- Squeeze the upper arm and shin into each other.
- If the hand does not clasp the wrist behind the back, hold the opposite hand or fingers, or use a strap.
- Squeeze the elbows in. Lift the shoulders up.
- Lift the pelvic floor and tone the low belly.
- Round the back evenly.
- If the forehead does not reach the floor, place the forehead on the edge of a block. Adjust the height of the block as necessary.

refinement

The more complex the form, the more single-pointed the mind must become. The depth of awareness and focus rather than the degree of difficulty is one of the boons of advanced poses.

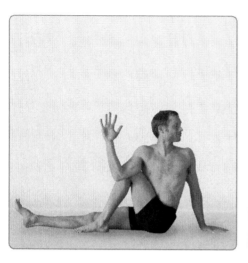
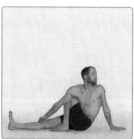

marichyasana 3 prep
Sage Marichi's pose 3

shape
(from *dandasana*)

1. Bend the left knee. Place the heel just in front of the left sit bone. Point the knee up.
2. Press the hands down. Lift the hips up and forward. Bring the left sit bone against the left heel. Lower the hips to the floor.
3. Curve the low back in and up. Place the left hand on the floor a few inches behind the sacrum. Straighten the arm.
4. Inhale, lift the right arm vertical.
5. Exhale, turn the torso to the left and place the right elbow or upper arm on the outer left knee. Bend the elbow—forearm and fingers pointing up, palm facing out.
6. Inhale, lengthen the spine. Exhale, turn the torso away from the leg and look past the shoulder. Hold the pose and breathe.
7. To come out, inhale, look forward. Release the hands to the floor next to the hips. Straighten the bent leg.

Repeat on the second side.

safety

- If the low back rounds, sit on one or more blankets and/or step the foot of the bent leg forward.
- Engage the extended leg. Press the back of the knee down.
- Flex the front foot—flare the outer two toes.
- Squeeze the bent knee to completely close the knee.
- If the outer shoulder does not come to the outer knee, hold the outer knee with the hand or inner elbow.
- Move the base of the sternum back and lift the chest.
- Move the shoulders back.
- Lift the pelvic floor and tone the low belly.

refinement

For a more challenging variation of this pose, straighten your front arm and press your palm into the outer shin of your extended leg.

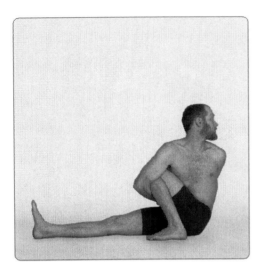

marichyasana 3
Sage Marichi's pose 3

shape
(from *marichyasana 3* prep)

1. Straighten the top arm and point the elbow forward to wrap the right arm around the left leg.
2. Bring the back of the left hand to the right side of the torso.
3. Hold the right wrist with the left hand.
4. Inhale fully. Exhale, turn the abdomen to the left. Look straight back. Hold the pose and breathe.
5. To come out, inhale, look forward. Exhale, release the hands to the floor next to the hips and straighten the legs.

Repeat on the second side.

safety
- If the low back rounds, sit on one or more blankets and/or step the foot of the bent leg forward.
- If the front arm does not wrap around the top knee, practice *marichyasana 3 prep* instead.
- If the hand does not clasp the wrist behind the back, hold the hand or fingers, or use a strap.
- Engage the extended leg. Press the back of the knee down.
- Flex the front foot—flare the outer two toes.
- Squeeze the bent knee to completely close the knee.
- Move the base of the sternum back and lift the chest.
- Move the shoulders back.
- Lift the pelvic floor and tone the low belly.

refinement
This pose can also be practiced with the left heel next to the left hip. This variation decreases the difficulty in binding the hands and creates a more stable foundation in the legs and hips. The torso will also lean back, which requires more strength in the abdomen and hip flexors.

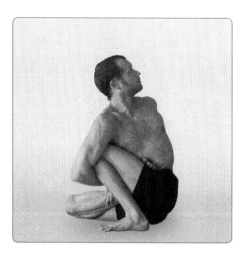

marichyasana 4
Sage Marichi's pose 4

shape
(from *dandasana*)

1. Bring the right palm to the inner right knee.
2. Pull the knee as far right and back as possible so that the legs come into an obtuse angle—outer leg and knee to floor.
3. With the hands, lift the right foot and place the outer right foot on the upper inner left thigh at the crease of the groin. Point the right knee forward and lower the leg.
4. Lean to the left and place the left hand on the inner right thigh—fingers between the calf and thigh. As the hip lowers to the floor, spin the thigh down with the left hand and pull the right glutes back with the right hand.
5. Keep the right knee on the floor and place the left heel just in front of the left sit bone—knee pointing up.
6. Inhale, lift the right arm vertical. Exhale, twist the torso to the left to place the right elbow to the outside of the left knee. Pause and breathe.
7. Inhale fully. Exhale, lower the right shoulder to the outer left knee.
8. Wrap the right arm around the leg.
9. Swing the left arm behind the back and clasp the right shin with the left hand and the left wrist with the right hand.
10. Inhale, look forward. Exhale, turn the head to the left and look past the shoulder. Hold the pose and breathe.
11. To come out, inhale, look forward. Exhale, release the hands next to the hips. Straighten both legs.

Repeat on the second side.

safety
- If the outer shoulder does not reach the outer knee, bring the outer elbow to the knee and the other hand to the floor behind the sacrum.
- Push the top of the lifted foot and toes into the thigh. Spread the toes.
- Push the top heel into the abdomen.
- Squeeze the knee to engage the *ardha padmasana* leg.
- Pull both shoulders toward the spine.
- Lift the pelvic floor.

refinement

If you need additional leverage to come into *marichyasana 4*, try placing your left hand on the floor behind your hips. Keep your torso upright, twist to the left and lift your right knee and hip away from the floor to balance on your left foot and left hand. Round your back over your left hip and place your right elbow on your outer left thigh just below your knee. Place your left hand on your outer left thigh and push your thigh to bring your right shoulder to the outside of your left knee. Balancing only on your left foot slowly wrap your right arm around your left leg. Then lower your hip to the floor.

For several years I practiced the primary series of Ashtanga Yoga, often practicing the four *marichyasanas* six times per week. These poses—especially when practiced regularly and frequently, prepare the body for a wide range of advanced forward folds, hip openers, and twists.

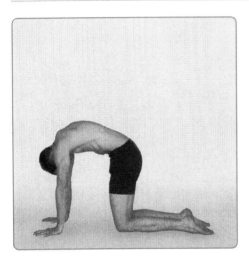

marjarasana
cat pose

shape
(from *bharmanasana*)

1. Inhale fully. Exhale, press the hands down, squeeze the elbows straight, and round the back.
2. Bring the chin to the chest and move the tailbone down and forward.
3. Look past the tip of the nose. Hold the pose and breathe.
4. To come out, inhale, bring the spine to a neutral position.

safety

- Press the fingertips and the roots of the index fingers down.
- Press the tailbone down and lift the low belly.
- Lift the base of the sternum up.
- Point the toes straight back and flare the outer two toes.
- Squeeze the heels in until they are vertical to the floor.
- If there is discomfort in the knees, place a blanket underneath the knees for additional padding.

refinement

The tendency is for the outer edge of the hands to take the majority of the upper body weight. To protect and strengthen the wrists, it is essential to evenly distribute the weight of the body on the perimeter of your palms and fingertips. This, of course becomes even more critical when practicing advanced arm balances. In many arm balances, you will need to press the index knuckles down so strongly that the outer edges of the hands lift up off the floor, which will tone the forearms.

Marjarasana is often practiced and taught in tandem with *bitalasana*. When cat and cow poses are performed together, practitioners exhale into cat pose and inhale into cow pose, which only allows for half a breath in each pose. I recommend that you hold cow pose for at least five breaths as a way to warm up your back and spine at the start of your practice. Then, hold cat for five breaths before moving into the cat-cow cycle.

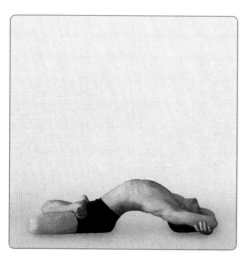 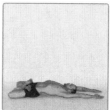 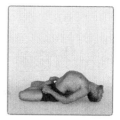

matsyasana
fish pose

shape
(from *padmasana*)

1. Place the hands behind the hips, lean back and lower the forearms and then the torso to the floor.
2. Place the hands on the floor by the head—thumbs facing in and fingers pointing toward the feet. Point the elbows up.
3. Press the hands down, and inhale, lift the head and torso away from the floor to come into a backbend in the upper back. Exhale, lower the top of the head to the floor.
4. Release the hands and hold the right elbow with the left hand and the left elbow with the right hand. Exhale, lower the forearms to the floor.
5. Look at the tip of the nose. Hold the pose and breathe.
6. To come out, inhale, lift the forearms away from the floor and place the elbows on the floor beside the chest. Press the elbows down and lower the torso to the floor. Use the hands to lift the torso vertical.

Repeat on the second side—switch the cross of the legs.

safety

- If the legs cannot fold into *padmasana*, practice this pose with the legs in *sukhasana* instead.
- Clamp the knees closed and press the outer edges/tops of the feet into the thighs.
- Press the sit bones and head down.
- Lift the low back and chest. Tone the low belly and do not push out through the abdomen.
- Extend the shoulders toward the floor.
- If there is any pain or discomfort in the neck, keep the back of the head on the floor and extend the arms overhead.
- If there is pain or discomfort in the shoulders or if the forearms do not reach the floor, place a folded blanket underneath the forearms for extra padding.

refinement

This is a backbend that promotes inner calm and quiet. Another variation of *matsyasana* is to keep the top of your head on the floor and hold your feet with your hands. This variation requires more strength in the neck but it is pacifying due to the connection between the hands and feet.

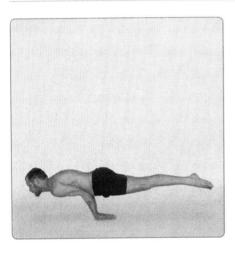
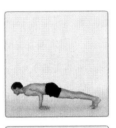
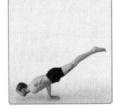
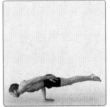

mayurasana
peacock pose

shape

1. Come onto the hands and knees.
2. Bring the outer edge of the hands together with the wrists pointing forward.
3. Point the fingers straight back. Separate the fingers slightly.
4. Bend the elbows and lean forward. Place the abdomen on the elbows so they are just below the sternum. Bring the forearms vertical and press the inner elbows together.
5. Lean forward even more to bring the weight into the hands and to walk the feet back. Extend the left leg, then the right leg, straight back. Curl the toes under. Pause and breathe.
6. Walk the feet toward the hands to reach forward through the head. This will straighten the arms slightly.
7. Lower the chin toward the floor and lift the feet. Pause and breathe.
8. Slowly lift the head and lower the feet until the body is parallel to the floor.
9. Look straight ahead. Hold the pose and breathe.
10. To come out, lower the feet, bend the knees, and lift to kneel on the shins.

safety

- Press the fingertips and the perimeter of the palms down into the floor with equal pressure. Press the tips of the thumbs down and in.
- Straighten and strengthen the legs. Engage the glutes.
- Press the tailbone down and lift the low belly.
- Do not allow the elbows to press into the ribs.
- If the feet cannot lift off the floor, practice the pose with the feet against a wall and walk the feet up the wall to an appropriate height. Or practice lifting one leg, then the other leg. Alternatively, bend the knees and join the soles of the feet into *baddha konasana* legs and lift the head.

refinement

This pose is said to transmute poison into nectar. It must do so in a homeopathic manner because this pose feels more like poison than nectar.

Advanced practitioners can enter this pose from *sirsasana 3*. Keeping the legs lifted, exhale, lower your abdomen onto your elbows. Slowly lower your legs toward the floor as you lift your head. Hold the pose and breathe for 15 to 60 seconds. To come out, exhale, lower the top of your head to the floor and lift your legs vertical to return to *sirsasana 3*. This transition from *sirsasana 3* into *mayurasana* requires a great deal of balance.

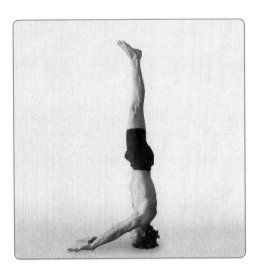

mukta hasta sirsasana
free hands headstand pose

shape
(from *baddha hasta sirsasana*)

1. Extend down through the head and in one movement, straighten the arms and place the backs of the hands on the floor—shoulder-width apart in front of the face.
2. Point the palms up. Look forward. Hold the pose and breathe.
3. To come out, either lower the legs to the floor and rest with the hips and forehead down in *balasana*, or continue with *prasarita hasta sirsasana* in the *sirsasana* sequence.

safety
- Press the hands down and lift the shoulders up.
- Stretch up through the legs and feet.
- Press the inner feet, ankles, and knees together.
- Engage the glutes and abdomen.
- Move the base of the sternum back and the tailbone forward.
- Breathe as evenly as possible.
   If the balance is difficult, practice against or near a wall.

refinement
If moving from *baddha hasta sirsasana* into *mukta hasta sirsasana* proves to be too difficult, start in *vajrasana*. Any of these headstand variations can also be approached from *sirsasana 1* or *2*.

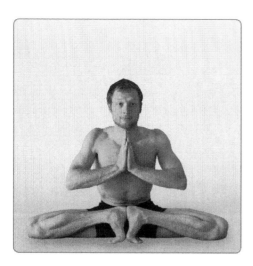

mulabandhasana
root lock pose

shape
(from *baddha konasana,* torso upright)

1. Bring the feet a few inches away from the pubic bone.
2. Press the feet into each other, but pull the toes back away from each other.
3. Lift the heels off the floor and hold the outsides of the feet with the hands.
4. Lift the heels vertical and in toward the hips. Bring the mounds of the toes to the floor.
5. Place both hands to the floor behind the hips. Lift the hips up and forward until the feet are vertical.
6. Lower the hips and knees to the floor.
7. Place the palms together in front of the chest. Look forward. Hold the pose and breathe.
8. To come out, release the hands next to the hips. Use the hands to lift the hips and release the feet.

safety

- If the hips cannot lower to the floor once the feet are in place, sit on a block or on one or more folded blankets.
- If the knees cannot lower to the floor once the feet are in place, place a folded blanket underneath the knees.
- When lowering the hips to the floor, press the heels together, move the toe mounds apart, and roll the inner thighs down toward the floor.
- Slide the hips forward as close to the feet as possible.
- Lift the pelvic floor and tone the low belly.

refinement

Do not attempt this pose unless you are already a proficient practitioner of *baddha konasana* and *ardha mulabandhasana.*

This pose requires as much force as it does flexibility. Interestingly, even if you have the flexibility to do *mulabandhasana* you might not have the strength to hold the pose. The heels will press together like a vice. It takes me five to seven sets to get into this pose. In between sets, I do *supta virasana* to reset the thighs.

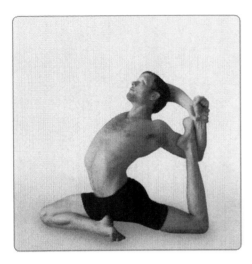

naginyasana 1
mermaid pose 1

shape
(from *adho mukha svanasana*)

1. Inhale fully. Exhale, bend the right knee and place the knee to the right of and just behind the right wrist. Lower the hips and the outer right leg to the floor with the right heel touching the front of the left hip.
2. Slide the hips back slightly so the front of the back leg touches the floor.
3. Inhale, lift the torso upright and bend the back knee.
4. Reach the left arm back and catch the back foot with the crease of the elbow.
5. Inhale, lift the right arm vertical. Exhale, bend the right elbow and hold the left wrist with the right hand or vice versa. Square the torso and hips to the top of the mat.
6. Press the head into the top arm and look up. Hold the pose and breathe.
7. To come out, exhale, release the hands to the floor in front of the top shin, shoulder-width apart, and lower the back foot. Curl the toes under and press the hands down and forward to push the hips up and back. Step the front foot back.

Repeat on the second side.

safety
- Press the outer edge/top of the front foot down.
- Clamp the front knee closed.
- Center the weight in the hips and pelvis. The weight tends to lean into the hip of the bent leg, which will cause the back knee to widen.
- Isometrically squeeze the knees toward each other and lift the hips slightly.
- Tone the back leg and rotate the inner thigh up.
- Press the tailbone down and lift the low belly.
- Engage the glutes of the back leg.
- Press the back foot and elbow into each other.
- Stretch the spine and chest up.
- If there is pain or discomfort in the low back or to reduce the intensity of the stretch in the back quads, lift the hips slightly and/or place a blanket or block underneath the sit bone of the front leg.

refinement

The compression on the sides of the torso that *indudalasana* requires is essential to taking the hand/foot position in poses such as *naginyasana 1, eka pada rajakapotasana,* and *mandalasana.*

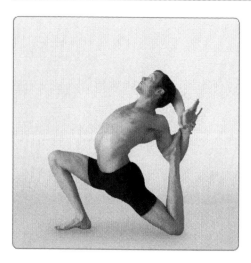

naginyasana 2
mermaid pose 2

shape
(from *lunge pose*)

1. With the right leg forward, lower the back knee to the floor. Lift the back foot and bend the knee to capacity.
2. Place the right hand on the right thigh. Inhale, lift the torso upright and reach the left arm back.
3. Hold the inner edge of the back foot with the left hand and bring the inner heel toward the outer edge of the hip. Slide the back foot to the crease of the elbow.
4. Inhale, lift the right arm vertical. Exhale, bend the elbow and hold the left wrist with the right hand or vice versa.
5. Press the head into the top arm.
6. Inhale, tone the low belly. Exhale, lower the hips down and forward.
7. Lift the chest and look up. Hold the pose and breathe.
8. To come out, exhale, release the clasp of the wrist and lower both hands to the floor shoulder-width apart. Lower the back foot and curl the toes under. Straighten the leg.

Repeat on the second side.

safety

- Square the torso and hips to the top of the mat.
- Press the inner edge of the front foot down.
- Isometrically squeeze the front foot and back knee toward each other.
- Tone the back leg and rotate the inner thigh up.
- Press the tailbone down and lift the low belly.
- Engage the glutes of the back leg.
- Press the back foot and elbow into each other.

- Press the top arm and head together.
- Stretch the spine and chest up.
- If there is pain or discomfort in the low back or to reduce the intensity of the stretch in the back quads, lift the hips slightly and/or hold the back foot with the hand instead of the elbow.

refinement

Naginyasana 2 is both a good preparatory and alternate pose for *eka pada rajakapotasana 1* and *2*.

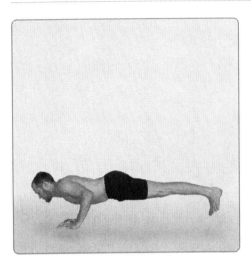

nakrasana
crocodile pose

shape
(from *chaturanga dandasana*)

1. Inhale, lift the hands and feet off the floor and lunge the whole body a foot forward.
2. Repeat four more times, and then hop the body back five times.
3. To come out, exhale, lower the front body to the floor.

safety

- Lift the pelvic floor and tone the low belly.
- Contract the glutes and press the tailbone down.
- Spread the fingers and press the index knuckles firmly into the floor between jumps.
- Tighten the kneecaps and make the legs stiff and unbendable.
- Keep the body as parallel to the floor as possible.

refinement

This pose has teeth! It will bite, strike, and devour weakness in your entire body. If you practice *nakrasana* on a regular basis, it will make you feel as strong as a crocodile. Before even attempting this pose, first become proficient in performing *chaturanga dandasana*.

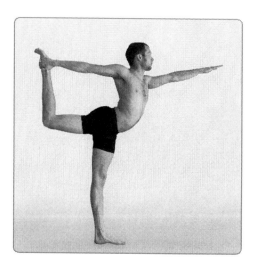

natarajasana
baby dancer pose

shape
(from *tadasana*)

1. Place the left hand on the left hip.
2. Kick the right foot back and hold the outside of the right foot with the hand. Point the foot, then flare the outer two toes.
3. Square the hips and shoulders to the top of the mat.
4. Lift the left arm parallel to the floor in front of the torso—biceps up, palm down.
5. Inhale, tone the standing leg and lift the chest.
6. Exhale, lift the right foot up and back until the thigh is parallel to the floor—shin vertical. Keep the torso upright.
7. Lift the chin and look straight ahead. Hold the pose and breathe.
8. To come out, lower the lifted leg and release the hands by the sides.

Repeat on the second side.

safety

- Lock the standing leg into a straight position and lift the kneecap.
- Move the tailbone down and draw the low belly in.
- Lower the hip of the lifted leg.
- Move the hip of the standing leg back.
- Pull the shoulders up and back to promote a backbend in the upper back.

refinement

Extend your top knee back. Kick your foot into your hand, pull your foot with your hand. Lift and expand your chest—especially the top of your sternum. Extend your head away from your hips and stretch your entire spine. There are two variations of *natarajasana*. In this variation, the upper body is similar in shape to *dhanurasana*. Bring your upper body into a deep backbend and keep your chest lifted. The other variation emphasizes the lift of the back leg by allowing the torso to come parallel to the floor.

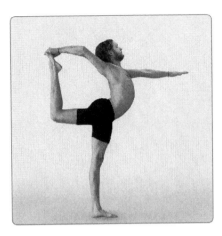

natarajasana 1
Lord of the Dance pose 1

shape
(from *tadasana*)

1. Bend the right knee and point the kneecap straight down. Flex the foot and turn the foot out.
2. Turn the torso to the right and reach the right hand underneath the back foot. Wrap the thumb around the outer edge of the foot—palm facing up.
3. Lift the right knee, shorten the right side of the torso, and turn the hand to point the elbow up.
4. Inhale fully. Exhale, lean the torso forward and bend the back knee to a 90-degree angle— back thigh parallel to the floor.
5. Hold the inner edge of the top foot with the left hand and change the clasp of the right hand to hold the big toe with the first two fingers and thumb.
6. Extend the left arm forward—arm parallel to the floor, palm facing down.
7. Lift the chin slightly and look straight ahead. Hold the pose and breathe.
8. To come out, inhale, lift the torso vertical. Release the right arm and lower the right leg to the floor.

Repeat on the second side.

safety
- To make this pose more accessible, wrap a strap around the ankle of the lifted foot. Hold the strap instead of the foot, and slowly walk the hands closer to the foot to deepen the stretch.
- Straighten and tighten the knee of the standing leg.
- Tone and lift the inner thigh of the top leg.
- Press the tailbone down, engage the glutes, and lift the low belly. Tone the pelvic floor.
- Kick the top foot up and back. Engage the foot and flare the toes.
- Move the shoulders up and back.
- Move the base of the sternum back and stretch the spine and chest up.

refinement
This pose symbolizes the yogin's desire to attain a mental and emotional state that is undisturbed by the twists and turns of life. A film can turn a tragedy into a beautiful and meaningful experience, with a soundtrack that awakens the soul for the viewer. Yoga invites us to observe the good, the bad, the beautiful, and the ugly aspects of our lives in the same way.

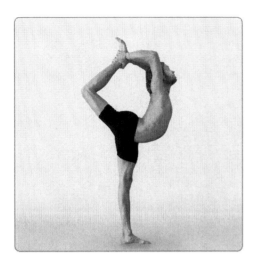

natarajasana 2
Lord of the Dance pose 2

shape
(from *tadasana*)

1. Bend the right knee and point the kneecap straight down. Flex the foot and turn the foot out.
2. Turn the torso to the right and reach the right hand underneath the back foot—thumb up, palm facing out. Wrap the thumb around the inner edge of the big toe mound—palm facing up.
3. Lift the right knee, shorten the right side of the torso, and turn the hand to point the elbow up.
4. Inhale fully. Exhale, lean the torso forward and bend the back knee to a 90-degree angle— back thigh parallel to the floor.
5. Reach the left hand up and back and hold the right forearm with the left hand. Walk the hand down the forearm and hold the foot with the hand.
6. Clasp the ankle with both hands. Flex the foot.
7. Inhale fully. Exhale, lean the torso forward to lift the top heel directly above the bottom heel. Bring the forearms parallel to the floor.
8. Look up. Hold the pose and breathe.
9. To come out, inhale, lift the torso to vertical. Exhale, release the clasp of the hands. Inhale, stretch the arms overhead and lower the right foot to the floor next to the left foot. Exhale, lower the arms.

Repeat on the second side.

safety

- To make this pose more accessible, wrap a strap around the ankle of the lifted foot. Hold the strap instead of the foot, and slowly walk the hands closer to the foot to deepen the stretch.
- Straighten and tighten the knee of the standing leg.
- Kick the top foot up and back.
- Pull the top foot up with the hands.
- Press the tailbone down, engage the glutes, and lift the low belly. Tone the pelvic floor.
- Move the shoulders up and back.
- Move the base of the sternum back and stretch the spine and chest up.

refinement

Natarajasana 2 can also be practiced with the back thigh and forearms parallel to the floor. Every form is malleable. And yet, what is essential is that you are seeking a particular form instead of just getting into the form that you happen to get into. There is no true *ananda* (bliss) without some kind of aim.

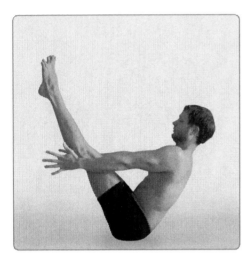

navasana
boat pose

shape
(from *dandasana*)

1. Bend the knees and roll back slightly onto the backs of the sit bones.
2. Point the feet and place the toes on the floor halfway toward the sit bones.
3. Curve the low back in, tone the low belly, and lift the chest.
4. Keep the spine long and lift the feet off the floor. Bring the shins and arms parallel to the floor—palms facing in.
5. Straighten the legs. Look straight ahead. Hold the pose and breathe.
6. To come out, exhale, release the arms and legs. Place the hands next to the hips.

safety

- To reduce the intensity of the pose, bend the knees slightly or hold the legs with the hands for support.
- Do not allow the low back to round or the chest to collapse.
- If there is discomfort in the sit bones, place a blanket under the hips for padding.
- Tighten the knees and tone the thighs.
- Press the inner feet, ankles, and knees together.
- Squeeze the elbows straight. Extend the hands forward to empower the abdomen.
- If this pose tightens or tweaks the hip flexors, squeeze the legs and torso closer toward each other to bring the legs as vertical as possible.

refinement

Navasana is another pose that is similar in shape to *dandasana* and *adho mukha svanasana*. (See *dandasana* refinement.) This pose is meant to emphasize and develop abdominal strength.

However, if the legs are kept straight and the low back rounds, the benefit of developing core strength is greatly diminished. These benefits go beyond vanity or physical beauty. A strong core is essential to keeping the entire spine healthy, particularly the low back region, a common area of pain. If the low back rounds in *navasana*, bend the knees to shift the focus from the hamstrings to the low belly. In B. K. S. Iyengar's *Light on Yoga*, *dandasana*, *adho mukha svanasana*, and *navasana* are grouped together.[1]

---

[1]   B. K. S. Iyengar, *Light on Yoga* (New York: Schocken Books, 1977) pp. 110-114.

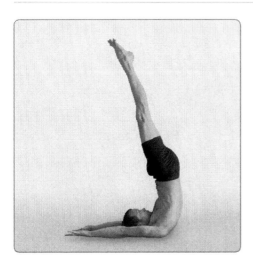

niralamba sarvangasana 1
unsupported shoulderstand pose 1

shape
(from *niralamba sarvangasana 2*)

1. Extend the arms overhead and place the backs of the hands on the floor shoulder-width apart.
2. Look past the tip of the nose. Hold the pose and breathe.
3. To come out, bring the hands to the floor behind the back and lower the legs.

safety

*   Press the shoulders down, in toward each other, and forward toward the head.
*   Center the head and press the head down. Bring the chin vertical—do not allow the chin to drop toward the floor.
*   Press the backs of the hands and arms down into the floor.
*   Engage the glutes and legs. Squeeze the inner knees, ankles, and feet together.
*   Move the hips and tailbone forward in the direction of the face. Extend the heels up and back.
*   Stretch up through the spine and legs.
*   Relax the jaw, eyes, and face.
*   Breathe as evenly as possible.

refinement

For a more doable entry into this pose, from *halasana* extend the arms overhead onto the floor. Lift one leg at a time into *niralamba sarvangasana 1*. The most difficult aspect of this pose is balance. Nearly falling out of this pose is a sign that you are in it. Practice makes potential palpable.

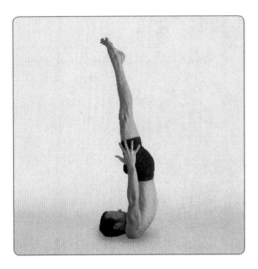

niralamba sarvangasana 2
unsuported shoulderstand pose 2

shape
(from *sarvangasana 2*)

1. Keeping the arms straight, release the hands and lift the arms vertical.
2. Look past the tip of the nose. Hold the pose and breathe.
3. To come out, lower the hands behind the back and place the hands as low on the back as possible to return to *sarvangasana 1*, or continue with *niralamba sarvangasana 1* in the *sarvangasana* sequence.

safety

- Press the shoulders down, in toward each other, and forward toward the head.
- Center the head and press the head down. Bring the chin vertical—do not allow the chin to drop toward the chest.
- Engage the glutes and legs. Squeeze the inner knees, ankles, and feet together.
- Move the hips and tailbone forward in the direction of the face. Extend the heels up and back.
- Stretch up through the spine, arms, and legs.
- Relax the jaw, eyes, and face.
- Breathe as evenly as possible.

refinement

For a more doable entry into this pose, from *halasana* lift the arms vertical. Lift one leg at a time into *niralamba sarvangasana 2*.

The most difficult aspect of this pose is balance. Move your feet above your head to hold the balance. This pose requires a strong back to resist the legs falling forward, and a strong core to resist the legs falling backward. If it is not difficult for you to balance, chances are you are not vertical enough. When you are consistently on the verge of falling out of this pose, you will know that you are indeed in it.

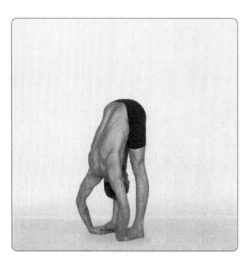

padahastasana
foot to hand pose

shape
(from *tadasana*)

1. Separate the feet hip-width apart. Inhale fully. Exhale, fold the torso over the legs.
2. Without bending the knees or lifting the heels off the floor, lift the bottoms of the feet one at a time and slide the hands underneath the feet—palms up, tips of toes against the wrists.
3. Press the toes into the hands.
4. Bend the elbows out to the sides.
5. Inhale fully. Exhale, pull the torso toward the legs—face between shins.
6. Lean the hips forward so the legs are completely vertical from outer hip to knee to ankle. Hold the pose and breathe.
7. To come out, inhale, lift the head. Release the hands, one at a time, to the floor on either side of the feet. Inhale, lift the torso to stand.

safety
- Lift the kneecaps and lock the legs into a straight position.
- Press the tailbone down and draw the low belly in.
- Squeeze the feet and legs toward each other.
- To reduce pressure on the low back and backs of the legs, or if the wrists cannot meet the toes, bend the knees and rest the torso on the thighs.

refinement
Press your fingers into the floor. Stretch your shoulders and spine toward the floor. This is a deeper and more intense forward fold than *uttanasana*. Before performing this pose, establish proper alignment in *uttanasana*. Many poses are modifications, variations, or continuations of other poses, which can be differentiated by their degree of difficulty. Do not confuse more difficult with more benefits. The more challenging poses do not necessarily offer more. In fact, if you are ill-prepared, they can offer much less! Practice with awareness and safety.

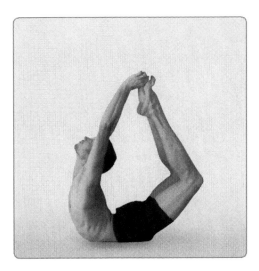

padangustha dhanurasana
big toe bow pose

shape

1. Bring the front body to the floor.
2. Bend the knees and lift the shins vertical. Flex the feet and turn the feet out as much as possible.
3. Hold the inner edges of the big toes with the fingers.
4. Inhale, lift the legs and torso. Exhale, rotate the arms to point the elbows forward.
5. Wrap the fingers and thumbs around the big toes.
6. Inhale, kick the feet up and back to capacity—straighten the arms.
7. Lift the chin. Look up. Hold the pose and breathe.
8. To come out, exhale, lower the arms and legs to the floor.

safety

- Lift and tone the inner thighs.
- Press the tailbone down, engage the glutes, and lift the low belly. Tone the pelvic floor.
- Kick the feet into the hands and pull the feet up with the fingers.
- Lock the elbows into a straight position.
- Stretch the shoulders and arms up and back.
- Move the base of the sternum back and stretch and strengthen the entire spine.
- If it is not possible to simultaneously rotate both arms to attain the hand-to-foot position, begin in *bhujangasana 1* with bent elbows. Bend one knee and hold the inner edge of the big toe. Rotate the arm to point the elbow forward. Repeat on the second side.
- To make the entry even more accessible, wrap a strap around both ankles and lower onto the front body. Lift the arms overhead and walk the hands down the strap toward the feet.

refinement

I have always felt that the form of *padangustha dhanurasana* is beautiful. When I take the form of *padangustha dhanurasana*, the beauty of the form invokes a *bhavana* (uplifted mood) in my heart.

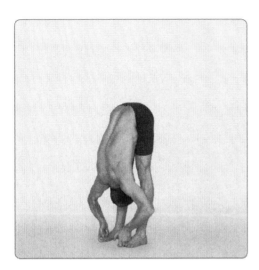

padangusthasana
big toe pose

shape
(from *tadasana*)

1. Separate the feet outer hip-width apart.
2. Inhale fully. Exhale, fold the torso over the legs.
3. Hold the big toes with first two fingers and thumbs.
4. Inhale, straighten the legs and arms, and look up.
5. Exhale, pull the torso into the legs—face between shins.
6. Bend the elbows out to the sides.
7. Bring the weight forward until the hips come directly over the heels. Hold the pose and breathe.
8. To come out, inhale, lift the head. Exhale, release the hands to the floor on either side of the feet. Inhale, lift the torso to stand.

safety

- Lift the kneecaps and lock the legs into a straight position.
- Squeeze the feet and legs toward each other.
- Lift the toes with the fingers and press the toes into the fingers.
- To reduce the pressure on the low back and hamstrings, bend the knees slightly and rest the torso on the thighs.
- Move the tailbone down and draw the low belly in.

refinement

Engage your abdomen to pull your torso toward your legs. This is a more intense variation of *uttanasana* because the fingers, hands, and arms pull the torso deeper into the forward fold, where as *uttanasana* depends largely on the pull of gravity. This hand-to-foot position, called "yogi toe lock," develops a strong connection between the lower and upper body and its respective energies. It also establishes strength in the fingers and hands and is especially beneficial for those who spend a lot of time typing or mousing. Before performing this pose, establish proper alignment in *uttanasana*.

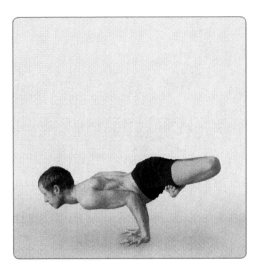

padma hamsasana
lotus swan pose

shape
(from *padmasana*)

1. Place the hands in front of the legs and lift the hips.
2. With the weight on the hands and knees, walk the hands forward until the thighs and arms are vertical.
3. Place the tips of the thumbs together. Spread the fingers and point the index fingers straight ahead.
4. Bend the elbows, lean forward, and place the elbows as close to the waistline as possible.
5. Lean forward until the elbows are forward of the wrists.
6. Transfer all of the weight onto the hands and lift the knees. Curl the head back. Look forward. Hold the pose and breathe.
7. To come out, exhale, lower the knees. Push the hands down and forward to lift the hips up and back. Slowly lower the hips to the floor.

Repeat on the second side—switch the cross of the legs.

safety
- Press the fingertips and the perimeter of the palms—especially the mounds of the index fingers—down into the floor with firm and equal pressure. Do not attempt this pose if you have a wrist injury.
- Press the tailbone down and lift the low belly. Engage the abdomen.
- Engage the glutes.
- Bend the knees to capacity. Press the outer edges/tops of the feet into the thighs.

refinement
Padma hamsasana is much more doable than *hamsasana* itself. Therefore *padma hamsasana* makes for an excellent preparatory pose for *hamsasana*. For me, *hamsasana* is the most challenging arm balance to perform.

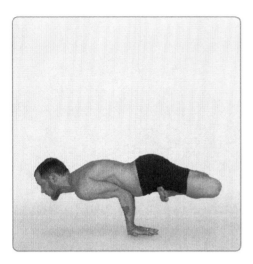

padma mayurasana
lotus peacock pose

shape
(from *mayurasana*)

1. Swing the legs into *padmasana*. Bring the legs parallel to the floor. Hold for five breaths.
2. Release and recross the legs. Hold for five breaths.
3. To come out, release the legs, lower the feet, and walk the feet forward to release the hands.

safety

- Press the fingertips and the perimeter of the palms down with equal pressure. Press the tips of the thumbs down and in.
- Engage the glutes and abdomen.
- Do not allow the elbows to press into the ribs.
- Squeeze the knees closed. Press the outer edges/tops of the feet into the thighs.
- If the legs cannot fold into *padmasana*, practice the pose with the legs in *siddhasana* or *baddha konasana*.

refinement

If you can do full lotus, *padma mayurasana* is easier to perform than *mayurasana*. Another point of entry is from *padmasana* seated. Place your hands in front of your legs and lift your hips. With the weight on your knees, walk your hands forward and turn your fingers back to join the outer wrists. Bend your elbows and place your torso on your upper arms. Lift your legs.

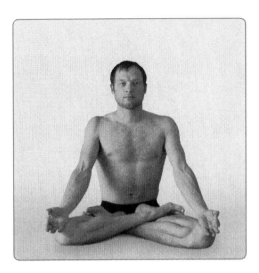

padmasana
lotus pose

shape
(from *dandasana*)

1. Bring the left palm to the inner left knee.
2. Pull the knee as far left and back as possible so that the legs come into an obtuse angle.
3. With the hands, lift the left foot and place the outer foot on the upper inner right thigh at the crease of the groin. Point the knee forward and lower the leg.
4. Bend the right knee out to the side and bring the heel to the front of the left shin. Point the foot.
5. Hold the left shin with the left hand. Hold the right foot with the right hand.
6. Lift the right knee slightly higher than the left knee. Flex the right foot and place the heel on the left shin.
7. If optimal, slide the right foot over the left shin and thigh and bring the outer edge of the foot to the crease of the left groin. Lower the right knee.
8. Lean to the right and use the left hand to pull the glutes back. Repeat on the other side.
9. Place the hands on the knees, palms up. Straighten the arms. Look straight ahead. Hold the pose and breathe.
10. To come out, lift the knee of the top leg and flex the foot. Use the hands to slowly slide the top foot off the shin. Release the other leg and straighten both legs. Bring the arms by the sides.

Repeat on the second side—switch the cross of the legs.

safety

- If there is any discomfort or pain in the knees, exit from the pose immediately.
- Do not attempt full *padmasana* until you can do *ardha padmasana* with the knee touching the floor.
- If the hips are tight or if there is pain or injury in the knees, do not lift the top foot up and over the shin, as that can strain the knee.
- Press the outer edges/tops of the feet down.
- Push the heels into the low belly.
- Lift the pelvic floor and tone the low belly.
- To bring the knees in toward each other, flex, as opposed to point, the feet.

refinement

Over a decade ago I read Swami Muktananda's *Play of Consciousness*. The following is a passage from this book that had a strong impact on me: "Remember that when you sit in lotus posture for 3 hours, the 720 million *nadis* are completely purified." Swami Muktananda also says, "It is said that only when a yogi can hold this posture for three hours has he really mastered it."[1] After reading those passages I decided to give it a try. I made a flyer for a 3-hour lotus practice, included the above quotes, and posted it at YogaOasis, the studio that I direct. Amazingly about 12 people showed up! Unfortunately, the night before the practice I got the flu and only slept for 2 hours.

The next day, I started the workshop by saying, "I just want you to know my stance on this: I will stay in lotus for three hours or die trying." I had no idea what I was in for. The longest that I had held full lotus up to that point was 15 minutes! And to top it off, I didn't even warm up—I just went into the pose! Thirty minutes later I knew I was in trouble because my knees were aching and my ankles were burning. At one hour I was in definite pain. I spoke up and said, "I don't think I can do this."

One by one people came out of the pose. Milo held the pose for 90 minutes, and then switched legs after falling out from headstand. When I hit 90 minutes, I knew there was absolutely no escape or reprieve from the pain. I spontaneously went into *simhasana* (which is done in full lotus) and roared and roared like a lion. One woman, still in lotus pose, opened her eyes and said, "Holy Cow! Somehow that gave me the strength to make it to 2 hours." By 2 hours I was soaking with sweat. There was nothing but bastard brutal pain. And yet I had resolved by this time to stay in no matter what.

When I hit 2.5 hours I was convinced my knees and ankles would be permanently damaged. I picked up my watch and did a 30-second count down. I said, "I can stay in for 30 more seconds." I did that 59 times in a row. The only way I could cope was to stay in the pose for 30 seconds at a time. When the final minute hit I cried and cried because I knew the pain would be gone and that I was about to achieve a 3-hour lotus. Amazingly in that last 30 seconds I felt no pain. I realized later that the most difficult thing to deal with was not the pain but rather the aversion to pain.

In the end, three of us completed the entire 3-hour lotus, and each of us had different reactions to the intensity of this endeavor. I cried and couldn't stand or walk for some time (and was unable to teach my next class which was scheduled for 15 minutes after this so-called workshop); another woman thought she had broken her ankle, and another woman began chanting with fervor.

I think my 720 million *nadis* were more pulverized than purified. I had not, and never will, master *padmasana*; the pose had mastered me! The one benefit of staying in lotus for 3 hours was that by the time I left the studio, I no longer had the flu. Even so, I would rather take 3 days to recover from the flu than spend 3 hours in lotus pose. A few months later I read another of Swami Muktananda's books on meditation. In this book he says, "When you sit in lotus posture for 1.5 hours, the 720 million *nadis* are completely purified."[2] I thought, dharma damn, I wish I had read this book first!

---

[1]   Swami Muktananda, *Play of Consciousness: A Spiritual Autobiography* (Fallsburg, NY: Siddha Yoga Publications, 2000) p. 238.

[2]   Swami Muktananda, *Meditate* (Fallsburg, NY: Siddha Yoga Publications, 1991).

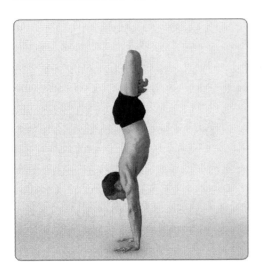

padmasana in adho mukha vrksasana
lotus in downward-facing tree pose

shape
(from *adho mukha vrksasana*)

1. Move the right leg back slightly.
2. With momentum, swing the left foot into *ardha padmasana*.
3. Move the left knee back slightly.
4. With momentum, swing the right leg into *padmasana*.
5. Hold the pose and breathe for five breaths. Release and recross the legs to move into *padmasana* on the other side. Hold the pose and breathe for five breaths.
6. To come out, release the legs to a vertical position to return to *adho mukha vrksasana*.

safety
• Do not attempt this pose if the legs cannot fold into *padmasana*.
• Be prepared to fall out of the pose and release the legs as quickly as possible so, like a cat, you always land on your feet.

refinement
In *tadasana* practitioners balance without any conscious effort. The same can eventually occur in *padmasana in adho mukha vrksasana*—the balance is no longer hit or miss. The way to achieve such balance is by practicing *adho mukha vrksasana* on a daily basis away from the wall. Think of balance as a commodity, as something you can have more or less of. Through this practice you can generate more balance, and unlike many things, the more you use it the more you have.

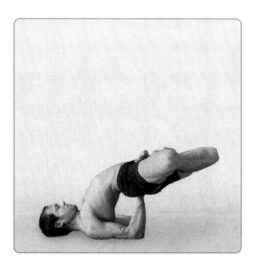

padmasana in parsva sarvangasana
lotus in turned shoulderstand pose

shape
(from *sarvangasana 1*)

1. Move the right leg back slightly.
2. With momentum, swing the left foot into *ardha padmasana*.
3. Move the left knee back slightly.
4. With momentum, swing the right leg into *padmasana*.
5. Inhale fully. Exhale, lower the knees toward the head to round the low back. Place the right palm on the sacrum and lower the legs away from the head—fingers pointing in the same direction as the knees.
6. Bring right forearm vertical and the thighs parallel to the floor.
7. Place the weight of the hips and legs on the right palm.
8. Look past the tip of the nose. Hold the pose and breathe for to 15 to 60 seconds.
9. To come out, inhale, lift the legs and torso vertical. Release and straighten the legs.

Repeat on the second side—switch the cross of the legs.

safety

- If the legs cannot fold into *padmasana*, do *parsva sarvangasana* instead.
- Press both shoulders down toward the floor and in toward the spine.
- Center the head and press the head down. Bring the chin vertical—do not allow the chin to drop toward the floor.
- To reduce pressure on the wrist, press the fingertips into the body.
- Press the outer edges/tops of the feet into the thighs and squeeze the heels toward the hips.
- Relax the jaw, eyes, and face.
- Breathe evenly and deeply.

refinement

To stabilize the pose, hold the outer edge of the mat with your free hand. Lift your outer left hip and extend out through your thighs and knees. To reduce discomfort or soreness in the wrist when exiting the pose, press your hand and fingers into the back as you slide your palm down your back to a *sarvangasana 1* hand position. To reduce difficulty in the balance, press your opposite shoulder down and reach your knees down.

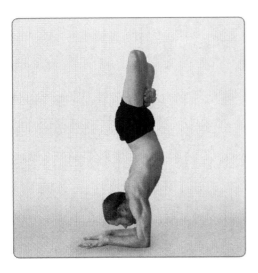

padmasana in pincha mayurasana
lotus in peacock feather pose

shape
(from *pincha mayurasana*)

1. Move the right leg back slightly.
2. Bend the left knee out to the side and place the outer edge/top of the foot on the front of the right quad at the crease of the groin.
3. Move the left knee back slightly and bend the right knee out to the side. Place the outer right ankle against the shin and slide the outer edge of the foot to the crease of the groin.
4. Hold the pose and breathe for five breaths. Release and recross the legs to move into *padmasana* on the other side. Hold the pose and breathe for five breaths.
5. To come out, release the legs to a vertical position.

safety

*   Do not attempt this pose if the legs cannot fold into *padmasana*.
*   Be prepared to fall out of the pose and release the legs as quickly as possible so, like a cat, you always land on your feet.

refinement

There is a considerable amount of backbending required for *padmasana* in *pincha mayurasana*, even to point the knees directly up. To enhance the balance, press the edges/tops of your feet into the thighs and squeeze your knees in toward each other. Keep your low belly toned to avoid falling backward.

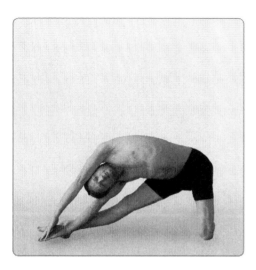

parighasana
gate keeper pose

shape

1. Come into an upright kneeling position.
2. Extend the right leg out to the side—foot in line with knee. Point the foot to the right.
3. Inhale, bring the arms out to the sides, parallel to the floor. Exhale, fold the torso to the right and place the back of the right hand on the floor just inside the right foot.
4. Inhale, stretch the left arm up. Exhale, reach the arm to the right and place the left palm onto the right palm.
5. Straighten the arms.
6. Bring the chin to the chest and pull the head through the arms.
7. Rotate the left shoulder above the right shoulder. Look up. Hold the pose and breathe.
8. To come out, exhale, look down. Inhale, lift the torso upright and stretch the arms out to the sides. Bring the arms by the sides and join the knees.

Repeat on the second side.

safety

- Move the hips back until the left thigh is perfectly vertical.
- Engage the extended leg. Tone the thigh and tighten the knee.
- Isometrically squeeze the right foot and left shin toward each other.
- Squeeze the elbows straight.
- Press the hands down and away from the foot. Move the top shoulder back.
- Lift the pelvic floor and tone the low belly.
- Turn the abdomen up.

refinement

Pull this dusty pose off the shelf and practice it. What I like about *parighasana* is that it is a humbling pose. No matter how flexible or strong you are, *parighasana* feels awkward and incomplete. Offer up your weakness, defects, limitations, and so on and so forth to the gate-keeper of yoga! The yoga gatekeeper might just receive and transmute them!

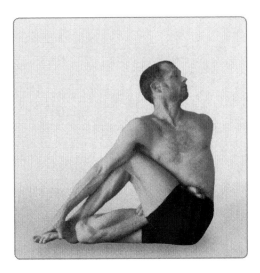

paripurna matsyendrasana
full Lord of the Fishes pose

shape
(from *ardha matsyendrasana 3*)

1. With the fingers of the back hand, crawl the hand toward the shin. Clasp the shin with the fingers.
2. Turn the head and look straight back. Hold the pose and breathe.
3. To come out, inhale, look forward. Release the hands next to the hips and straighten the legs.

Repeat on the second side.

safety

- If it is not possible to clasp the shin with the hand, use a strap or practice *ardha matsyendrasana 3* instead.

refinement

Ardha matsyendrasana 3 and *paripurna matsyendrasana* are nearly identical. The difference is in *ardha matsyendrasana 3,* the back of the back hand is at the waistline just above the right hip. In *paripurna matsyendrasana* the back hand clasps the inner shin. That subtle difference requires significant effort. *Paripurna matsyendrasana* is far more difficult to get into than *ardha matsyendrasana 3*; and in *Light on Yoga,* B. K. S. Iyengar even describes a different entry into the pose in order to clasp the shin.[1]

---

[1]   B. K. S. Iyengar, *Light on Yoga* (New York: Schocken Books, 1977) pp. 273–274.

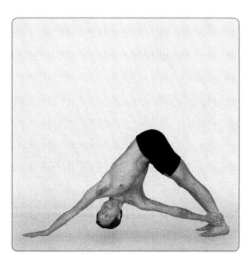

parivrtta adho mukha svanasana
revolved downward-facing dog pose

shape
(from *adho mukha svanasana*)

1. Bend the left knee slightly and hold the outer left ankle with the right hand. Straighten the leg.
2. Turn the torso to the left and pull the right hip back to square the hips.
3. Turn the chin toward the left armpit. Look up. Hold the pose and breathe.
4. To come out, place the right hand on the floor in line with the left hand, hands shoulder-width apart. Stretch the spine.

Repeat on the second side.

safety

- Press the front hand down and forward. Do not attempt to point the biceps in toward each other like in *adho mukha svanasana*. Instead, allow the twist of the torso to internally rotate the front arm, which will point the biceps down slightly.
- Squeeze the front elbow straight and lock it into a straight position.
- Lean a little to the left and put more weight on the left foot than the right foot.
- If holding the ankle is too intense, hold the outer shin and/or bend the knee.

refinement

Parivrtta adho mukha svanasana can serve as a sufficient warm up for more advanced poses requiring shoulder and arm strength. This pose is a valuable addition to a *surya namaskar* sequence.

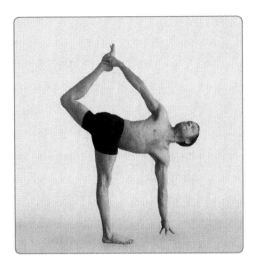

parivrtta ardha chandrachapasana
revolved half moon bow pose

shape
(from *tadasana*)

1. Inhale fully. Exhale, fold the torso over the legs.
2. Inhale, lift the chest. Place the fingertips on the floor directly below the shoulders.
3. Lift the left leg parallel to the floor.
4. Point the top foot, then flare the outer two toes.
5. Bend the standing leg slightly.
6. Bend the lifted leg and hold the inside of the foot with the right hand.
7. Lift the top thigh parallel to the floor and kick the top foot up to capacity.
8. Rotate the top shoulder over the bottom shoulder.
9. Straighten the standing leg.
10. Look up. Hold the pose and breathe.
11. To come out, exhale, look down. Release the foot and place both hands on the floor under the shoulders. Straighten and lower the back leg. Inhale, lift the torso to stand. Bring the arms by the sides.

Repeat on the second side.

safety
- Strengthen the standing leg.
- Turn the thigh of the standing leg out until the kneecap points straight ahead. Pull the hip back.
- Level the hips and squeeze both thighs toward the midline.
- Point the biceps of the lower arm toward the top of the mat.
- Move the tailbone down and draw the low belly in.
- Turn the abdomen up.
- Engage the top foot—do not sickle the top ankle.

refinement
Extend your top knee, foot, and hand away from your hips. Pull your foot with your hand and kick your foot into your hand. Lengthen your entire spine.

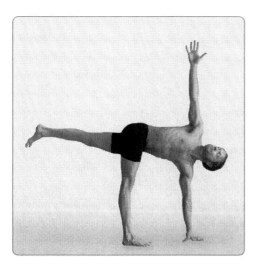

parivrtta ardha chandrasana
revolved half moon pose

shape
(from *tadasana*)

1. Inhale fully. Exhale, fold the torso over the legs.
2. Inhale, lift the chest. Place the fingertips on the floor directly below the shoulders.
3. Lift the left leg back, parallel to the floor. Point the back foot.
4. Place the left hand on the floor directly under the face and the right hand on the right hip.
5. Without lowering the right hip, exhale, rotate the right shoulder over the left shoulder.
6. Tone the low belly and turn the abdomen and ribs to the right.
7. Lift the right hand up—arm vertical, palm facing out.
8. Look up. Hold the pose and breathe.
9. To come out, exhale, look down. Place the right fingertips on the floor and bring both hands directly below the shoulders. Lower the lifted leg. Inhale fully. Exhale, fold the torso over the legs. Inhale, lift the torso to stand. Bring the arms by the sides.

Repeat on the second side.

safety

- Engage the standing leg, especially the quads and hamstrings. Lift the kneecap.
- Point the kneecap of the lifted leg straight down.
- Lift the hip of the upper leg and pull the hip of the standing leg back.
- Move the tailbone down and draw the low belly in.
- Move the top shoulder back.
- Point the biceps of both arms toward the top of the mat.
- To reduce the intensity of the hamstring stretch, place the bottom hand on a block and/or slightly bend the standing leg.
- If the spine is stiff or if there is discomfort in the chest or shoulders, keep the upper hand on the hip.

refinement

Press your lower fingertips down. Extend your top hand up. Reach your top foot and head away from your hips. Center your head, hips, and back leg (the torso and back leg tend to sway in opposite directions).

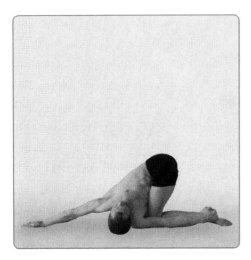

parivrtta balasana
revolved child's pose

shape
(from *vajrasana*)

1. Place the left hand on the left thigh.
2. Inhale, lift the right arm vertical.
3. Exhale, bring the right shoulder to the outside of the left knee. Hold the left heel with the right hand.
4. Place the left fingertips in front of the face.
5. Inhale, lift the hips and reach the left arm forward toward the front of the mat—palm facing up. Straighten the arm.
6. Bring the back of the head to the floor—point the top of the head toward the long edge of the mat.
7. Reach the left shoulder toward the floor.
8. Tone the low belly and turn the abdomen to the left. Look up. Hold the pose and breathe.
9. To come out, inhale, lift the left arm vertical. Exhale, place the hand on the floor next to the head. Inhale, lift the head and chest. Exhale, sit upright on the heels and bring both hands to rest on the thighs.

Repeat on the second side.

safety
- If the shoulder and knee do not connect, do not proceed further into this pose; practice *parsva balasana* or *vajrasana*.
- The right knee tends to move forward of the left knee. Bring the knees together and keep them together by continually squeezing the feet, ankles, and knees together.
- Press the right knee down and evenly distribute the weight of the body onto both knees.
- Press the tailbone down, tone the pelvic floor, and lift the low belly.
- Point the chin up.
- Do not overly stretch the back of the neck.

refinement

Press your right shoulder into your left knee. There should be no space between your torso and legs. Isometrically press the back of your front hand down and out (toward the thumb side of your hand) as you move your bottom shoulder down and in toward the floor. *Parivrtta balasana* stretches the back of the neck more than most twists. Exercise caution when twisting at the neck and top of the spine, particularly if you are also bearing weight in the neck or shoulders as in this pose.

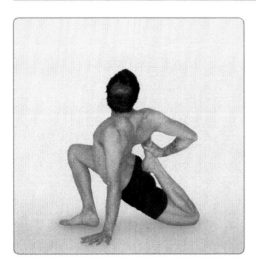

parivrtta eka pada rajakapotasana 2 prep

revolved one leg king pigeon pose 2

shape

(from *lunge pose*)

1. Lower the back knee to the floor.
2. Turn the front foot out 30 degrees and tilt the knee out slightly.
3. Move the hips down and forward until the back thigh is at a 45-degree angle.
4. Move the left hand forward and out slightly away from the left shoulder.
5. Press the left palm flat on the floor and turn the hand out 30 degrees.
6. Bend the back knee and lift the back foot. Hold the outer edge of the back foot with the right hand—thumb pointing up.
7. Point the back foot, then flare the outer two toes.
8. Pull the back heel towards/to the left hip. Lift the elbow and spin the hand so the fingers point forward toward the top of the mat.
9. Rotate the right shoulder over or even beyond the left shoulder.
10. Backbend in the upper back.
11. Look over the top shoulder. Hold the pose and breathe.
12. To come out, exhale, look forward, and release the back foot to the floor. Place both hands on the floor on either side of the front foot. Curl the back toes under and lift the hips.

Repeat on the second side.

safety

- If there is pain or discomfort in the back knee, place a blanket under the knee for padding. Technically it is not the back kneecap but the top of the thigh that is on the floor or blanket.
- If the hamstrings cramp when the back foot lifts off the floor, lean most of the weight onto the

front hand before lifting the back foot. Or, wrap a strap around the back foot and pull the foot up via the strap.
- If the hand-to-foot clasp causes discomfort or pain, hold the outer edge of the foot with the back hand.
- Move the hips down and forward toward the front of the mat to stretch the front of the thigh.
- Isometrically draw the front foot and back knee toward each other and draw the legs toward the midline of the body.
- Point the bottom bicep forward.
- Move the tailbone down and draw the low belly in.
- Turn the abdomen to the right.
- Move the base of the sternum back and lift the chest.
- Shrug the shoulders up and back.

refinement

Parivrtta eka pada rajakapotasna 2 prep, also known as "twisted monkey," is a radical pose—it is a thigh stretch, twist, and backbend all in one. To move deeper into the backbend, lower your left forearm to the floor and bring your left shoulder down the back, away from your ear. Rotate your chest up away from your lower hand. Lift your chest, and curl your chest and head back. Look back.

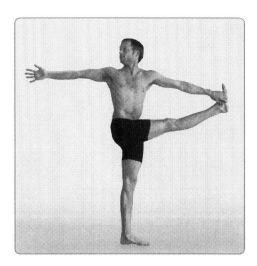

parivrtta hasta padangusthasana
revolved hand to big toe pose

shape
(from *tadasana*)

1. Place the right hand on the right hip.
2. Balancing on the left foot, lift the right foot and hold the outside of the foot with the left hand.
3. Twist the torso to the right and extend the right arm back—arm parallel to the floor and long edge of the mat.
4. Point the right bicep and thumb up.
5. Stand upright and lift the top shin parallel to the floor.
6. Inhale, straighten the leg.
7. Exhale, turn the abdomen to the right. Look past the right thumb. Hold the pose and breathe.
8. To come out, inhale, look forward. Exhale, release the foot and bring the arms by the sides.

Repeat on the second side.

safety
- Straighten the standing leg and lock it into a straight position.
- Pull the foot with the hand, push the foot into the hand.
- Extend the inner edge of the top foot forward and move the hip of the standing leg down.
- Move the base of the sternum back and stretch the spine.
- To reduce the intensity of the hamstring stretch, keep the top knee bent.

refinement
Japanese proverb: *Fall down seven times, get up eight.* Just as falling apart can be part of the path, falling over is part of the practice.

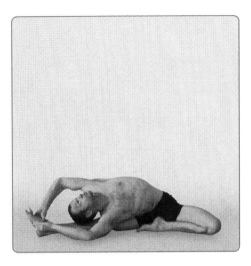

parivrtta janu sirsasana
revolved head to knee pose

shape
(from *dandasana*)

1. Bring the left hand to the inner left knee—palm facing out. Pull the knee as far back as possible, creating an obtuse angle with the legs.
2. Move the foot to the groin—heel to pubic bone. Lift the heel and point the left foot. Spin the top of the foot down to the floor. Point the heel up.
3. Lean to the right and place the right hand to the inner left thigh—fingers between calf and thigh. As the hip lowers to the floor, spin the thigh down with the right hand and pull the left glutes back with the left hand. Repeat on the other side.
4. Turn the torso to the left.
5. Inhale, lengthen the spine.
6. Exhale, place the right shoulder on the floor to the inside of the right knee. Hold the inner edge of the right foot with the right fingers—thumb across the top of the foot. Rest the right elbow and forearm on the floor inside the right shin.
7. Look at the right foot. Inhale, lift the left arm vertical. Exhale, stretch the arm forward and hold the outer edge of the right foot with the hand—thumb across top of the foot.
8. Bring the chin to the chest. Move the head forward between the space of the arms. Stretch the elbows away from each other, press the lower elbow into side of the knee, and revolve the chest and torso up. Look up. Hold the pose and breathe.
9. To come out, exhale, look down. Inhale, lift the left arm vertical. Exhale, lift the torso. Straighten the leg and place the hands next to the hips.

Repeat on the second side.

safety

- If the upper hand cannot reach the foot, place a strap around the front foot. Hold the strap with the top hand and walk the hand along the strap toward the foot. Lift the top elbow and twist the torso.
- To reduce the intensity of the twist, straighten the top arm overhead toward the top of the mat rather than holding the outer edge of the front foot. If the pose is still too intense, place the lower forearm on top of the shin, bend the top arm, and place the head into the hand. Move the elbow back and revolve the chest.

- Squeeze the calf of the bent leg into the thigh.
- Engage the front leg. Press the knee down.
- Extend the front foot forward into the hands and push the foot down into the floor.
- Push the inner edge of the front foot forward and pull the outer edge of the foot back.
- Rotate the top shoulder over the bottom shoulder.
- Tone the pelvic floor and lift the low belly.

refinement

The following are good preparatory poses for *parivrtta janu sirsasana*, which may or may not be practiced in sequence: *indudalasana, baddha parsvakonasana, baddha trikonasana, parighasana,* and *surya yantrasana*. Many twists require that you bring the shoulder to the opposite knee in order to achieve the twist, such as *ardha matsyendrasana 1* and *3* and *marichyasana 3*. These types of twists are considered "closed twists" because the abdomen compresses in order to perform the twist. In *parivrtta janu sirsasana*, however, the shoulder and knee of the same side come together before twisting. This type of twist is considered an "open twist" because the abdomen expands and stretches to yield a deep stretch in the obliques.

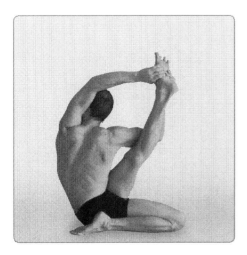

parivrtta krounchasana
revolved heron pose

shape
(from *dandasana*)

1. Bend the right knee and place the inner ankle against the right outer hip—shin and top of foot on floor. Point the foot back.
2. Lean to the left and pull the right glutes back with the right hand. Repeat on the other side.
3. Place the left foot on the floor in front of the left sit bone.
4. Flex the left foot—heel on the floor, toes lifted. Hold the foot with both hands.
5. Inhale, lengthen the spine. Exhale, lift and straighten the front leg.
6. Release the right hand and place the right upper arm on the outer shin. Hold the outer edge of the top foot with the right hand.
7. Clasp the inner edge of the right foot with the left hand.
8. Point the left elbow up and back. Inhale, draw the top leg and torso into each other. Exhale, twist the torso to the left. Push the back of the head into the top upper arm and bring the chin toward the armpit. Look back. Hold the pose and breathe.

9. To come out, inhale, look forward and turn the torso to face the top of the mat. Exhale, release the hands and lower the leg. Straighten both legs.

Repeat on the second side.

safety

- If the low back rounds or if the bottom leg does not fold into *virasana*, sit on one or more blankets with the foot on the floor.
- Or, if there is still discomfort in the knee, practice with *baddha konasana* legs by bending the knee out to the side with the heel near the pubic bone.
- Tone the thigh of the lifted leg. Flex the foot and spread the toes.
- If the upper arm does not reach the outer shin, bring the elbow to the outer knee and hold the outer ankle instead of the foot.
- Press the foot into the hands and pull the foot with the hands.
- Lift the pelvic floor and tone the low belly.

refinement

The top foot tends to swing past the midline at the initiation of the twist. Push your top shin into your arm to bring your leg parallel to the long edge of the mat. Once your top leg is in place, push your top arm into your shin to twist your spine. The more complex the form, the more single-pointed the mind must become. That's one of the boons of advanced poses: not the degree of difficulty but rather the depth of awareness and focus they require.

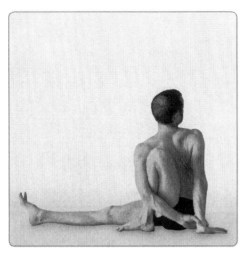
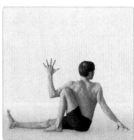

parivrtta marichyasana 1
revolved Sage Marichi's pose 1

shape
(from *dandasana*)

1. Bend the left knee. Place the heel in front of the left sit bone. Point the knee up.
2. Press the hands down. Lift the hips up and forward. Bring the left sit bone against the left heel. Lower the hips to the floor.
3. Curve the low back in and up. Place the right hand on the floor a few inches behind the sacrum. Straighten the arm.
4. Inhale, lift the left arm vertical. Exhale, twist the torso to the right and place the outer left shoulder on the inner left knee.
5. Lean the torso forward and wrap the left arm around the leg. Place the back of the hand on the outer left hip.
6. Swing the right arm behind the back and hold the right wrist with the left hand.
7. Straighten the right arm and place the palm flat on the floor.
8. Turn the torso away from the bent leg. Look over the right shoulder. Hold the pose and breathe.
9. To come out, inhale, look forward. Release the hands to the floor next to the hips. Straighten the bent leg.

Repeat on the second side.

safety

- Engage the extended leg. Press the back of the knee down.
- Flex the front foot—flare the outer two toes.
- Squeeze the bent knee to completely close the knee joint.
- If the outer shoulder does not come to the inner knee, press the outer elbow into the inner knee, and place the other hand a few inches behind the sacrum.
- Move the shoulders back.
- Lift the pelvic floor and tone the low belly.
- If the back palm does not reach the floor behind the hips, clasp the opposite wrist with the hand and bind.

refinement

Parivrtta marichyasana 1 with the back arm straight is an intense shoulder stretch. It serves as an excellent preparatory pose to *pasasana*. This twist, along with other "open twists" in which the abdomen is exposed rather than compressed, is an appropriate pose for pregnant women. Widen the legs hip-width apart and bind the hands.

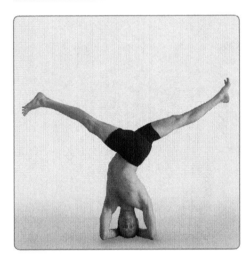

parivrtta pada sirsasana
revolved legs headstand pose

shape
(from *sirsasana 1*)

1. Extend the left leg back and the right leg forward like in *hanumanasana*, and move into a slight backbend. Keep the hips squared.
2. Inhale fully. Exhale, turn the hips to the left. Look forward. Hold the pose and breathe.
3. To come out, exhale, return to center. Inhale, lift the legs vertical.

Repeat on the second side.

safety

- Press the forearms and wrists down. Lift the shoulders up.
- Extend down through the head.
- One shoulder tends to push forward and the other back in order to achieve the twist. Keep the shoulders squared and facing forward.
- Engage the abdomen, and move the base of the sternum back and tailbone forward.
- Straighten and strengthen the legs. Extend out through the legs.
- Spin the back, inner thigh down to lower the leg. Lift the front, outer thigh to move the leg up.
- Breathe evenly. Soften the eyes and jaw.

refinement

Parivrtta pada sirsasana is a good preparatory pose for *eka pada viparita dandasana 1* and its variations. In general, *sirsasana* and variations are a great way to prepare for many, if not most, backbends. To do *sirsasana 1* after backbends, however, could be problematic because by then you might be too fatigued to maintain safe alignment.

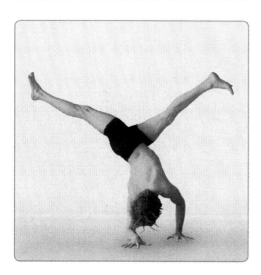

parivrtta pada visama pincha mayurasana
revolved legs uneven peacock feather pose

shape
(from *visama pincha mayurasana*)

1. Inhale fully. Exhale, twist the torso to the left.
2. Keeping the legs straight, extend the right leg to the left and the left leg back and to the right. Bring the feet equidistant to the floor.
3. Hold the pose and breathe for five breaths. Return to center and bring the legs together.
4. Attempt to return to *pincha mayurasana* and then switch sides.

Repeat on the second side.

safety

*   Straighten and strengthen both legs.
*   Engage the feet—flare the toes.
*   Engage the glutes and abdomen.
*   Press the tailbone in.
*   Press the forearm down.
*   Stretch the shoulders, spine, and legs up.

refinement

This pose develops agility in the superlative. Regular practice of *parivrtta pada visama pincha mayurasana* will make the arm variations in *sirsasana* seem easy. Advanced practitioners can attempt this pose with the left arm straight.

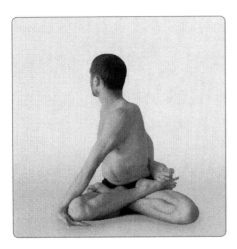

parivrtta padmasana
revolved lotus pose

shape
(from *padmasana*, right foot on top)

1. Lean back, lift the knees, and balance on the hips.
2. Hold the outside of the right thigh with the right hand.
3. Flex the left hand and place the back of the left hand under the right knee—fingers parallel to the top of the mat.
4. Lower the knees to the floor. Press the front palm down.
5. Swing the right arm behind the back and hold the right big toe with the first two fingers and thumb.
6. Inhale fully. Exhale, twist the torso to the right and look over the right shoulder. Hold the pose and breathe.
7. To come out, inhale, look forward. Exhale, release the hands and sit upright.

Repeat on the second side—change the cross of the legs.

safety
- If the legs do not fold into *padmasana*, practice the pose in *sukhasana* instead.
- If the front hand does not reach the floor underneath the knee or if the underside of the forearm is tight, place a folded towel or a thin blanket below the wrist. Or, hold the outer thigh instead.
- If the back hand does not reach the back foot, use a strap to hold the foot, or place the hand a few inches behind the sacrum.
- Press the outer edges/tops of the feet down.
- Press the front wrist down and the forearm into the thigh/knee.
- Engage the feet and pull the right foot back with the right hand.
- Move both shoulders back. Lift the chest.
- Press the tailbone down, tone the low belly, and lift the pelvic floor.

refinement
Spread the fingers of your lower hand and press the pads of your fingers into the floor. The stretch on the underside of the forearm acts as a counter pose for intense arm balances in which the hands bear the weight of the body. It can also bring relief to those who spend a lot of time on the computer typing or mousing. *Parivrtta padmasana* is a great pose to prepare the legs, chest, and shoulders for *yoga mudrasana* and *supta vajrasana*.

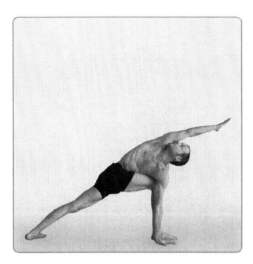

parivrtta parsvakonasana
revolved side angle pose

shape
(from *lunge pose*)

1. Pivot the back heel down to the floor and turn the foot in 60 degrees.
2. Hold the upper right thigh with the right hand—thumb on top of thigh, fingers on outer quads.
3. Inhale, lift the torso and left arm vertical.
4. Exhale, twist the torso to the right, and place the left shoulder on the outer right knee.
5. Place the left palm on the floor to the outside of the front foot. Straighten the left arm.
6. Turn the abdomen to the right and rotate the right shoulder over the left shoulder.
7. Extend the right arm up and forward across the face. Straighten the arm.
8. Look up, and turn the chin toward/to the armpit. Point the top palm down. Hold the pose and breathe.
9. To come out, look down. Inhale, lift the upper arm vertical. Exhale, place both hands on either side of the front foot. Lift the back heel.

Repeat on the second side.

safety

- To make the pose more doable, lift the back heel vertical.
- If it is still too intense, press the palms together in front of the chest and practice twisted lunge pose.
- Lengthen the stance as necessary to create a straight line from the outer left ankle all the way to the outer right wrist.
- Do not allow the front knee to move beyond the front heel.
- Do not allow the front shin to tilt in.
- Move the right hip back.
- Press the tailbone down and move the low belly in.
- Move the shoulders back.
- If looking up is too intense for the neck and jaw, look down.

refinement

Although keeping your back heel down on the floor in this pose makes for a much deeper twist, it is actually less intense on the left hip flexors. Extend your back foot, front knee, and top hand away your hips. Tighten your back knee and top elbow, and extend them in opposite directions. Press your left arm into your front leg and your leg into your arm to deepen the twist. Keep your head and hips centered. The head tends to swing to the right, the hips to the left.

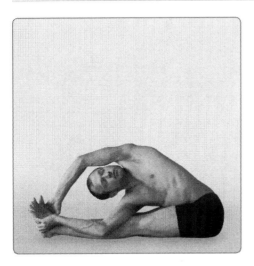

parivrtta paschimottanasana
revolved back stretched out pose

shape
(from *dandasana*)

1. Hold the right elbow in front of the face with the left hand.
2. With the left hand, pull the right elbow to the left—right shoulder under chin.
3. Point the palm up.
4. Inhale fully. Exhale, fold the torso over the legs.
5. Place the right elbow on the outside of the left shin.
6. Keep the palm facing up, spin the thumb down and hold the outer edge of the left foot with the right hand.
7. Press the right forearm into the left shin.
8. Inhale, lift the left arm vertical. Exhale, hold the outer edge of the right foot with the left hand.
9. Twist the torso to the left and rotate the left shoulder over the right shoulder. Rotate the left elbow over the head. Reach the chest and head between the arms.
10. Look up. Hold the pose and breathe.
11. To come out, lower the left elbow and release the hands. Inhale, lift the torso vertical. Place the hands next to the hips.

Repeat on the second side.

safety

- To reduce the stretch in the hamstrings, separate the feet outer hip-width apart. (This will make the twist more difficult.)

- Straighten and strengthen the legs—tighten the knees, tone the thighs, and press the backs of the knees down.
- Squeeze the inner feet, ankles, and knees together.
- Lift the pelvic floor and tone the low belly.
- Pull the feet with the hands. Stretch the shoulders forward.
- Extend the elbows forward and apart. Use the pulling action of the hands to fully stretch the spine.
- If the elbow does not reach the outer shin, slide the elbow back toward/to the knee and reach the left arm forward, toward the top of the mat.
- If the lower hand does not clasp the outer edge of the foot, wrap a strap around both feet and hold the strap with the right hand. Walk the hand down the strap as close to the feet as possible.

refinement

Keep the inner edges of your feet together. The right leg tends to extend forward as the left leg moves back. You can actually turn this tendency into an advantage as you come into this pose. As the right leg moves forward, it will bring the left knee closer to the right elbow. Once you've clasped the feet with the hands, bring the inner edges of your feet back together by pulling your right leg back. *Parivrtta paschimottanasana* is a unique twist due to the symmetry of the legs. In most twists, the legs are asymmetrical which offers more leverage. Asymmetrical twists usually twist one part of the spine more than another. This twist turns the spine evenly.

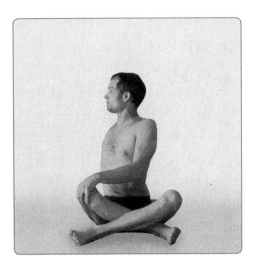

parivrtta sukhasana
revolved easy pose

shape
(from *sukhasana*)

1. Place the left hand on the right knee.
2. Place the right fingertips on the floor directly behind the sacrum.
3. Inhale fully. Exhale, twist the torso to the right and look over the right shoulder. Hold the pose and breathe.
4. To come out, inhale, look forward and return the head and torso to center.

Repeat on the second side.

safety

- Keep the hips squared to the front of mat. The hips tend to turn with the twist.
- Press the outer edges of the feet down.
- Isometrically squeeze the feet toward the hips.
- Use the hands to deepen the twist—pull the right knee with the left hand and press the right knee down and forward.
- Pull the right hand toward the thumb to twist further.
- Lift the right shoulder up and back.
- Extend the knees out. Stretch your spine up and lift the top of the sternum.

refinement

The more doable poses reveal essential insights into the more difficult and complex poses.

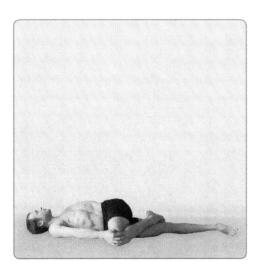

parivrtta supta padangusthasana
revolved reclined big toe pose

bent knee

shape
(from *supta tadasana*)

1. Bend the left knee and place the sole of the foot on the floor to the inside of the right knee.
2. Move the hips to the left a few inches and bring the outer right hip, foot, and leg to the floor.
3. Line up the hips and right foot with the head.
4. Extend the left arm out to the side—wrist in line with shoulder, palm facing up.
5. Hook the back of the right knee with the left foot. Keep the left shoulder on the mat and lower the knee to the floor.
6. Place the right hand on the outside of the left knee. Straighten the arm.
7. Look up. Hold the pose and breathe.
8. To come out, release the arms, straighten the leg, and lie on the back.

Repeat on the second side.

safety
- If the top knee does not reach the floor, place the knee on a block of appropriate height. Keep both shoulders on the floor.
- Engage the feet.
- Strengthen the extended leg.
- Press the tailbone in and tone the low belly.
- Turn the abdomen to the left.
- Move the base of the sternum back.

refinement
To increase the twist, look past your left shoulder. To bring a sense of calm and ease to the pose, drop your tongue into your lower palate away from the roof of your mouth. Relax your jaw and breathe deeply. *Parivrtta supta padangusthasana* looks like a relatively benign pose. It is actually a demanding twist, especially if you keep both shoulders down as the knee lowers to the floor.

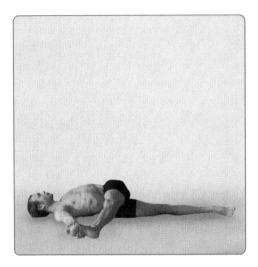

parivrtta supta padangusthasana
revolved reclined big toe pose

shape
(from *supta tadasana*)

1. Bring the left arm out to the side—wrist in line with shoulder, palm facing up.
2. Lift the left leg vertical and hold the inside of the foot with the right hand.
3. Push the right heel down and shift the hips a few inches to the left.
4. Inhale fully. Exhale, roll onto the outer right hip and lower the left foot and right hand to the right and to the floor.
5. Bring the outer right hip, leg, and foot in line with the head.
6. Straighten the arms and legs. Look up. Hold the pose and breathe.
7. To come out, inhale, lift the leg and arm vertical. Return the hips to center.
   Exhale, release the leg and arm.

Repeat on the second side.

safety
- If the top foot does not reach the floor, place it on a wall at an appropriate height, or rest the leg on a block or bolster. Keep both shoulders on the floor.
- Engage the arms and legs and lock them into a straight position.
- Push the foot into the hand and push the hand into the foot.
- Extend out through the inner edge of the bottom foot. Flare the outer two toes.
- Isometrically squeeze the feet toward each other.
- Rotate the lower leg away from the floor so that the heel moves toward the floor.
- To reduce the intensity of the hamstring stretch, use a strap and/or lower the top foot toward the bottom foot. Keep the leg straight.

refinement
Parivrtta supta padangusthasana is a good preparatory pose for *parivrtta hasta padangusthasana*, fallen sage, and *eka pada koundinyasana 1.*

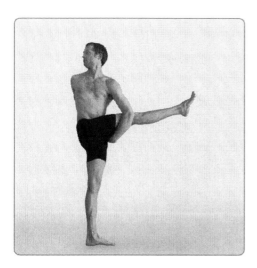

parivrtta svarga dvijasana
revolved bird of paradise pose

shape
(from *lunge pose*)

1. Hold the upper right thigh with the right hand.
2. Inhale, lift the torso and left arm vertical.
3. Exhale, twist the torso to the right and place the left shoulder on the outer right knee.
4. Swing the left arm under the hips and place the back of the hand on the left side of the torso.
5. Swing the right arm around the back. Hold the right wrist with the left hand.
6. Look down.
7. Step the left foot forward next to the right foot—feet outer hip-width apart.
8. Balancing on the left foot, lift the right foot off the floor. Keep the standing leg bent and lift the torso to stand upright.
9. Straighten the standing leg.
10. Lift the right shin parallel to the floor.
11. Twist the torso to the right and straighten the right leg.
12. Look back past the right shoulder. Hold the pose and breathe.
13. To come out, exhale, look forward. Bend the top knee and lower the right foot next to the left foot. Step the left foot back and take a long stance. Release the hands and place them on either side of the front foot.

Repeat on the second side.

safety
- If the shoulder does not reach the knee, do not proceed further into this pose. Instead, press the palms together and perform twisted lunge pose or *parivrtta hasta padangusthasana*.
- If clasping the wrist is not accessible, hold the hand or fingers.
- Strengthen the standing leg—lift the kneecap.
- Before straightening the top leg, engage the arm and shrug the left shoulder up and back. Engage the top leg.
- Press the right wrist into the left hand.
- To reduce the intensity of the hamstring stretch, keep the lifted knee bent.
- Press the left elbow into the right knee to protect the inner shoulder.
- If the balance is difficult, keep the gaze forward.

refinement

Turn your navel away from your foot. Drop the hip of your lifted leg down. Bring your lifted foot into a position halfway between flexed and pointed. Flare your outer two toes. Extend your head away from your hips—stretch your entire spine. This is a good preparatory pose for *marichyasana 4, pasasana, parsva bakasana,* and *dwi pada koundinyasana.*

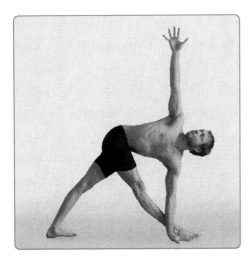

parivrtta trikonasana
revolved triangle pose

shape
(from *lunge pose*)

1. Hop the back foot forward slightly. Pivot the back heel down, turn the foot in 60 degrees.
2. Line up the middle of the back arch with the front heel.
3. Straighten the front leg.
4. Square the hips to the top of the mat—right hip back, left hip forward.
5. Lift the left hip up slightly so the hips are parallel to the floor.
6. Keeping the head and hips centered, place the left palm or fingertips on the floor just outside of the right foot.
7. Press the inner edge of the right foot down; move the right hip back. To empower this action, hold the right hip with the right hand—thumb across crease of hip, fingers on outer hip. With the hand, pull and extend the right hip back.
8. Turn the abdomen up and rotate the right shoulder over the left shoulder.
9. Extend the right hand up—arm vertical to floor.
10. Point the biceps toward the top of the mat.
11. Look up. Hold the pose and breathe.
12. To come out, look down and place both hands on either side of the front foot. Bend the front knee, step the back foot back, and lift the back heel.

Repeat on the second side.

safety

- Press the front foot down.
- Contract the quads, tighten the kneecaps and hamstrings.

- Press the back foot down.
- Simultaneously move the inner edge of the back leg and the outer edge of the front leg back.
- Engage the left glutes.
- Move the tailbone down and the low belly in.
- To reduce the intensity of the hamstring stretch, place the bottom hand on the floor, or on a block, inside of the front foot.
- If looking up is too intense for the neck or jaw, look down.

refinement

Once your hips are aligned, keep them steady and still. If the hips distort and follow the twist, the shoulders will turn more but the spine will twist less; the twist must happen in the spine, not the hips. Press your feet down and apart. Press your left hand/fingertips into the floor. Stretch your right hand up. Lock your knees and elbows into straight position. Extend your head away from your hips to lengthen the spine. Due to the demands of the pose, the tendency is for the hips and legs to disengage as soon as you initiate the twist. Practice won't necessarily reverse problematic patterns but gives us the opportunity to align with what is optimal.

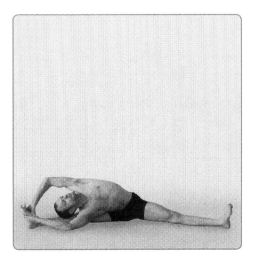

parivrtta upavishta konasana
revolved seated angle pose

shape
(from *dandasana*, facing long edge of mat)

1. Widen the legs to a 90-degree angle or beyond.
2. Press the hands down and lift the hips off the floor slightly.
3. Move the top of the pelvis forward and the sit bones back. Lower the hips.
4. Keep the hips down and flex and point the feet in rapid succession to widen the legs. Press the calves into the floor and lift the heels as the feet flex. Press the heels into the floor as the feet point. This action will drag the hips, glutes, and hamstrings back. (See *ardha baddha padma paschimottanasana*.)
5. Inhale fully. Exhale, place the right shoulder on the floor to the inside of the right knee. Hold the inner edge of the right foot with the right fingers——thumb across the top of the foot. Rest the right elbow and forearm on the floor inside the right shin.
6. Inhale, lift the left arm vertical. Exhale, stretch the arm over head to the right. Hold the outer

edge of the right foot with the left fingers—-thumb across the top of the foot.

7. Bring the chin to the chest. Move the head forward through the space between the arms. Stretch the elbows away from each other, press the lower elbow into the side of the knee, and revolve the chest and torso up.
8. Look up. Hold the pose and breathe.
9. To come out, exhale, look down. Inhale, lift the left arm vertical. Exhale, lift the torso vertical. Place the hands next to the hips and join the legs.

Repeat on the second side.

safety

- To reduce the intensity of the twist, straighten the left arm overhead rather than holding the outer edge of the right foot. If the pose is still too intense, bring the right elbow to the inner right knee and point the forearm perpendicular to the leg—palm facing up.
- Engage the right leg. Press the right knee down until there is little to no space between the back of the knee and the floor.
- If the upper hand cannot reach the foot, wrap a strap around the front foot and hold the strap as close to the foot with the arm overhead.
- Extend the right foot forward into the hands and push the foot down into the floor.
- Push the inner edge of the right foot forward and pull the outer edge back.
- Rotate the left shoulder over the right shoulder.
- Press the left side of the face into the top arm.
- If possible, place the back of the head on the shin.
- Tone the pelvic floor and lift the low belly.
- Once deeply into the twist, it is likely the left sit bone will lift off the floor slightly.

refinement

Parivrtta upavishta konasana is a good preparatory pose for *visvamitrasana*.

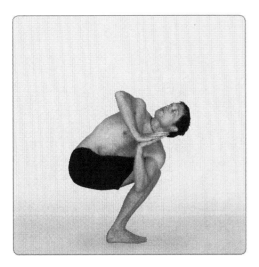

parivrtta utkatasana
revolved powerful pose

shape
(from *tadasana*)

1. Inhale, lift the arms overhead. Exhale, bend the knees and lower the hips until the thighs are parallel to the floor.
2. Place the right hand on the right thigh.
3. Momentarily move the knees to the left and twist the torso to the right. Lower the left shoulder to the outer right knee.
4. Bring the knees back to center. Keep the head in line with the hips.
5. Press the palms together in front of the chest.
6. Rotate the top shoulder over the bottom shoulder. Point the top elbow up.
7. Tone the low belly and turn the abdomen up. Look over the top shoulder.
   Hold the pose and breathe.
8. To come out, exhale, look down. Inhale, lift the torso to stand, release the arms by the sides.

Repeat on the second side.

safety
- Press the inner edges of the feet, ankles, and knees together.
- Move the tailbone down and draw the low belly in.
- Press the arm into the leg, leg into the arm.
- Move the shoulders back.
- For a more accessible variation, lift the hips and place the outer elbow on the outer knee.

refinement
Move your left hip back and right hip down to square your hips. Bring your left knee in line with your right knee. Stretch your spine. With each inhalation, expand your torso and deepen the twist. With each exhalation, turn inward and focus. To deepen the twist, place the fingertips of your bottom hand on the floor outside of your right foot. To twist even more, bring your top arm behind your back and hold your right inner thigh with your left hand. Pause here and breathe. Then release your hand from the inner thigh. Bring your bottom hand under your shins and clasp your hands.

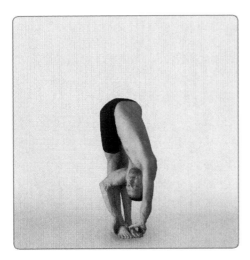

parivrtta uttanasana
revolved forward fold pose

shape
(from *tadasana*)

1. Lift the left forearm in front of the face.
2. Hold the left forearm just above the elbow with the right hand. With the right hand pull the left elbow to the right—bring the left shoulder underneath the chin.
3. Point the thumb forward and the outer edge of the hand back so the palm faces up.
4. Inhale fully. Exhale, fold the torso forward. Bend the left knee, keep the right leg straight.
5. Place the left elbow outside of the right shin.
6. Spin the hand toward the top of the foot and grab the outer edge of the right foot with the left fingertips. Press the thumb into the arch of the foot.
7. Press the left arm against the right shin.
8. With the right fingertips, grab the outer edge of the left foot—press the thumb into the arch of the foot.
9. Rotate the right elbow to the left until it is in line with the left leg.
10. Bring the right ear against the upper right arm, pull the head through the arms.
11. Keeping the hips square, twist the torso to the right and look forward.
12. Turn the abdomen to the right. Hold the pose and breathe.
13. To come out, release the hands and torso. Pause in *uttanasana*. Inhale, lift the torso to stand.

Repeat on the second side.

safety
- To reduce the stretch and create a more stable foundation, separate the feet outer hip-width apart. While this creates a more stable foundation, it increases the difficulty of the twist.
- Squeeze the feet and legs together.
- Straighten and strengthen the legs—lock them into a straight position and squeeze the kneecaps up.
- Press the big toes down, spread the toes.
- Move the right hip back to keep the hips square.
- Move the tailbone down and the low belly in.
- If it is not possible to move the head and torso through the arms for the twist, place the right hand on a block about twelve inches in front of the feet. Press the hand into the block and twist.

refinement

Pull your feet with your hands. Extend your shoulders toward the floor. Extend your elbows out to deepen the twist. *Parivrtta uttanasana* is a unique twist because the legs are symmetrical. The symmetry of the legs with square hips is what makes this twist difficult—it gives little leverage. When the legs are asymmetrical, one part of the spine will twist more than another. In *parivrtta uttanasana*, hatha-however, the spine twists evenly.

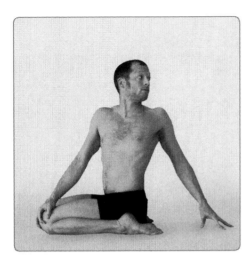

parivrtta virasana
revolved hero pose

shape
(from *virasana*)

1. Place the right hand on the left knee and the left fingertips on the floor behind the sacrum.
2. Inhale fully. Exhale, twist the torso to the left and look over the left shoulder. Hold the pose and breathe.
3. To come out, inhale, return the torso and head to center. Place the hands on the legs.

Repeat on the second side.

safety
- If there is pain or discomfort in the knees, separate the knees and/or place a folded blanket under the sit bones, between the feet. Sit on the edge of the blanket with most of the blanket behind the back and keep the feet on the floor/mat.
- To reduce the intensity on the ankles, put one or two rolled-up blankets underneath the bottom of the shins at the level of the ankles. Over time, work toward removing the blankets.
- Clamp the knees closed to engage the hamstrings.
- Keep the thighs parallel and point the toes straight back.
- Squeeze the heels in until they are vertical.
- Lift the pelvic floor and tone the low belly.
- Move the base of the sternum back and lift the chest.
- Lower the left shoulder back and down away from the ear.

refinement
Extend your left thigh forward. Press your right hand into your leg and your left hand down and out to deepen the twist. Revolve your torso along the midline and keep your head centered over your pelvic floor.

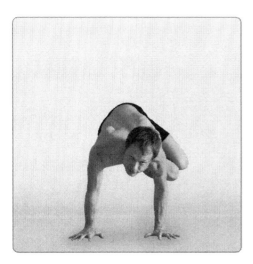

parsva bakasana
turned crane pose

shape

1. Come into a squat position—legs and feet together.
2. Place the hands on the floor behind the hips and lean back.
3. Inhale, squeeze the legs together and lift the left arm vertical.
4. Exhale, twist the torso to the right and place the left shoulder on the outside of the right knee.
5. Place the hands shoulder-width apart on the floor outside of the right hip.
6. Separate the fingers and rotate the hands out until the index fingers are parallel.
7. Lift the heels and balance on the toes. Lean forward and place the outer left knee on the left upper arm.
8. Bend the elbows slightly and transfer the weight of the body from the feet to the hands.
9. Lift the hips up and to the right. Press the outer right knee into the left arm and lift the feet as high as possible.
10. Straighten the left arm and keep the right arm slightly bent.
11. Look straight ahead. Hold the pose and breathe.
12. To come out, exhale, bend the elbows and lower the feet to the floor. Place the hands on the floor in front of the legs.

Repeat on the second side.

safety

- Press the fingertips and the perimeter of the palms into the floor with equal pressure. Equalize the weight between the hands as much as possible.
- Move the shoulders back.
- Squeeze the inner knees and ankles together.
- Attempt to keep the knees flush. The top knee will tend to move forward.
- Move the top hip back. Turn the abdomen away from the legs.
- Tone the pelvic floor and low belly.
- To reduce the pressure on the wrists, place the heels of the palms on the mat and the knuckles and fingers off the mat. (This will only be effective if you have a thick mat.)
- If there is still pain or discomfort in the wrists, keep the elbows bent to bring the elbows directly over the wrists and reduce the angle of the arms.

refinement

Advanced practitioners can come into *parsva bakasana* from *sirsasana 2*. Bend your knees completely and bring your thighs into your abdomen. Twist to the left and lower your right knee onto your left upper arm. Lower your hips toward the floor to transfer the weight from your head to your hands. Slowly lift your head and come into *parsva bakasana*. Hold for five breaths, then lower your head and lift your legs into *sirsasana 2*. Repeat *parsva bakasana* on the other side, and return to *sirsasana 2*. Drop your feet back and straighten your arms into *urdhva dhanurasana 1* for five breaths. Kick your feet up and over into *adho mukha svanasana*.

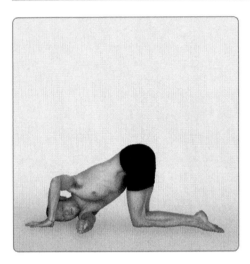

parsva balasana
turned child's pose

shape
(from *bharmanasana*)

1. Bring the knees, ankles, and big toes together. Point the toes straight back.
2. Inhale, lift the right arm out to the side.
3. Exhale, swing the right arm under the torso. Lower the outer right arm to the floor—outer shoulder in line with the right knee.
4. Keep the right arm straight and make a fist with the right hand—pinky side of hand on floor.
5. Bend the left elbow to 90 degrees—forearm vertical to floor. Place the right side of the face on the floor.
6. Tone the low belly and turn the abdomen to the left. Hold the pose and breathe.
7. To come out, push the left hand down to lift the head, chest, and arm. Place the right hand below the right shoulder and separate the knees hip-width apart.

Repeat on the second side.

safety

- For a more steady foundation, separate the knees outer hip-width apart—shins parallel.
- Squeeze the knees and feet together.
- Isometrically lift the feet away from the floor to engage the hamstrings.
- Press the tailbone down and lift the low belly.
- Tone the pelvic floor.

- Move the base of the sternum back and reach the chest forward.
- Isometrically pull the right arm back and press the left hand out.
- Move the top shoulder back.

refinement

Keep your hips over your knees. Squeeze your legs together and lift your outer ankles so the ankles do not sickle. Push your right hip back away from your shoulder and lift your right hip. Press your left hand into the floor to empower the twist. *Parsva balasana* works well as both a warm up and cool down pose.

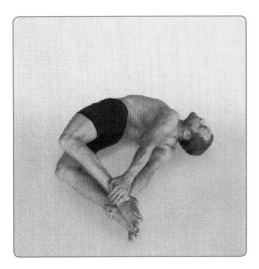

parsva dhanurasana
sideways bow pose

shape
(from *dhanurasana*)

1. Inhale fully. Exhale, roll onto the right side of the body.
2. Keep the knees outer hip-width apart and bring the inner edges of the feet together.
3. Turn the head to look up over the top shoulder or down past the bottom shoulder. Hold the pose and breathe.
4. To come out, inhale, roll onto the hips and abdomen.

Repeat on the second side.

safety

- Press the hips and tailbone forward, lift the pelvic floor, and tone the low belly.
- Engage the glutes.
- Kick the feet into the hands and pull the feet with the hands.
- Lock the arms into a straight position. Squeeze the shoulder blades together toward the spine.
- Lift the shoulders up and back.
- Lengthen the spine.

refinement

As you roll into and out of the pose, it is likely that you will come out of the backbend. To keep the backbend as you enter the pose, kick your feet back, extend your hips forward, and move your bottom shoulder back so that the entire outer right ribcage rests on the floor (instead of your outer shoulder resting on the floor). To keep the backbend as you exit the pose, lift your lower foot faster than your top foot to return to center.

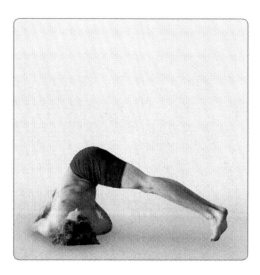

parsva halasana
turned plow pose

shape
(from *halasana*)

1. Walk the feet to the right in line with the head.
2. Bring the feet and legs together.
3. Look past the tip of the nose. Hold the pose for 30 to 60 seconds and breathe.
4. To come out, walk the feet back to center.

Repeat on the second side.

safety

- Keep the seventh cervical (the bony protrusion at the base of the neck) off the floor. If your seventh cervical touches the floor in *halasana*, place folded blankets below the torso and shoulders as described in *sarvangasana 1*.
- Press the shoulders down, in toward each other, and forward toward the head.
- Center the head and press the head down. Bring the chin vertical.
- Squeeze the inner knees, ankles, and feet together.
- Extend the left hip up in line with the right hip.
- Engage the biceps and press the hands into the torso.
- Extend the hips and spine up.
- Breathe evenly.

refinement

To increase core strength, release your hands, straighten your arms and interlace your fingers. To deepen the pose, attempt to keep your heels flush. Because *parsva halasana* is an asymmetrical twist, the tendency is for one hip to drop, which shortens the torso on that side of the body. Like in *sarvangasana 1*, lower your hands to lift your hips.

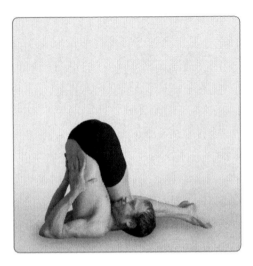

parsva karnapidasana
turned ear pressure pose

shape
(from *halasana*)

1. Walk the feet to the right, bend the knees, and bring the left knee to the right ear.
2. Point the feet.
3. Look up. Hold the pose for 30 to 60 seconds and breathe.
4. To come out, straighten the legs and walk the feet back to center.

Repeat on the second side.

safety
- Keep the seventh cervical (the bony protrusion at the base of the neck) off the floor. If your seventh cervical touches the floor in *halasana*, place folded blankets below the torso and shoulders as described in *sarvangasana 1*.
- Press the shoulders down, in toward each other, and forward toward the head.
- Center the head and press the head down. Bring the chin vertical—do not allow the chin to drop toward the chest.
- Push the torso with the hands to move the hips forward and the knees down.
- Engage the biceps and press the hands into the torso.
- Extend the hips and spine up.
- Breathe evenly.

refinement
Yoga requires that we do what we would not normally do and in doing so hopefully access better results. As G. I. Gurdjieff says, "The evolution of man can be taken as the development in him of those powers and possibilities which never develop by themselves, that is, mechanically. Only this kind of development, only this kind of growth, marks the real evolution of man. There is, and there can be, no other kind of evolution whatever."[1]

---

[1]   P. D. Ouspensky, *In Search of the Miraculous* (New York: Mariner Books, 2001) p. 56.

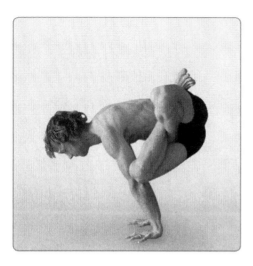

parsva kukkutasana
turned rooster pose

shape
(from *sirsasana 2*)

1. Extend the inner edge of the right leg back and move the tailbone in.
2. With momentum, swing the left foot into *ardha padmasana*.
3. Move the left knee back slightly.
4. With momentum, swing the right leg into *padmasana*.
5. Twist the torso to the left.
6. In one swift movement, lower the right outer knee onto the left arm just above the elbow.
7. Transfer the weight onto the hands and slowly lift the head off the floor.
8. Move the hips down and to the right slightly.
9. Straighten the right arm, then the left arm.
10. Look down. Hold the pose and breathe.
11. To come out, bend the elbows and lower the head to the floor, then lift the hips and bring the spine and legs vertical. Uncross and lift the legs.

Repeat on the second side—switch the cross of the legs.

safety
- Press the fingertips and the perimeter of the palms into the floor with firm and equal pressure.
- Press the outer edges/top of the feet into the thighs. Squeeze the heels towards the hips to clamp the knees closed.
- Flare the toes.
- Engage the abdomen. Move the tailbone forward.
- Lift the pelvic floor.

refinement
There are two ways to switch sides in *parsva kukkutasana*. The more doable approach is to switch the cross of your legs while seated in *padmasana*, then move to the other side. The more challenging approach is to stay in *padmasana* as you move from one side to the other. In this case, the second side is far more difficult to do than the first. Be prepared to fall onto your hips as you lift your head off the floor. If you cannot fall softly, put a folded blanket under your hips for padding.

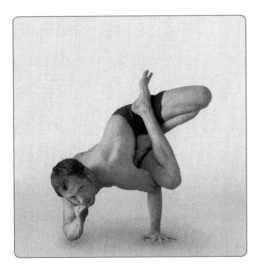

parsva kukkutasana
turned rooster pose

hand to chin

shape
(from *sirsasana 2*)

1. Extend the inner edge of the right leg back and move the tailbone in.
2. With momentum, swing the left leg into *ardha padmasana*.
3. Move the left knee back slightly.
4. With momentum, swing the right leg into *padmasana*.
5. Twist the torso to the left.
6. In one swift movement, lower the left outer knee onto the left arm just above the elbow.
7. Place the right forearm on the floor—right elbow in line with the left hand.
8. Transfer the weight onto the left hand and right forearm. Slowly lift the head off the floor.
9. Place the right hand on the right side of the face. Look straight ahead. Hold the pose and breathe for five breaths.
10. To come out, release the hand from the face and lower the head to the floor. Lift the right elbow and place the right hand on the floor in line with the left hand. Lift the hips vertical and bring the spine back to a neutral position. Uncross and lift the legs.

Repeat on the second side—switch the cross of the legs.

safety
- Press the fingertips and the perimeter of the left hand into the floor with firm and equal pressure.
- Press the outer edges/top of the feet into the thighs. Squeeze the heels toward the hips to clamp the knees closed.
- Flare the toes.
- Engage the abdomen and tone the pelvic floor.

refinement
This is much more doable than *parsva kukkutasana* since, in this variation, the center of gravity is lower. Bringing one forearm to the floor makes *astavakrasana* more accessible as well.

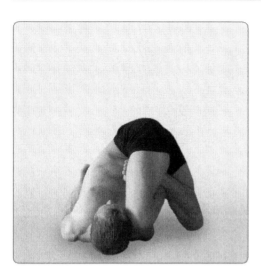

parsva pindasana
turned embryo pose

shape
(from *sarvangasana 1*)

1. Move the right leg back slightly.
2. In one movement, bring the left leg into *ardha padmasana*.
3. Move the left knee back slightly and in one movement, bring the right leg into *padmasana*.
4. Lower both knees to the floor to the right of the head. Look past the tip of the nose. Hold the pose and breathe.
5. To come out, inhale, lift the legs and torso vertical.

Repeat on the second side—switch the cross of the legs.

safety
*   Press the shoulders down, in toward each other, and forward toward the head.
*   Center the head and press the head down. Bring the chin vertical.
*   Press the outer edges/tops of the feet into the thighs and squeeze the heels toward the hips.
*   Press the knee into the ear.
*   Attempt to press both shoulders into the floor with equal weight.
*   If there is any pain or discomfort in the neck, do not lower the legs.

refinement

A prerequisite for this pose is the ability to do *parsva halasana* without your seventh cervical touching the floor. This is an extremely deep forward fold and twist in which the shoulders and head bear a decent amount of the body's weight. If your aim is to perform the more advanced asanas, give yourself many years to work on them. Progressing too fast in asana is dharma-dangerous.

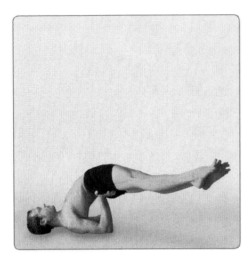

parsva sarvangasana
turned shoulderstand pose

shape
(from *sarvangasana 1*)

1. Lower the legs forward—toward the head—and place the right hand on the sacrum, fingers pointing out.
2. Lift the chest, lower the hips, and bring the legs vertical. Place the full weight of the hips on the right hand. Keep the left hand connected to the torso.
3. Inhale fully. Exhale, reach the left hip away from the shoulder and lower the legs parallel to the floor. Point the legs out to the right.
4. As the legs lower to a horizontal position, slide the base of the palm just above the tailbone. If the hand is higher, it will strain the wrist.
5. Look up past the tip of the nose. Hold the pose and breathe.
6. To come out, inhale, lift the legs vertical. Push the hand into the sacrum and lift the hips. Place both hands on the back as low to the ground as possible and bring the legs vertical.

Repeat on the second side.

safety

- If your seventh cervical (the base of your neck) touches the floor, do not perform this pose. Folded blankets will not offer a solid enough foundation.
- Press the shoulders down, in toward each other, and forward toward the head.
- Press the right shoulder down toward the floor.
- Center the head and press the head down. Bring the chin vertical—do not allow the chin to drop toward the chest.
- Engage the legs and glutes.
- Press the inner feet, ankles, and knees together.
- Push the hands into the torso.
- Engage the biceps and press the hands into the torso.
- Extend the hips and spine up.
- Breathe evenly.

refinement

To avoid falling over sideways straighten your left arm and hold the outer edge of your mat. Pull the mat out with your hand.

Advanced practitioners can keep the legs straight and lower the feet an inch or so above the floor. Hold this pose without holding your breath. Keep all effort out of the face. This might be regarded as "pose face," as opposed to "poker face." Many poses require the full capacity of our effort. Yet, in order to be of benefit, they also require that we soften and release rather than generate tension.

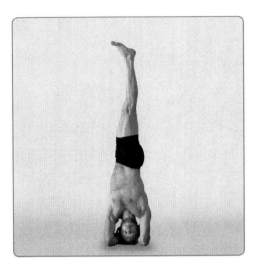

parsva sirsasana
turned headstand pose

shape
(from *sirsasana 1*)

1. Inhale fully. Exhale, turn the hips to the left. Hold for 30 to 60 seconds. Keep the feet centered directly over the head.
2. Inhale, return to center.
3. Exhale, turn the hips to the right. Hold for 30 to 60 seconds.
4. Inhale, return to center.

safety

- Press the forearms and wrists down. Lift the shoulders up.
- Extend down through the head.
- One shoulder tends to push forward and the other back in order to achieve the twist. Keep the shoulders squared and facing forward.
- Engage the abdomen, and move the base of the sternum back and the tailbone forward.
- Press the inner feet, ankles, and knees together.
- Straighten, strengthen, and stretch the legs up.
- Breathe evenly. Relax the eyes and jaw.
- If the balance is difficult, practice against or near a wall.

refinement

Advanced students can move into a slight backbend.
A friend of mine who practices Iyengar Yoga once led me through the following sequence:
1. Inhale fully. Exhale, *parsva sirsasana* to the left for four minutes. Inhale back to center.
2. Exhale, *parsva sirsasana* to the right for four minutes. Inhale back to center.
3. Exhale, *parsva sirsasana* to the left for four minutes. Inhale back to center.
4. Exhale, *parsva sirsasana* to the right for four minutes. Inhale back to center.
5. Exhale, *balasana*.
That was the first and last time I did that dharma damn difficult sequence. This friend of mine would often lead me through crazy or uncommon practices. For example, I remember doing *tadasana* for ten minutes. Difficult! Holding poses for long periods definitely builds stamina, which is an essential asset in any kind of *sadhana* (spiritual practice).

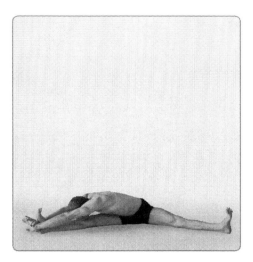

parsva upavishta konasana
lateral seated angle pose

shape
(from *dandasana,* facing long edge of mat)

1. Widen the legs to a 90-degree angle or beyond.
2. Press the hands down and lift the hips off the floor slightly.
3. Move the top of the pelvis forward and the sit bones back. Lower the hips.
4. Flex and point the feet in rapid succession to move the legs into an obtuse angle.
   (See *ardha baddha padma paschimottanasana.*)
5. Point the kneecaps and feet up.
6. Place the hands on the floor on either side of the right leg.
7. Inhale fully. Exhale, twist the torso to the right and fold over the right leg. Line up the center of the sternum with the right kneecap.
8. Stretch both hands beyond the right foot and hold the back of the left hand with the right hand.
9. Place the forehead on the right kneecap and/or the chin on the shin. Hold the pose and breathe.
10. To come out, bring the hands underneath the shoulders. Inhale, use the hands to lift the torso upright. Place the hands next to the hips and join the legs.

Repeat on the second side.

safety
- Before folding forward, tilt the pelvis forward and curve the low back in. If the low back rounds, sit up on one or more blankets.
- Engage the legs. Press the backs of the knees down.
- If clasping the hands is not possible, hold the foot, ankle, or calf with both hands, or use a strap around the front foot.
- To emphasize the twist, hold the inner edge of the right foot with the left hand and place the right fingertips on the floor about one foot outside of the right knee. Use this hand position to lengthen, twist, and fold the torso.
- Press the right foot into the hands and pull the foot with the hands.
- Extend the inner edge of the right foot forward. Pull the outer edge of the left foot back.
- Press the right heel down into the floor and point the toes straight up.

- Extend the elbows out to the sides as the fold deepens.
- Lift the pelvic floor and tone the low belly.
- Breathe into and inflate the right waist and ribcage.
- Lift the shoulders up.

refinement

While it is easy to emphasize the stretch of the left side of the torso in *parsva upavishta konasana*, it is often done at the expense of compressing the right side of the torso. Avoid this tendency by consciously twisting your navel over the right thigh before folding forward. Take several breaths to focus on the twisting action as you lower.

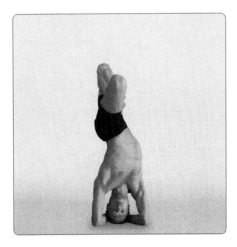

parsva urdhva padmasana in sirsasana
turned raised lotus in headstand pose

shape
(from *urdhva padmasana in sirsasana*)

1. Inhale fully, exhale, turn the torso and hips to the right. Hold for 30 to 60 seconds.
2. Inhale, return to center.
3. Exhale, turn the torso and hips to the left. Hold for 30 to 60 seconds.
4. Inhale, return to center.

safety

- Press the wrists and forearms down. Lift the shoulders up.
- Extend down through the head. Push the thighs up and back.
- One shoulder tends to push forward and the other back in order to achieve the twist. Keep the shoulders squared and facing forward.
- Engage the abdomen and move the base of the sternum back. Press the tailbone forward.
- Squeeze the knees in toward each other to tighten the legs.
- Press the outer edges/tops of the feet into the thighs and squeeze the heels toward each other.
- Avoid holding the breath or clenching the jaw.
- If the balance is difficult, practice against or near a wall.

refinement
Parsva urdhva padmasana in sirsasana is an important preparatory pose for *parsva kukkutasana*.

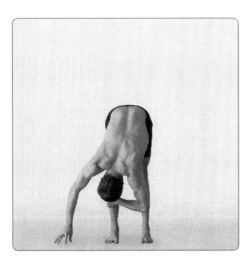

parsva uttanasana
lateral forward fold pose

shape
(from *tadasana*)

1. Separate the feet outer hip-width apart.
2. Inhale fully. Exhale, fold the torso forward, and place the hands on the floor outside of the feet.
3. With the left hand, hold the outer right shin.
4. Laterally slide the torso to the right, and bring the forehead in line with the right leg. Slide the right hand out about 12 inches.
5. With the left hand and right fingertips, pull the torso toward the right leg. Bring the forehead toward/to the right shin.
6. Bring the weight forward until the hips are directly over the heels. Hold the pose and breathe.
7. To come out, release the hands to the floor outside of the feet. Inhale, lift the torso to stand.

Repeat on the second side.

safety

- Squeeze the feet and legs toward each other.
- Straighten and strengthen the legs, especially the backs of the legs.
- Lift and lock the kneecaps into a straight position.
- To reduce the intensity of the hamstring stretch, keep the knees bent.
- Press the tailbone down and lift the low belly.
- Keep the hips square—the left hip tends to move forward, while the right hip tends to move back.

refinement

Keep the free leg strong and straight. This is a lateral forward fold, not a spinal twist. Keep equal weight on both of your feet. Before practicing this pose, establish optimal alignment in *uttanasana*.

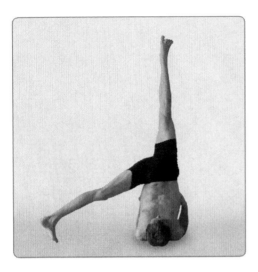

parsvaika pada sarvangasana
one leg turned out shoulderstand pose

shape
(from *sarvangasana 1*)

1. Turn the left foot out 90 degrees—heel to arch of right foot.
2. Inhale fully. Exhale, lower the left foot to the floor in line with the head.
3. To come out, lift the lower leg vertical.

safety

- If the lower foot does not reach the floor in line with the head, allow the leg to come forward, beyond the head. Do not distort the hips in order to lower the foot in line with the head.
- Press the shoulders down, in toward each other, and forward toward the head.
- Center the head and press the head down. Bring the chin vertical—do not allow the chin to drop toward the chest.
- Press the hands into the torso.
- Extend the inner edge of the top leg back so the kneecap points straight ahead.
- Extend the outer edge of the bottom leg up. Lift the hip up and toward the top leg.
- Engage the glutes and move the hips and tailbone forward.
- Do not allow the hips or top leg to sway to the side.
- Stretch the spine and top leg up. Spread the toes and center the foot over the hips.
- Relax the jaw, eyes, and face. Breathe evenly.

refinement

If you practice *supta padangusthasana 2, utthita hasta padangusthasana 2*, and *vasisthasana* on a regular basis you will be well prepared for *parsvaika pada sarvangasana*. All the insights and breakthroughs you attain in one pose become an immediate asset to your overall practice. The benefits of this practice are exponential.

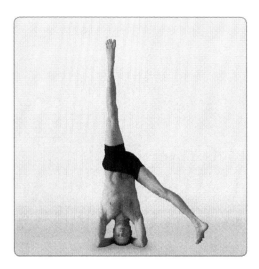

parsvaika pada sirsasana
one leg turned out headstand pose

shape
(from *sirsasana 1*)

1. Turn the right foot out 90 degrees—heel to arch of foot.
2. Inhale fully. Keep your top foot directly above your hips. Exhale, lower the right foot out to the right side.
3. Keep the hips and top foot directly above the head. Look forward. Hold the pose and breathe.
4. To come out, inhale, lift the leg vertical.

Repeat on the second side.

safety

- If there is limited rotation in the hips, the foot will not be able to lower directly out to the side. Allow the bottom foot to lower to the side organically rather than distorting the hips or top leg to get the lower foot in line with the head, as this will not be possible for most people.
- If the bottom foot cannot reach the floor, place the foot against a wall at an appropriate height.
- Press the forearms and wrists down. Lift the shoulders up.
- Extend down through the head. Straighten, strengthen, and stretch the top leg up.
- Move the inner edge of the top leg back so the kneecap points straight ahead. Press the tailbone forward.
- Lift the outer edge of the bottom thigh and the outer hip. Lift the sit bone of your lower leg.
- Engage the glutes of the lifted leg.
- Engage the abdomen.
- Breathe evenly, and relax the eyes and jaw.
- If the balance is difficult, practice against or near a wall.

refinement

An effective way to attain the form of inverted poses is to perform them in front of a mirror. You may think your top leg, bottom leg, and hips are doing one thing when in fact they are doing another. The mirror will reflect where you are in relation to your aim.

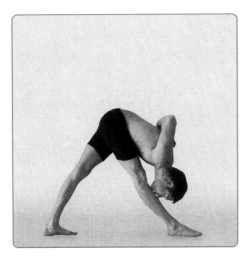

parsvottanasana

side stretched out pose

shape
(from *tadasana*, facing long edge of mat)

1. Inhale, bend the knees.
2. Exhale, take a stance shorter than *trikonasana*.
3. Inhale, lift the arms overhead.
4. Exhale, swing the arms down and behind the back. Place the hands as high up on the back as possible. Start with the backs of the hands together, then rotate the wrists and press the palms together.
5. Turn the left foot in 60 degrees, right foot out 90 degrees. Pivot the hips to face the same direction as the front foot—right hip back, left hip forward.
6. Move the tailbone down and forward. Inhale, curl the head and torso back.
7. Exhale, fold the torso over the front leg.
8. Turn the abdomen to the right until the center of the torso is in line with the front leg.
9. Take the chin toward/to the shin. Hold the pose and breathe.
10. To come out, inhale, lift the head and torso vertical. Exhale, turn the hips toward the long edge of the mat and parallel the feet. Bring the feet together and lower the arms.

Repeat on the second side.

safety
- Press the top of the front foot down to engage the calf.
- Press the inner edge of the front foot down and move the right hip back.
- Without moving the foot, turn the front quad out until the knee is in line with the foot. If the front kneecap still falls in (and/or down), turn the front foot out slightly until the knee faces forward.
- Straighten the back leg and lock it into a straight position without hyperextension.
- Squeeze the kneecaps up.
- Engage the back glutes.
- Press the tailbone down and tone the low belly.
- Engage the arms and move the shoulders up and back.
- If it is not possible to bring the hands together on the upper back due to tightness or injury, or if there is pain or tension in the wrists or shoulders, hold opposite elbows with opposite hands.

- Round the back evenly. Do not overly round any single part of the spine (a common tendency is to overly round the lower back), in order to compensate for tight hamstrings. Instead, come only halfway down and breathe. While this is more taxing on the legs, it is safer for the back. Otherwise, practice *parsvottanasana* with the hands on blocks to work on maintaining length in the spine and a safe stretch in the hamstrings.

refinement

Press your feet down and apart. Fully lengthen your spine. It is through the forms of the yoga poses that practitioners can access their functions. And yet, be careful not to attain the form of the pose for the sake of the form. In gymnastics form is paramount. A gymnast is expected to attain the form often at the expense of the body. In yoga, however, you may have to compromise the so-called final form that you see in these photos, to access its benefits. To attain the form at the expense of your body goes against one of the founding precepts of yoga called *ahimsa*, or nonviolence. Yoga is generous. As long as you honor yourself and others, no matter how limited you are in your pose, this practice will offer you all of its benefits.

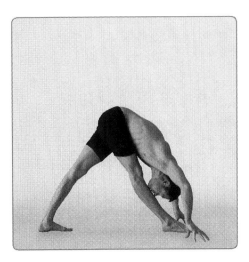

parsvottanasana
side stretched out pose

hands to floor

shape
(from *tadasana,* facing long edge of mat)

1. Inhale, bend the knees.
2. Exhale, take a wide stance slightly shorter than *trikonasana*. Place the hands on the hips.
3. Turn the left foot in 60 degrees, right foot out 90 degrees. Line up the middle of the back arch with the front heel.
4. Inhale, pivot the hips to face the same direction as the front foot—right hip back, left hip forward.
5. Exhale, fold the torso over the front leg.
6. Place the hands on the floor and walk the hands forward. Bend the elbows out to the sides.
7. Lift the left hip until the sacrum is parallel to the floor.
8. Take the chin toward/to the shin. Hold the pose and breathe.
9. To come out, place the hands on the hips. Inhale, lift the torso. Exhale, parallel the feet. Bring the feet together and lower the arms.

Repeat on the second side.

safety
- To reduce the intensity of the hamstring stretch, straighten the arms and lift the torso parallel to the floor, or place the hands on blocks or even a chair.
- If it is difficult to square the hips to the top of the mat or if there is discomfort at the front of the left hip/groin, line up the back heel with the front heel, or even widen the stance as much as hip-width apart.
- Engage the legs.
- Straighten the back leg with precision and strength. Precision means not hyperextending the back knee. It is common for practitioners to hyperextend the back leg in standing poses.
- Engage the left glutes.
- Press the front foot down to strengthen hamstrings.
- Press the top of the front foot down to engage the calf. Lift the kneecap up.
- Press the inner edge of the front foot down and move the right hip back.
- Press the tailbone down and tone the low belly.

- Turn the abdomen to the right.
- Line up the middle of the torso with the front leg.

refinement

Press your feet down and apart. Press your fingertips down and forward, and move the top of your right thigh back. Stretch your spine. The distance between the feet (the length of your stance) depends on your body type and range of motion. In general, the stance in *parsvottanasana* is shorter than the stance of *trikonasana*. In *parsvottanasana*, what will determine how far apart to separate your feet is your ability to square your hips to the front of the mat while keeping your back heel down and both legs straight. A shorter stance can accommodate tight hamstrings or calves, while a longer stance may be optimal if you have a short torso and long legs. In *parsvottanasana*, prioritize squared hips and straight legs.

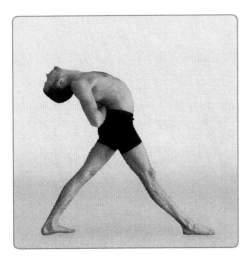

parsvottanasana
side stretched out pose

hands in reverse anjali mudra, backbend variation

shape
(from *tadasana*, facing long edge of mat)

1. Inhale, bend the knees.
2. Exhale, take a stance shorter than *trikonasana*.
3. Inhale, lift the arms overhead.
4. Exhale, swing the arms down and behind the back. Place the hands as high up on the back as possible. Start with the backs of the hands together, then rotate the wrists and press the palms together.
5. Turn the left foot in 60 degrees, right foot out 90 degrees.
6. Pivot the hips to face the same direction as the front foot.
7. Inhale, curl the head and torso back.
8. Look up. Hold the pose and breathe.
9. To come out, inhale, lift the head and torso vertical. Look forward. Exhale, turn the hips toward the long edge of the mat and parallel the feet. Bring the feet together and lower the arms.

Repeat on the second side.

safety
- Press the top of the front foot down to engage the calf and lift the kneecap up.
- Press the inner edge of the front foot down and move the right hip back.
- Straighten the back leg and lock it into a straight position without hyperextension.
- Press the tailbone down and tone the low belly.
- Engage the back glutes.
- Engage the arms and move the shoulders up and back. This minimal movement will create maximum stability for the shoulders.
- To get the hands higher up the back, lift the right wrist with the left hand and the left wrist with the right hand. Attempt to bring the knuckles in line with the lower tips of the shoulder blades.

- If it is not possible to bring the hands together on the upper back due to tightness or injury, or if there is pain or tension in the wrists or shoulders, hold opposite elbows with opposite hands.

refinement

Press your feet down and apart. Fully lengthen your spine. Lift your chest. Keep your low belly toned as you use your breath to deepen the backbend. Use your inhalations to lift your chest and use your exhalations to curl your chest back.

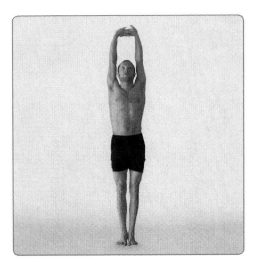

parvatasana
mountain pose

tadasana

shape
(from *tadasana*)

1. Inhale, extend the arms overhead. Interlace the fingers above the head; point the palms up.
2. Point the elbows out to the sides.
3. Squeeze the shoulder blades together on the back.
4. Straighten the arms.
5. Bring the arms vertical until the elbows are directly above the shoulders.
6. Look straight ahead. Hold the pose and breathe.
7. To come out, exhale, lower the arms.

safety

- Engage the legs.
- Squeeze the feet and legs together.
- Engage the glutes.
- Move the tailbone down and the low belly in.
- Move the base of the sternum back and lift the chest.
- Stretch the knuckles up—squeeze the wrists and elbows in.
- Stretch the arms up and back.

refinement

Stretch your arms up to capacity. Extend your feet and hands in opposite directions. *Parvatasana* is an optimal warm up for the shoulders. It is a great pose to practice before *indudalasana*, *vrksasana, surya namaskar,* and *adho mukha vrksasana.*

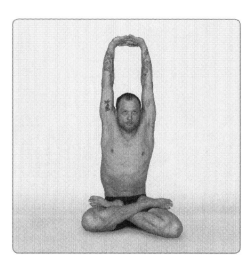

parvatasana
mountain pose

padmasana

shape
(from *padmasana*)

1. Interlace the fingers and place the backs of the hands on the crown of the head.
2. Inhale, straighten the arms overhead.
3. Point the elbows out to the sides.
4. Look straight ahead. Hold the pose and breathe.
5. To come out, exhale, bend the elbows and lower the backs of the hands to the crown of the head. Release the hands to the legs.

Repeat on the second side—switch the cross of the legs and fingers.

safety
- If the legs cannot not fold into *padmasana*, practice the pose with the legs in *sukhasana* instead.
- Press the outer edges/tops of the feet down.
- Clamp the knees closed by squeezing the heels toward the hips.
- Tone the pelvic floor and move the low belly toward the spine.
- Move the base of the sternum and arms back. Lift the chest.
- If the low back rounds, sit on one or more folded blankets.

refinement
Lift your ribcage away from your waist to lengthen your torso. Extend your arms and shoulder blades up. Squeeze your elbows in toward each other. Stretch evenly through the knuckles of your hands. Breathe evenly and deeply. Relax your jaw, throat, and eyes.

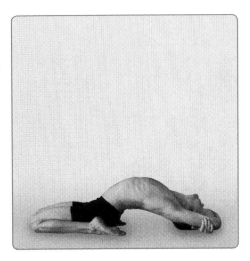

paryankasana
couch pose

shape
(from *supta virasana*)

1. Place the hands on the floor by the head—thumbs facing in and fingers pointing toward the feet. Point the elbows up.
2. Press the hands down, and inhale, lift the head and torso away from the floor to come into a backbend in the upper back. Exhale, lower the top of the head to the floor.
3. Hold the right elbow with the left hand and the left elbow with the right hand.
4. Lower the elbows and forearms to the floor. Look at the tip of the nose. Hold the pose and breathe.
5. Change the cross of the arms. Hold the pose and breathe.
6. To come out, release the elbows and place the hands next to the head. Straighten the arms slightly, lift the head, and lower the torso to the floor.

safety
- Point the toes straight back and squeeze the heels in toward the hips.
- Press the tops of the feet, hips, and head down.
- Lift the low back and chest up. Do not push out through the abdomen.
- Relax the shoulders.
- If there is any pain or discomfort in the low back, tone the low belly and/or rest the torso on a bolster.
- If there is pain or discomfort in the shoulders, or if the forearms do not reach the floor, place a folded blanket underneath the forearms for extra padding.

refinement
What is somewhat unique about this backbend is that it is calming and restorative, and that much of the bend happens in the neck. It also tends to be a peripheral pose, meaning it doesn't seem to be one that is practiced often. That is something I contemplate a lot these days, what makes one pose more popular than another? *Paryankasana* is far more doable than many of the staple or common backbends. What about it makes it a seldom-practiced asana? Well, you could change that today! Practice and keep practicing *paryankasana*!

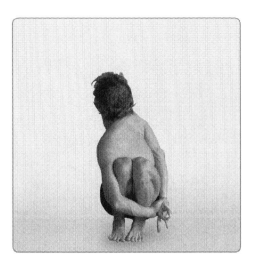

pasasana
noose pose

shape

1. Come to a squat position—feet and knees together, heels down.
2. Place the hands on the floor behind the hips.
3. Inhale, squeeze the legs together and lift the left arm vertical. Lean onto the back hand.
4. Exhale, twist the torso to the right and place the left shoulder outside of the right knee.
5. Wrap the left arm around both legs and place the back of the hand on the outer shin.
6. Lean forward and swing the right arm behind the back. Clasp the hands.
7. Turn the head and look back. Hold the pose and breathe.
8. To come out, inhale, look forward. Exhale, release the hands. Lower the hips and come to sit.

Repeat on the second side.

safety

- To reduce the intensity of the pose, sit on a block.
- If the heels do not lower to the floor, place one or more folded blankets below the heels.
- If the clasp is difficult, use a strap. Alternatively, move the left knee forward of the right knee and then clasp the hands. Once the hands are clasped, bring the shins and knees back together.
- Press the elbow into the leg and the leg into the elbow.
- Pull the front hand away from the back wrist and push the wrist into the hand.
- Bring the weight back into the heels, squeeze the legs together, and lift the chest.

refinement

As you progress in your asana practice, you will be able to come into the full form of this pose without lifting the heels. Ideally your knees will be flush. In order to keep the legs symmetrical and the heels down, *pasasana* requires exceptional balance.

I recommend waiting a minimum of four hours after a big meal before practicing deep twists like *pasasana*. Even a small cup of water may cause discomfort when attempting this pose. For this reason, reconsider drinking water during your yoga practice.

The moment you get into this pose your breath will likely be quick and shallow. Attempt to breath normally in *pasasana*. To do so you must become calm in the midst of discomfort.

And that is just one of the many skills this practice offers that applies off the mat. Again and again, these poses put us into stressful situations, and then require us to become calm and focused. It is an excellent skill to develop.

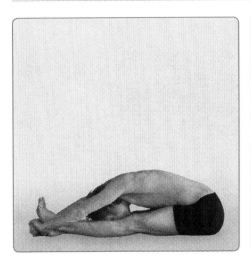
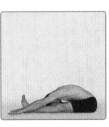
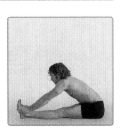
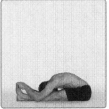
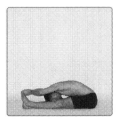

paschimottanasana
back stretched out pose

shape
(from *dandasana*)

1. Inhale fully. Exhale, lean the torso forward and hold the outer edges of the feet with the hands, or hold the big toes with the first two fingers and thumbs.
2. Straighten the legs, arms, and spine. Pause and breathe.
3. Inhale fully. Exhale, fold the torso over the legs. Bring the face toward/to the shins.
4. Stretch the hands beyond the feet and hold the back of the left hand with the right hand, or vice versa.
5. Round the back evenly. Hold the pose and breathe.
6. To come out, inhale, lift the head. Exhale, release the hands to the floor directly below the shoulders. Inhale, lift the torso vertical and place the hands next to the hips.

safety

- To reduce the intensity of the hamstring stretch, separate the feet outer hip-width apart, or, if needed, as wide as the mat.
- If the head does not reach the shins, separate the feet slightly and place the forehead on the edge of a block.
- Tighten the knees and tone the thighs.
- Press the backs of the knees down.
- Pull the feet with the hands and press the feet down and forward into the hands.
- Bend the elbows out to the sides.
- Use the arms to lengthen the spine.

refinement

There are two common approaches to practicing this pose. One way is to perform the pose pulling and fighting and struggling. Some students even "bounce" in the pose and make touching the feet or bringing the head to the legs the goal. The other way is to encounter the physical limitation of the body and cease all effort. This method often involves hanging the head over the torso and waiting for the pose to end. Don't choose between two bad options. Find a third option that will actually benefit your practice. In *paschimottanasana*, engage your legs and feet, lengthen your entire torso, gain as much space and length in your body, and then surrender into the experience of that effort. Every time your mind or body asks you to come out of the pose, confront your motivation. If it is due to laziness, boredom, or aversion to discomfort, realign with the third option.

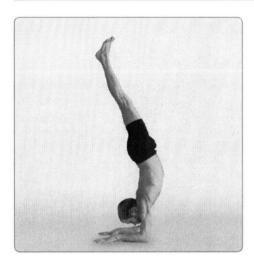

pincha mayurasana
peacock feather pose

shape

1. Come onto the hands and knees and place the forearms on the floor—elbows shoulder-width apart, forearms parallel, upper arms vertical.
2. Without moving the hands, move each forearm in a couple of inches. Press the forearms down and without lifting the arms, slide the forearms back into place. This will make the skin of the forearms taut, which will help to keep the forearms in place when kicking up into *pincha mayurasana*.
3. Separate the fingers and point the index fingers straight ahead. Isometrically press the fingers down and in.
4. Lift the knees and straighten the legs. Walk the feet forward and press the shoulders back toward the feet. Lift the hips up and back. Pause and breathe.
5. Keep backbending in the upper back and step one foot in. Kick the other leg up into a vertical position.
6. Move the inner edge of the top leg back. Lift the second leg to join the legs.
7. Extend the feet back slightly to imitate the shape of a peacock feather. Look down. Hold the pose and breathe.
8. To come out, lower one leg, then the other. Stretch the arms forward and lower the forehead to the floor. Pause and rest.

safety

- To avoid falling over, practice the pose against a wall.
- Do not allow the hands to move in or the elbows to move out.
- Keep the upper arms vertical. If the shoulders are tight, they will move forward beyond the elbows.
- Press the hands, forearms, and elbows down. Stretch the shoulders, spine, and legs away from the floor.
- Press the inner legs together and engage the feet—flare the outer two toes.
- Engage the glutes and abdomen, and press the tailbone in.
- Move the base of the sternum back.
- If the wrists and hands slide in and/or the elbows and forearms slide out, use a block between the hands to keep the forearms parallel and in place.

refinement

My mom balanced for the first time in *pincha mayurasana* away from the wall when she was 57 years old. My mom started practicing hatha yoga, and never stopped, 40 years ago. My mom is a great example of how one can always continue to explore and evolve in this practice. To this day, she starts her hatha yoga practice at four in the morning while my dad sits nearby and reads out loud from a wide variety of scriptures. Then they both meditate in their huts that my dad built down by the pond. Keep practicing and this practice will always offer more.

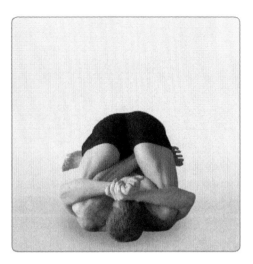

pindasana
embryo pose

shape
(from *sarvangasana 1*)

1. Move the right leg back slightly.
2. In one movement, bring the left leg into *ardha padmasana*.
3. Move the left knee back slightly and in one movement, bring the right leg into *padmasana*.
4. Inhale fully. Exhale, fold the legs into the torso and press the knees into the shoulders.
5. Release the hands and wrap the arms around the legs. Bind the hands.
6. Look past the tip of the nose. Hold the pose and breathe for 30 to 60 seconds.
7. To come out, release the hands. Inhale, lift the legs and torso vertical. Release and straighten the legs.

Repeat on the second side—switch the cross of the legs.

safety

- If the legs cannot fold into *padmasana*, do *karnapidasana* instead.
- Press the shoulders down, in toward each other, and forward toward the head.
- Center the head and press the head down. Bring the chin vertical.
- Press the outer edges/tops of the feet into the thighs and squeeze the heels toward the hips.
- Squeeze the legs with the arms.

refinement

A prerequisite of this pose is the ability to do *karnapidasana* without your seventh cervical touching the floor. Although complicated and difficult to get into, *pindasana* is deeply calming. This applies to the overall practice as well. Yoga asana is always challenging and difficult to one degree or another. And yet at the end of practice, there is a deep state of calm. Everything costs something. Is a state of calm worth the price of an hour or so of asana? The cost of not practicing is far more expensive than the cost of practicing, for me anyway. If you are reading this right now, my guess is that the same goes for you. Sri Pattabhi Jois used to say, "Practice and all is coming."

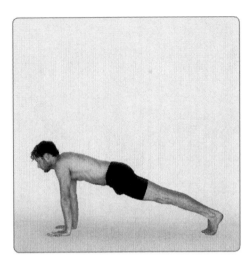

plank pose

shape
(from *adho mukha svanasana*)

1. Inhale, move the torso and shoulders forward until the arms are vertical.
2. Make a straight line from the heels to the hips and from the hips to the head.
3. Lift the chin slightly and look straight ahead. Hold the pose and breathe.
4. To come out, push the hands down and forward, and stretch the hips up and back.

safety
- Separate the hands slightly wider than the shoulders. Separate the fingers. Point the index fingers straight ahead.
- Evenly press the fingertips and the perimeter of the palms into the floor. To achieve this, press the mounds of the index fingers down, which tend to lift up.
- Lock the elbows and knees into a straight position. Tone the triceps and thighs.
- Press the tailbone down and lift the low belly. Move the base of the sternum up.
- Bring the heels directly over the toe mounds.
- If the hips sag, lower the knees to the floor and create a straight line from the hips to the head.

refinement
Plank pose is a great way to warm up your arms and your core. It is often used as a transitional pose when flowing through *surya namaskar*. Holding it for 30 seconds to a minute will help you develop strength and stamina that will serve you well in your practice. The hands bear a significant amount of weight, and as a result, this pose will prepare you for more challenging arm balances.

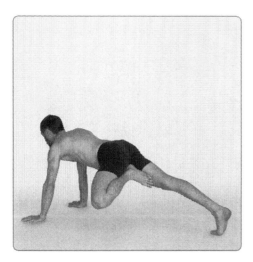

plank pose

leg in tree

shape

(from *vasisthasana*, legs together)

1. With the right hand and outer right foot on the floor, hold the top ankle with the top hand and place the sole of the foot on the inner thigh of the bottom leg.
2. Point the top knee up.
3. Rotate the front of the body to face down and place the top hand on the floor—hands outer shoulder-width apart.
4. Extend the bent knee directly out to the side.
5. Lift the chin and look forward. Hold the pose and breathe.
6. To come out, roll onto the right hand and the outer edge of the right foot. Release the top knee, straighten the leg, and stack the legs. Lift the top arm.

Repeat on the second side.

safety

- Place the foot of the bent leg above or below the knee—do not place the foot against the side of the knee.
- Press the fingertips and the perimeter of the palms into the floor with equal pressure.
- Squeeze the elbows straight.
- Tighten the kneecap and tone the quads of the straight leg.
- Lift the hips slightly to prevent collapsing in the low back. Bring the back heel into a vertical position.
- Press the foot into the thigh and press the thigh into the foot.
- Engage the glutes and abdomen.
- Press the tailbone down and lift the low belly.

refinement

Plank pose with the leg in tree is a great way to strengthen the abdomen. To strengthen the arms, lower into *chaturanga dandasana* with the leg still in tree. Advanced practitioners move into *nakrasana* with one leg in tree by hopping forward and backward five times.

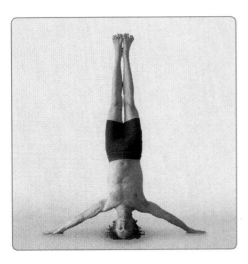

prasarita hasta sirsasana
spread hands headstand pose

shape
(from *baddha hasta sirsasana*)

1. Extend down through the head and in one movement, straighten the arms and extend the hands out to the sides.
2. Look forward. Hold the pose and breathe.
3. To come out, either lower the legs to the floor and rest with the hips and forehead down in *balasana*, or continue with *urdhva padmasana* in *prasarita hasta sirsasana* in the *sirsasana* sequence.

safety
*   Press the hands down and lift the shoulders up. Separate the fingers to aid the balance.
*   Stretch up through the legs and feet.
*   Press the inner feet, ankles, and knees together.
*   Engage the glutes and abdomen.
*   Move the base of the sternum back and the tailbone forward.
*   Keep the breath even and the eyes steady.
*   If the balance is difficult, practice against or near a wall.

refinement
If coming into *prasarita hasta sirsasana* from *baddha hasta sirsasana* proves to be too difficult, begin in *vajrasana*. Any of these headstand variations can also be approached from *sirsasana 1* or *2*.

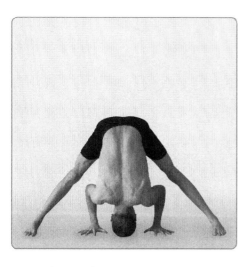
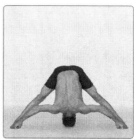

prasarita padottanasana
wide legs forward fold pose

shape
(from *tadasana*, facing long edge of mat)

1. Inhale, bend the knees. Exhale, take a wide stance.
2. Place the hands on the hips. Straighten the legs.
3. Inhale, press the hands down on the hips and stretch the spine up.
4. Exhale, fold forward.
5. Place the palms flat on the floor between the feet—shoulder-width apart.
6. Place the top of the head toward/to the floor. Hold the pose and breathe.
7. To come out, walk the hands forward and place the hands on the hips. Inhale, lift the torso to stand. Exhale, bring the feet together.

safety
- Squeeze the feet in.
- Engage the leg muscles: calves, quads, hamstrings. Lift the kneecaps up.
- Move the tailbone down and the low belly in.
- Lift the shoulders up, away from the ears.
- To reduce the intensity of the stretch, place the hands on the floor or on blocks directly below the shoulders. Straighten the arms.
- If there is pain in the outer ankles or feet, draw the outer ankles in and press the inner feet down.
- Avoid hyperextending the knees.
- Do not put any weight on the head.

refinement
Press your feet down and apart. To fold more deeply, engage your abdomen, press your hands down and forward, and place the top or the back of your head on the floor between your feet. If you have a long torso, you may need to shorten your stance in order to get the crown of your head to the floor between your feet. A wider stance will allow you to curl your head in and place the back of your head on the floor. If you have low blood pressure or feel dizzy or faint when you lift to stand, lift the torso parallel to the floor and pause for a few breaths before standing up.

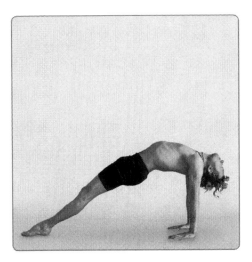

purvottanasana
front body stretched out pose

shape
(from *dandasana*)

1. Point the toes.
2. Lean the torso back and place the hands a foot and a half behind the hips. Lift the chest and bring the shoulders directly above the wrists.
3. Turn the hands out slightly and point the thumbs straight ahead.
4. Inhale, lift the hips and straighten the arms. Exhale, curl the head back.
5. Look between the eyebrows. Hold the pose and breathe.
6. To come out, keep the chest lifted and exhale, lower the hips. Place the hands next to the hips.

safety
- Lock the elbows and knees into a straight position.
- Press the fingertips and the perimeter of the palms into the floor with equal pressure.
- Press the hands down, lift the chest, and shrug the shoulders toward the head.
- Press the feet, especially the mounds of the big toes, down. Lift the hips and engage the glutes.
- If there is pain or discomfort in the neck or jaw, look up or straight ahead.

refinement
Eventually work toward turning the hands in so the fingers point forward toward the feet. In the full form of *purvottanasana,* in which there is a 90-degree angle between the arms and torso, it will likely require intense effort in the legs, hips, back, and arms. *Purvottanasana* is a great warm up for deep backbends. *Paschimottanasana* and *purvottanasana* are like two sides of the same coin—the one balances out the other. Other poses that are also like two sides of the same coin are *trikonasana* and *parivrtta trikonasana; parsvakonasana* and *parivrtta parsvakonasana; sirsasana* and *sarvangasana; urdhva mukha svanasana* and *adho mukha svanasana; marichyasana 1* and *marichyasana 3, marichyasana 2* and *marichyasana 4.*

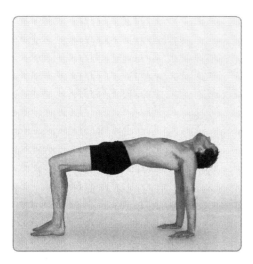

purvottanasana prep
front body stretched out pose

shape

1. Sit on the floor.
2. Bend the knees and place the feet flat on the floor about a foot and a half in front of the hips.
3. Separate the feet outer hip-width apart, point the knees up, and point the toes straight ahead.
4. Place the hands slightly wider than shoulder-distance apart about a foot behind the hips.
5. Separate the fingers, point the thumbs straight ahead, and straighten the arms.
6. Inhale, press the hands down to lift the chest. Pause and breathe. Inhale, lift the hips as high as the shoulders and knees. Keep the shins and arms vertical, which may require moving the feet back.
7. Exhale, curl the head back and look between the eyebrows. Hold the pose and breathe.
8. To come out, inhale, lift the head and look forward. Exhale, keep the chest lifted and lower the hips.

safety

- If there is pain or discomfort at the front of the shoulders, press the inner hands down and squeeze the shoulder blades together toward the spine to lift the chest. If there is still pain or discomfort, practice *purvottanasana* prep, forearms on floor, instead.
- Separate the fingers. Press the entire perimeter of the palms down, especially the mounds of the index fingers.
- Lock the elbows into a straight position.
- Extend the inner edges of the feet and thighs down.
- Contract the glutes.
- Lift the tailbone and hips.
- Shrug the shoulders toward the head and lift the chest.
- Isometrically squeeze the hands and feet toward each other.
- When curling the head back, engage the neck muscles (do not drop the head).
- If there is pain or discomfort in the neck or jaw, look up or forward.

refinement

If you keep your chest lifted from start to finish, you won't "lose" the pose once you elevate the hips to enter the pose, and you will prevent injury at the front of the shoulders once you lower the hips to exit the pose. Eventually work toward turning the hands in so the fingers point forward—toward the feet. *Purvottanasana prep* is an excellent way to warm up the quads and shoulders.

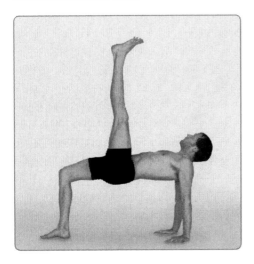

purvottanasana prep
front body stretched out pose

one leg lifted

shape
(from *purvottanasana prep*)

1. Inhale, lift and straighten the left leg. Center the heel directly over the hip.
2. Exhale, curl the head back and look between the eyebrows.
3. Hold the pose and breathe.
4. To come out, exhale, lower the lifted leg.

Repeat on the second side.

safety
- Separate the fingers. Press the entire perimeter of the palms down, especially the mounds of the index fingers.
- Lock the arms and top leg into a straight position.
- Keep the shins and arms vertical.
- Extend the inner edges of the bottom foot and thigh down.
- Engage the glutes of the bottom leg.
- Lift the tailbone, hips, and top foot.
- Shrug the shoulders toward the head and lift the chest.
- Isometrically squeeze the hands and feet toward each other.
- When curling the head back, engage the neck muscles (do not drop the head).
- If there is pain or discomfort in the neck or jaw, look up or forward.

refinement

Purvottanasana prep, one leg lifted, burns up the tension in my quads like no other pose. I perform this pose before going to sleep when I have excess tension in my legs. For the sake of your hip flexors, it is essential that your top leg is vertical to the floor. Bend your top knee as much as necessary to bring your thigh vertical to the floor.

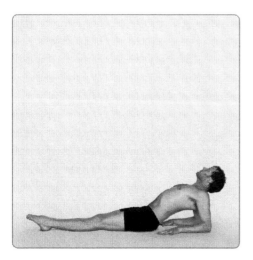

purvottanasana prep
front body stretched out pose

forearms on floor

shape
(from *dandasana*)

1. Point the feet.
2. Lean the torso back and bring the forearms to the floor—elbows directly below the shoulders.
3. Point the index fingers straight ahead.
4. Lift the low back and chest up to capacity.
5. Look straight ahead, up, or curl the head back and look between the eyebrows. Hold the pose and breathe.
6. To come out, inhale, push the hands and forearms down to lift the torso.

safety

- Straighten and strengthen the legs.
- Press the inner legs together and engage the glutes.
- Isometrically press the hands down and forward.
- Lift the chest up and back. Stretch the entire spine.
- Do not push the belly out to lift the low back.

refinement

Press your inner wrists down and keep your forearms parallel. *Purvottanasana prep* is a good counter pose for almost any forward fold and a good transition pose into *savasana*.

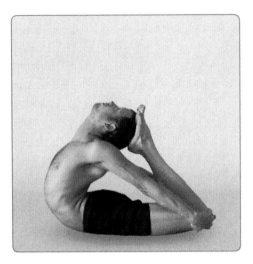

rajakapotasana
king pigeon pose

hands to knees

shape
(from *dhanurasana*)

1. Deepen the bend in the right knee and slide the right hand halfway down the shin toward the knee. Kick the right foot up and back until the shin is vertical to the floor. Repeat on the left side.
2. Slide the right hand farther down to the bottom of the shin just below the knee. Repeat on the left side.
3. Begin to straighten the legs to catch hold of the knees with the hands.
4. Once the hands are holding the knees, curl the head back and bend the knees. Press the soles of the feet onto the crown of the head.
5. Bring the inner edges of the feet together, including the heels.
6. Look between the eyebrows. Hold the pose and breathe.
7. To come out, inhale, lift the head and walk the hands up the shins. Clasp the feet or ankles.

safety
- Engage the feet and flare the outer two toes of each foot.
- Press the inner edges of the feet together.
- Isometrically squeeze the knees in and lift the inner thighs up.
- Engage the glutes and press the hips down.
- Tone the pelvic floor and low belly.
- Stretch and lengthen the entire spine; lift the chest up.
- Press the head and feet into each other.

refinement
The most difficult part of this pose is getting into it. Once you've clasped your knees with your hands and your head and feet are together it becomes much easier to expand and lengthen the spine. That is often the case with practice itself: often the most difficult part of practice is just showing up and getting onto the mat. That said, practice please practice.

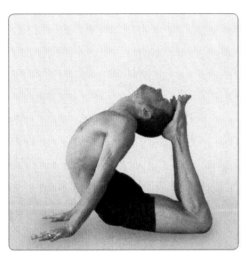
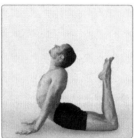

rajakapotasana
king pigeon pose

shape

1. Bring the front body to the floor.
2. Separate the legs outer hip-width apart and straighten the legs. Point the feet and bring the inner edges of the feet together.
3. Place the hands by the torso slightly wider than shoulder-distance apart.
4. Walk the hands back until the upper arms are parallel to the floor and forearms are vertical.
5. Bend the knees 90 degrees—heels over knees. Pause and breathe.
6. Inhale, lift the torso, straighten the arms, and curl the head back.
7. Flex the feet and place the crown of the head on the soles of the feet.
8. Look between the eyebrows. Hold the pose and breathe.
9. To come out, inhale, lift the head and bend the elbows. Lower the front body and legs to the floor.

safety

- Engage the feet—flare the outer toes.
- Press the inner feet together.
- Isometrically squeeze the knees toward each other.
- Tone the quads and lift the inner thighs up.
- Press the tailbone and hips down. Contract the glutes.
- Tone the pelvic floor and low belly.
- Isometrically press the hands down and back.
- Move the shoulders back and toward each other.
- Engage the upper back muscles, and move the shoulder blades and chest forward and up.
- Stretch and lengthen the entire spine.
- Press the head and feet together.

refinement

This is the gateway pose into all the other foot-to-head backbends. Before even attempting *kapotasana, eka pada rajakopotasana,* and *dwi pada viparita dandasana* variations, I recommend you first work toward getting your head to your feet in *rajakapotasana.* If you attempt these poses without a certain amount of flexibility in your spine, they could over stretch and strain your shoulders and/or low back. Similarly, students all too often cause strain on their shoulders because they do not twist deeply enough in *marichyasana 3* and *4* and *ardha matsyendrasana*.

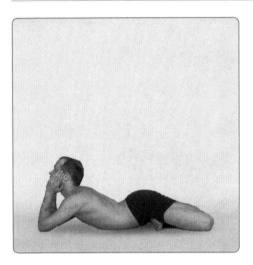

resting lion pose

shape
(from *padmasana*)

1. Place the hands in front of the shins.
2. Walk the hands forward to lift the hips. Continue to walk the hands forward and lower the front body to the floor.
3. Reach the arms forward and bend the elbows.
4. Rest the chin in the palms—fingers pointing out. Look straight ahead. Hold the pose and breathe.
5. To come out, release and lower the hands. Inhale, straighten the arms and lift the torso. Exhale, walk the hands back and lower the hips to the floor.

Repeat on the second side—switch the cross of the legs.

safety

- Engage the feet—flare the outer two toes of both feet.
- Press the outer edges/tops of the feet into the thighs.
- Squeeze the knees in toward each other.
- Press the tailbone down and tone the low belly.
- If there is pain or discomfort at the quads and/or if the hips cannot lower to the floor, place a bolster underneath the torso with the edge of the bolster at the pubic bone. Drape the legs over the bottom of the bolster.

refinement

Engage your abdomen and lift your knees away from the floor. This pose offers a safe stretch at the front of the neck. It is an especially welcome counter-pose after long-held shoulderstands and headstands and their variations.

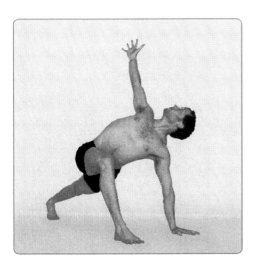

revolved lunge pose

shape
(from *lunge pose*)

1. Keeping the hips square, place the right hand on the right hip.
2. Inhale fully. Exhale, twist the torso to the right—rotate the right shoulder over the left shoulder.
3. Extend the right hand up.
4. Point the biceps toward the top of the mat, point the palm to the right.
5. Look up past the top thumb. Hold the pose and breathe.
6. To come out, inhale, look down at the floor. Exhale, lower the right hand to the outside of the right foot.

Repeat on the second side.

safety

-   Do not allow the front knee to move beyond the heel or to tilt in.
-   Move the back heel forward until it is vertical, lift the hips slightly.
-   Move the tailbone down and lift the low belly.
-   Move the right hip down, lift the back thigh up.
-   Move the base of the sternum back, stretch up through the chest.

refinement

Extend out through your back foot and front knee. Extend your head and back foot away from your hips. Stretch your entire spine. Extend your left hand down and reach your right hand up. Twists compress, release, and remove toxins from the abdominal organs. They also keep the spine strong and supple—a priceless asset.

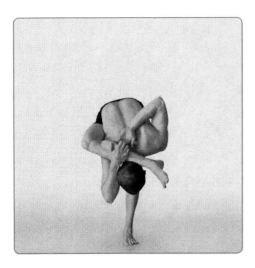

ruchikasana
Sage Ruchika's pose

hands clasped

shape
(from *kala bhairavasana,* right leg behind the head)

1. Place the left hand on the floor—shoulder-distance apart from the right hand.
2. Walk or jump the back foot forward to the inside of the left hand.
3. Bring the forehead to the left shin.
4. Balancing on the left foot, bind the hands behind the shoulders. Point the left elbow up. Point the right elbow down.
5. Look down. Hold the pose and breathe.
6. To come out, release the hands, bend the standing knee and come to sit.

Repeat on the second side.

safety
- Engage both feet, especially the top foot.
- Isometrically bend the top knee to engage the hamstrings.
- Straighten and strengthen the standing leg. Lift the left kneecap.
- Lift the pelvic floor and tone the low belly.
- If the hands do not clasp behind the back, use a strap.
- If it is difficult to balance, keep both hands on the floor directly below the shoulders, or keep the right hand directly below the shoulder and hold the calf with the left hand.

refinement
The only way to ensure complete safety in this pose, or any pose for that matter, is to not practice it. Every pose comes with both risks and rewards. If you want the rewards, you must accept the potential risks. Rajanaka Yoga founder Douglas Brooks once told me, "The world is never without scariness. The anti-forces of the world cannot be destroyed. They can be put in the right place but they cannot be eliminated. These anti-forces are in fact protected by Grace itself.

They are there to push back against us because unless we are challenged, we do not advance."[1] And so it goes with asana—risk can be put in the right place but it cannot be eliminated. The path of yoga requires that we navigate and not negate the inevitable risks. As Michael Corleone in *The Godfather, Part II* said, "Keep your friends close and your enemies closer."[2]

[1]   Personal communication with Douglas Brooks, Tucson, Arizona, April 2011.
[2]   The Godfather, Part II, Francis Ford Coppola, Paramount Pictures, 1974.

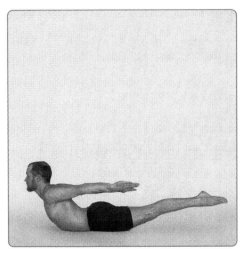 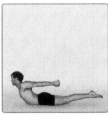 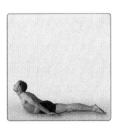

salabhasana
locust pose

shape

1. Bring the front body to the floor—arms alongside the torso. Point the palms up.
2. Straighten the arms and legs and bring the inner edges of the legs and feet together. Point the feet.
3. Inhale, lift the head, torso, hands and feet.
4. Lift the shoulders so the arms are parallel to the floor.
5. Look straight ahead. Hold the pose and breathe.
6. To come out, exhale, lower the torso, arms and legs.

safety

- If there is pain or discomfort in the low back, separate the feet outer hip-width apart.
- Lock the arms and legs into a straight position.
- Point the kneecaps straight down.
- Point the toes straight back and isometrically squeeze the ankles in.
- Press the tailbone down, engage the glutes, and lift the low belly.
- Stretch the spine forward and up.
- During menstruation, place a bolster below the front of the ribcage to lift the torso. This will reduce the upper back and core strength required while providing a stretch in the upper back.

refinement

The abdominal backbends such as *salabhasana*, *makarasana*, and *viparita salabhasana prep* are among the most beneficial poses for the low back. Abdominal backbends are also very heating for the body because of the strength that is required of the upper back to lift the torso and legs. I believe many students would benefit if their entire backbending syllabus were comprised of these abdominal backbends, along with *dhanurasana* and possibly *ustrasana*. Although all backbends offer potential benefits, they also come with risks that, like a crocodile, often bite.

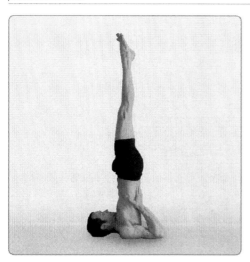

sarvangasana 1
shoulderstand pose 1

shape

1. Stack three folded blankets neatly on top of each other. If the blanket has frills, point the frills in the same direction.
2. Place the blankets flush with the top edge of the mat—frills pointing down. Fold the bottom of the mat three-quarters of the way up the blankets so that once in *sarvangasana* the shoulders will be on the blanket and the elbows will be on the mat.
3. Lie down with the head on the floor and the tops of the shoulders a few inches below the edge of the blankets.
4. Lift the legs and roll back to bring the feet to the floor behind the head shoulder-width apart.
5. Bring the hips directly above the shoulders until the spine is vertical.
6. Separate the feet as wide as the mat.
7. Straighten the arms and interlace the fingers.
8. One at a time, bring the shoulder blades toward the spine by walking the elbows toward the midline.
9. Bend the elbows and place the hands as low on the back as possible—fingers pointing up.
10. Squeeze the elbows in until they are shoulder-width apart, or slightly wider if necessary.
11. Bring the feet together and straighten the legs.
12. Inhale, lift the legs vertical until the chest, hips, and feet are in one vertical line. 1
13. Bring the feet halfway between a flexed and pointed position. Look up. Hold the pose and breathe.
14. To come out, exhale, lower the feet to the floor behind the head. Pause and breathe. Straighten the arms and slowly roll onto the back. Lower the legs to the floor and stretch the arms out to the sides. Slide the body in the direction of the head and pause as soon as the tops of the shoulders meet the floor. Move slowly to avoid overshooting the mark. Pause here and breathe. Roll to the side and come to sit.

safety

*   If there is pain or discomfort in the neck, cervical spine injuries or conditions, and/or loss of spinal curvature in the spine, do not lift the feet off the floor. Seek guidance from a skilled yoga instructor on modifications with chairs or against a wall.

- Do not practice inversions at any time during menstruation. Practice *supta baddha konasana* (a supine version of *baddha konasana*) on bolsters instead.
- Before lifting the legs vertical, make sure that the base of the neck is pressing into the blankets. If the boney protrusion at the base of the neck (called the "seventh cervical") has moved beyond the edge of the blankets, start again. This time come into the pose with the shoulders even farther away from the edge of the blankets.
- Once the shoulder blades are in place and the hands are supporting the back, the seventh cervical should lift away from the blankets. If it is still on the blanket, walk the shoulders even more in and up, use more blankets, or develop more flexibility in the shoulders before practicing this pose.
- Squeeze the shoulder blades toward each other like two strong magnets, and press the head, shoulders, upper arms, and elbows down.
- Shrug the shoulders toward the head to avoid over stretching the neck.
- Center the head. Once the legs are off the floor, do not turn the head from side to side. Bring the chin vertical—do not allow the chin to drop toward the chest.
- Press the hands and wrists into the torso.
- Engage the glutes and squeeze the inner knees, ankles, and feet together.
- Move the hips and tailbone forward in the direction of the face. Extend the feet up and back.
- Stretch up through the spine and legs.
- Relax the jaw, eyes, and face.
- Breathe evenly and deeply.
- To reduce the intensity or build endurance in the pose, bend the knees and place the feet on a wall, or practice *halasana* instead.

refinement

For a better grip, place your hands directly on the skin of your back as opposed to over clothing.

Ideally *sarvangasana* will resemble a still flame. Although the flame appears still, it constantly ascends. *Sarvangasana* done in poor form energetically looks like a wilting flower. *Sarvangasana* can be performed for one or more minutes. Build your *sarvangasana* capacity slowly. Take a few weeks or even months to build up to five minutes in this pose. Once you can hold *sarvangasana* in good form for five or more minutes, begin to explore the *sarvangasana* cycle.

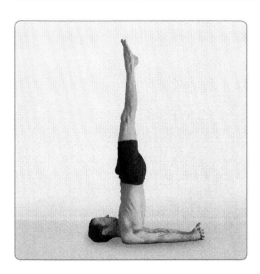

sarvangasana 2
shoulderstand pose 2

shape
(from *sarvangasana 1*)

1. Release the hands and straighten the arms. Lower the arms to the floor behind the torso.
2. Interlace the fingers and either bring the palms together or pull the wrists apart. Look past the tip of the nose. Hold the pose and breathe.
3. To come out, release the hands, bend the elbows, and place the hands as low on the back as possible.

safety

- Squeeze the shoulder blades toward each other like two strong magnets, and press the shoulders, upper arms, and elbows down.
- Shrug the shoulders toward the head to avoid over stretching the neck.
- Center the head and press the head down. Bring the chin vertical—do not allow the chin to drop toward the floor.
- Press the hands and wrists into the torso.
- Engage the glutes and squeeze the inner knees, ankles, and feet together.
- Move the hips and tailbone forward in the direction of the face. Extend the feet up and back.
- Stretch up through the spine and legs.
- Relax the jaw, eyes, and face.
- Gaze past the tip of the nose.
- Breathe evenly and deeply.

refinement

From *sarvangasana 1*, lower into *halasana* to reestablish proper alignment in the shoulders, and then return to *sarvangasana 2*. *Halasana* can serve as an alignment refuge for any of the *sarvangasana* variations. For a slightly more intense variation of *sarvangasana 2*, turn the palms out.

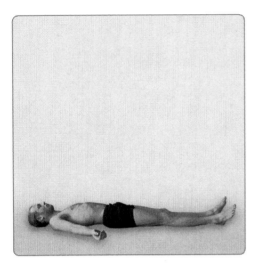

savasana
corpse pose

shape

1. Lie down on the floor.
2. Separate the feet outer hip-width apart. Relax the legs and allow the feet to turn out.
3. Bring the arms about 30 degrees away from the body. Straighten the arms and point the palms up. Relax the arms.
4. Close the eyes. Hold the pose and breathe normally.
5. To come out, be gentle and slow.

safety

- Remove eyeglasses and hair ties (which can force the head to turn to one side or the other). Center the head.
- Bring the shoulder blades onto the back away from the ears.
- Put a blanket under the body or head for extra padding.
- If the season is hot, lie directly on the floor without a mat and/or spread the arms and legs slightly wider.
- If the season is cool, bring the arms and legs slightly closer together and/or cover the body with a blanket.
- If the room is bright, dim or turn off the lights or cover the eyes with a cloth or eye pillow.
- Stay awake.
- Do not skip this pose. Practice this pose for 5-20 minutes depending on the length of the practice.

refinement

On November 21 and 22 of 2005, Milo photographed me doing all the photos in this book. On day one I performed all of the standing poses. On day two I performed everything else. Since then, we continued to replace many of these photographs with more refined expressions. The above photo was the last taken just after I finished doing all 400 poses. This photo is therefore significant to me. It was a moment of total dharma depletion and completion.

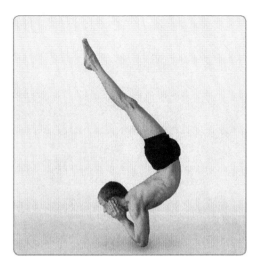

sayanasana
pose of repose

shape

1. Come onto the hands and knees and place the forearms on the floor—elbows shoulder-width apart, upper arms vertical.
2. Press the palms together.
3. Lift the knees and straighten the legs. Walk the feet forward and press the shoulders back. Lift the hips up and back. Pause and breathe.
4. Keep backbending in the upper back and step one foot in. Kick the other leg up to a vertical position. Join the legs and point the feet.
5. Bring the chin forward toward the hands. Move the feet beyond the head.
6. Lift the hands one at a time to support the chin. Look forward. Hold the pose and breathe.
7. To come out, release the hands and lower the legs.

safety

- If there is discomfort in the elbows, fold a mat into quarters and place it below the elbows to provide extra padding.
- Press the inner feet and legs together.
- Engage the glutes and abdomen.
- Press the tailbone in.
- Move the base of the sternum back.
- To avoid falling over, practice the pose against a wall.
- In order to stay balanced as the head and feet move forward, the hips must move back.

refinement

Luck is a definite factor both in life and in hatha yoga. To attain even momentary balance in *sayanasana* is as much a factor of luck as it is skill. The practice of yoga inspires us to make use of luck when it comes our way. There are ways to develop a relationship with luck. As it says in *Great by Choice*, "The critical question is not whether you'll have luck, but what you do with the luck you get."[1]

---

[1]   Jim Collins and Morten T. Hansen, *Great by Choice: Uncertainty, Chaos, and Luck—Why Some Thrive Despite Them All* (New York: HarperBusiness, 2011).

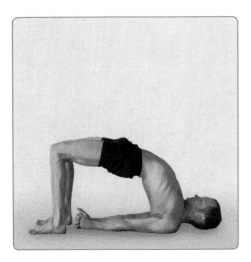

setu bandha sarvangasana
bridge pose

shape

1. Lie down on the back with the arms alongside the torso.
2. Bend the knees and bring the feet flat on the floor just in front of the hips—feet outer hip-width apart. Point the toes straight ahead.
3. Inhale, lift the hips and interlace the fingers below the sacrum. One at time, walk the shoulders up toward the head and in toward the spine. Do this several times until the chest is fully lifted.
4. Inhale, lift the hips. Adjust the feet so the heels are directly below the knees—thighs parallel to the floor and shins vertical.
5. Look up. Hold the pose and breathe.
6. To come out, release the hands and separate the arms shoulder-width apart. Exhale, lower the hips and straighten the legs.

safety

*   Bring the feet parallel and isometrically squeeze the knees in. The tendency is for the feet to turn out and the knees to widen beyond hip-distance.
*   Press the inner edges of the feet down and activate the outer two toes.
*   Tone the legs and spin the inner thighs down toward the floor.
*   Bring the shoulders toward the head to avoid overstretching the neck.
*   Press the feet, wrists, shoulders, and head down. Lift the chest and hips up and back—toward the head.
*   Center the head and avoid turning the head from side to side.
*   Keep the base of the chin vertical from start to finish.
*   If the shoulders are tight, hold the outer edges of the mat with the hands instead of interlacing the fingers. Separating the hands will help bring the shoulder blades together, which will prevent overstretching the neck.

refinement

Initiate the lift of your hips from your outer hips rather than pushing up through your pubic bone. For those with open shoulders, press your palms together. To discover a restful and restorative quality in the pose, place a block of appropriate height directly below your sacrum—along the width of the hips, block parallel to short edge of mat. Rest the weight of your hips on the block but continue to push your feet, wrists, shoulders, and head down to lift your chest. Stay for five to eight minutes.

Setu bandha sarvangasana is a unique backbend in that the neck is in a flexed position as it is in most forward folds. It can, therefore, be used to prepare for both backbends and *savasana*. *Setu bandha sarvangasana* is also a good preparatory pose for *uttana mayurasana, dhanurasana,* and *ustrasana*. It can also prepare the shoulders, spine and chest for *sarvangasana* and its variations.

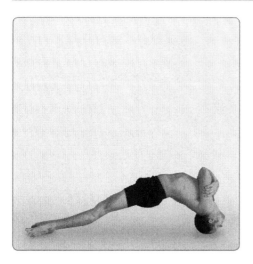

setu bandhasana
bridge building pose

shape

1. Lie down on the back.
2. Bend the knees and bring the feet about two feet in front of the hips.
3. Bring the inner heels together and point the toes out as far as possible. Widen the knees.
4. Place the hands next to the head—thumbs facing in and fingers pointing toward the feet. Point the elbows up. Use the hands to lift the head and bring the top of the head to the floor.
5. Cross the arms in front of the chest.
6. Press the head and feet down. Inhale, lift the hips and torso.
7. Straighten the legs. Look at the tip of the nose. Hold the pose and breathe.
8. Change the cross of the arms. Hold the pose and breathe.
9. To come out, exhale, release the arms to the floor and lower the body. Bend the knees and walk the feet back toward the head.

safety

- If there is a cervical spine injury or condition, do not practice this pose.
- To provide additional support to the neck, keep the hands by the head with the thumbs facing in and the fingers pointing toward the feet.
- Straighten and strengthen the legs.
- Press the inner heels and legs together.
- Lift the tailbone, and engage the glutes and low belly.
- Lift the shoulders away from the floor.
- Engage the neck muscles from start to finish.

refinement

This pose requires a strong neck. To lift your hips higher, continue to roll forward, toward the hairline. Make sure this pose serves to build and not burn your bridges, so to sadhana-speak.

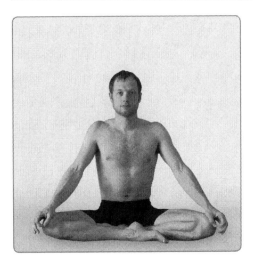

siddhasana
accomplished one pose

open

shape
(from *dandasana*)

1. Bend the left knee and place the left heel against the perineum. Lower the top of the foot and shin to the floor.
2. Bend the right knee and place the right foot in front of the left foot—outer right heel on top of the left ankle.
3. Place the hands on the knees. Straighten the arms. Look straight ahead. Hold the pose and breathe.
4. To come out, straighten the legs and place the hands next to the hips.

Repeat on the second side—change the cross of the legs.

safety

*   Press the outer edges of the feet down.
*   Tilt the pelvis forward—curve the low back in. To achieve this, one at a time pull the flesh from underneath the sit bones back with the hands. If the low back still rounds, sit up on one or more folded blankets.
*   Squeeze the elbows straight—engage the triceps.
*   Lift the pelvic floor and tone the low belly.
*   Move the base of the sternum back and lift the chest.
*   Level the shoulders and center the crown of the head over the pelvic floor. Lift the chin slightly.

refinement

If placing your hands on your knees pulls your shoulders forward, slide your hands slightly back to widen your collarbones and open across your chest. Keep your arms straight.

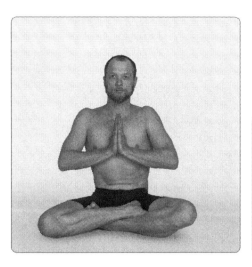
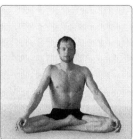

siddhasana
accomplished one pose

shape
(from *dandasana*)

1. Bend the left knee and place the left heel against the perineum. Lower the top of the foot and shin to the floor.
2. Bend the right knee and use the hands to lift the right foot off the floor.
3. Press the right heel into the middle of the upper inner left thigh.
4. Point the foot down at a 45-degree angle and point the toes. Wrap the toes around the left thigh.
5. Lift the right knee and, with the right hand, reach between the calf and thigh and hold the left foot.
6. Use the right hand to pull the left foot through the space of the leg.
7. Still holding the foot with hand, use the left hand to press the right knee down as you pull the left toes up through the calf and thigh of the right leg.
8. Place the hands on the knees and straighten the arms.
9. Look straight ahead. Hold the pose and breathe.
10. To come out, straighten the legs one at a time and place the hands next to the hips.

Repeat on the second side—change the cross of the legs.

safety
- If there is pain or discomfort in the ankles, perform the open variation of *siddhasana* instead.
- Lift the pelvic floor and tone the low belly.
- Move the base of the sternum back and lift the chest.
- Level the shoulders and center the crown of the head over the pelvic floor. Lift the chin slightly.
- Lengthen the spine.
- Straighten the elbows.

refinement
Siddhasana might as well be translated to mean "occasional pose" instead of "accomplished pose" because it is so seldom taught or practiced (at least in my experience). Consider doing this one as you sit at the computer or while reading at home. Another variation of *siddhasana*, as described below, is an optimal pose to practice *pranayama* (breath control techniques) and meditation:

1. Bend the left knee and place the left heel against the perineum. Lower the top of the foot and shin to the floor.
2. Bend the right knee.
3. Use the right hand to pull the knee higher than the foot and point the toes down. Insert the right toes and top of the foot between the left thigh and calf.
4. Keeping the right knee lifted, with the left hand reach between the right calf and thigh. Pull the top of the left foot up.
5. With the right hand, bring the right knee down to the floor.
6. Place the hands on the knees and straighten the arms.
7. Look straight ahead. Hold the pose and breathe.
8. To come out, straighten the legs and place the hands next to the hips.

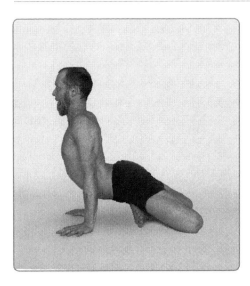

simhasana 2
lion pose 2

shape
(from *padmasana*)

1. Keep the legs in full lotus and come onto the hands and knees with the arms vertical.
2. Separate the hands shoulder-width apart and walk the hands forward to lower the hips toward the floor. Keep the arms straight.
3. Inhale fully. Exhale audibly and completely through the mouth and extend the tongue as far out as possible. Pause and retain the breath.
4. Look up between the eyebrows. Repeat three to five times.
5. To come out, inhale, withdraw the tongue, walk the hands back toward the knees, and lower the hips.

safety
- Evenly press the fingertips and perimeter of the palms into the floor.
- Straighten and strengthen the arms.
- Move the shoulders back, stretch the spine, and lift the chest up.
- Tone the low belly to prevent pain or discomfort in the low back.

• Press the outer edges/tops of the feet into the thighs and clamp the knees closed.

refinement

If you tend to hold tension in your jaw, consider this pose mandatory. Opening the jaw and extending the tongue out releases the jaw muscles. I once had an injury on the left side of my jaw that caused me intense suffering. *Simhasana* was among the most important healing exercises for me. Extend your tongue out to the right and left as well to remove even more tension from your jaw.

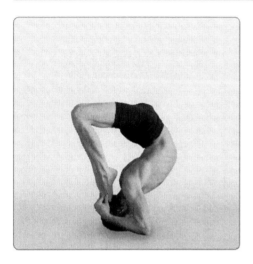

sirsa padasana
head feet pose

shape
(from *sirsasana 1*)

1. Bend the knees.
2. Move the chest forward while simultaneously moving the feet toward the back of the head.
3. As the chest moves forward, begin to lift the head to roll toward the forehead.
4. One at a time, catch the feet with the hands and pull them to the head.
5. Look straight ahead. Hold the pose and breathe.
6. To come out, release the hands and interlace the fingers behind the head. Root down through the head and the forearms, and inhale lift the legs vertical.

safety

• Press the inner edges of the feet together and flare the outer two toes.
• Tone the legs and extend the inner edges of the thighs down.
• Engage the glutes and lift the tailbone.
• Contract the low belly and move the base of the sternum forward.
• Squeeze the shoulders toward each other.
• Extend the upper back and chest toward the floor.
• Stretch the knees and chest in opposite directions—away from the hips.
• Strengthen the entire spine.

refinement

Why would you want to do this pose? If you don't have a burning desire to do it, I highly recommend that you don't! I have little interest in advanced asana these dharma-days. That said, it served me like nothing else when I used to practice that way. Although I'm no longer into it, I'm also all for it. I tell practitioners who are passionate about advanced asana to accomplish what they can, not while they still can, but while they still care. And I tell them to keep in mind that advanced asana is a gamble. You may get *ananda*, you may get agony… and you may get both.

One of the difficult aspects of this pose is the fact that the head is on the floor. Take a look at *vrischikasana 1* and notice how much higher the head is than in *sirsa padasana*. The feet must descend a foot or so farther to reach the head in *sirsa padasana* than in *vrischikasana 1*. Another difficulty is the balance. Once the feet reach the head you can push them into your head to support the balance. But to get the feet to the head without falling over is very difficult. Everything about this pose is challenging.

After I'm finished with this project, I'll go back to practicing and teaching poses that benefit the majority of practitioners. I don't plan on practicing advanced asanas again. Advanced poses were essential to my path for over a decade, which is why I'm willing to write about them. Even if the instructions for the advanced poses in this book only serve four or five people, it will be worth it to me.

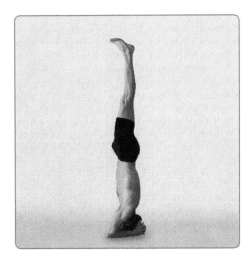

sirsasana 1
headstand pose 1

shape
(from *bharmanasana*)

1. Bring the elbows to the floor directly below the shoulders.
2. Interlace the fingers and pull the wrists apart. Point the thumbs up.
3. Place the top of the head on the floor in front of the hands and the back of the head in the palms against the thumb pads.
4. Curl the toes under, lift the knees, and straighten the legs.
5. Walk the feet toward the head and transfer most of the body weight onto the head and forearms.

6. Lift the heels above the toe mounds and the hips above the head. Keep the upper back vertical.
7. Bend the right knee and lift the heel toward the right sit bone. Bend the left knee and lift the foot toward the left sit bone. Balance on the forearms and top of the head. Pause and breathe.
8. Keeping the knees bent, lift the thighs vertical and point the knees up. Straighten the legs.
9. Bring the spine and legs vertical to the floor. Look forward. Hold the pose and breathe.
10. To come out, exhale, lower the feet to the floor, bend the knees, and place the sit bones on the heels. Reach the arms forward and lower the head between the arms. Pause to rest. Then lift to sit.

safety

- If there is pain or discomfort in the neck, cervical spine injuries or conditions, and/or loss of spinal curvature in the neck, do not lift the feet off the floor. Keep as little weight on the head as possible and seek guidance from a skilled yoga instructor on modifications with blocks, chairs, or even supine.
- Do not practice inversions at any time during menstruation. Practice *supta baddha konasana* (a supine version of *baddha konasana*) on bolsters instead.
- If the upper back rounds before lifting the feet off the floor, do not proceed into the pose. Instead, keep the feet on the floor and lift the head away from the floor. Extend the hips up and back like in *adho mukha svanasana* to open the shoulders in preparation for *sirsasana 1*.
- For extra padding, place a folded blanket on top of the mat or fold the mat into thirds or quarters. More padding than this will compromise the foundation and make the balance difficult.
- Initially, use a wall to develop balance in *sirsasana 1*. Practice with interlaced fingers no more than four inches away from the wall to prevent neck injury if balance is lost. Practice with both heels against the wall, and then lift one foot away from the wall. Eventually, bring both feet away from the wall.
- Press the forearms and wrists down. Lift the shoulders up.
- Extend down through the head and up through the legs.
- Press the inner feet, ankles, and knees together. Engage the glutes.
- Bring the feet halfway between a pointed and flexed position. Spread the toes and reach up through the inner feet.
- Do not allow the legs to move forward, back, or to the sides. Do not allow the hips to turn even slightly to the right or left.
- Engage the abdomen, and move the base of the sternum back and tailbone forward.
- Breathe evenly. Relax the eyes and jaw.

refinement

Sirsasana 1 can be performed for less than one minute and for up to seven minutes and beyond. If you do *sirsasana 1* and cycle, it can take anywhere from 12 to 25 minutes. In general, I do not recommend spending more than 5 to 7 minutes in *sirsasana 1*, even for advanced practitioners. My feeling is that you can gain many of the rewards that *sirsasana 1* has to offer in 5 to 7 minutes, and the longer you stay, the more risky the risks become. I also believe that the rewards of *sirsasana 1*, and *sarvangasana* for that matter, are excellent but not essential. It is often said that *sirsasana* and *sarvangasana* offer more benefits than any other pose. And yet, a full spectrum practice can provide similar benefits to these two poses. So if you cannot practice *sirsasana* and/ or *sarvangasana* for some reason, don't sweat it. Paramount to this practice is profit. In other words, you must walk away from your practice with more than you came with.

Advanced practitioners can come into and out of *sirsasana 1* with straight legs.

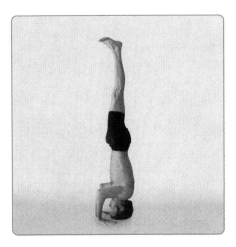

sirsasana 2
headstand pose 2

shape
(from *sirsasana 1*)

1. Keep the abdomen and legs toned and place the hands flat on the floor just in front of the head slightly wider than shoulder-width apart—wrists directly below elbows.
2. Point the index fingers straight back. Look forward. Hold the pose and breathe.
3. To come out, exhale, lower the feet to the floor, bend the knees, and place the sit bones on the heels. Reach the arms forward and lower the head between the arms. Pause to rest. Then lift to sit.

safety
- Press the hands down and lift the shoulders up.
- Extend down through the head. Straighten, strengthen, and stretch the legs.
- Move the tops of the thighs back and center the heels directly above the crown of the head.
- Press the inner feet, ankles, and knees together.
- Bring the feet halfway between a pointed and flexed position. Spread the toes and reach up through the inner feet.
- Engage the glutes and abdomen.
- Move the base of the sternum back and the tailbone forward.
- Breathe steadily. Relax the eyes and jaw.
- If the balance is difficult, practice against or near a wall.

refinement
If moving from *sirsasana 1* into *sirsasana 2* is too difficult, start seated in *vajrasana*, then:
- Lower your forehead to the floor just in front of your knees.
- Lift your hips to roll to the top of your head.
- Place your hands flat on the floor slightly wider than shoulder-width apart.
- Point your index fingers away from your feet. Bring your forearms perfectly vertical.
- Curl your toes under, lift your knees off the floor, and straighten your legs.
- Bring your hips directly over your head, bend your knees, and lift your heels to your sit bones. Hug your thighs against your torso so your knees point down.
- Lift your thighs and point your knees up. Lift your legs vertical and straighten your legs.
- Exit in the same way you entered.

Sirsasana 2 is an excellent entry point to many of the arm balances for advanced practitioners.

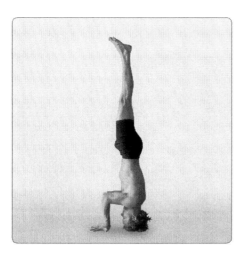

sirsasana 3
headstand pose 3

shape
(from *sirsasana 2*)

1. Extend down through the head and in one movement, bring the outer edges of the hands together in front of the face—elbows at a 90-degree angle.
2. Point the thumbs out and flare the outer two toes to promote balance.
3. Look forward. Hold the pose and breathe.

safety

- Press the tips of the fingers down and lift the shoulders up.
- Push the inner edges of the elbows together.
- Stretch up through the legs and engage the glutes.
- Move the tops of the thighs back and center the heels directly above the crown of the head.
- Press the inner feet, ankles, and knees together.
- Bring the feet halfway between a flexed and pointed position. Spread the toes and push the inner feet up.
- Engage the abdomen, and move the base of the sternum back and the tailbone forward.
- If the balance is difficult, practice against or near a wall.

refinement

If you start to fall backwards, flex your feet. If you start to fall forward, point your feet. To stay in the balance, never disengage your feet. This technique can be applied to any inversion. It is especially useful when learning how to balance in *adho mukha vrksasana*. In *sirsasana 3*, you are more likely to fall over sideways because the surface area is so narrow. This makes the hands more crucial than the feet for balance. If you start to fall to the left, press the right fingertips and thumbs into the floor. If you start to fall to the right, press the left fingertips and thumb into the floor. *Sirsasana 3* is among the most difficult inverted balancing poses in hatha yoga. To learn the balance required in *sirsasana 3*, start with the hands and elbows separated shoulder-width apart. If moving from *sirsasana 2* into *sirsasana 3* proves to be too difficult, start in *vajrasana* as described in *sirsasana 2*.

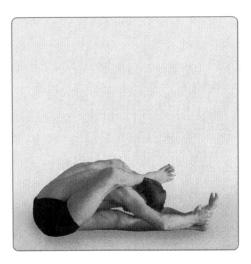

skandasana
War God pose

shape
(from *eka pada sirsasana*)

1. Inhale fully. Exhale, fold the torso over the extended leg.
2. Hold the front foot with both hands.
3. Place the forehead on the kneecap of the extended leg. Pause and breathe, then bring the forehead to the shin. Hold the pose and breathe.
4. To come out, release the hands and lift the torso vertical.

Repeat on the second side.

safety
- Engage both feet, especially the top foot.
- Isometrically bend the top knee to engage the hamstrings.
- Press the hands down, lift the shoulders up.
- Straighten and strengthen the extended leg. Tone the thigh and tighten at the knee. Press the back of the knee down.
- Lift the pelvic floor and tone the low belly.

refinement
A good way to prepare the back and spine for the leg-behind-the-head variations is to hold *paschimottanasana* for a full five minutes. To prepare the hamstrings, practice *krounchasana*, and to prepare the hips, hold *agnistambhasana* and/or *yogadandasana* for three minutes on each side.

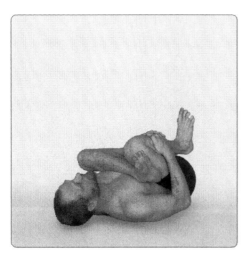
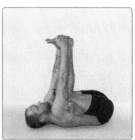

sucirandhrasana
eye of the needle pose

shape
(from *supta tadasana*)

1. Bend both knees and bring the feet to the floor in front of the sit bones.
2. Lift the feet and bring the outer left ankle onto the right thigh just below the knee. Flex both feet.
3. Reach the left arm through the space between the legs and interlace the fingers around the right shin.
4. Inhale fully. Exhale, bend the elbows out to the sides and bring the top shin toward/to the chest. Reach the left knee away from the shoulder.
5. Look up. Hold the pose and breathe.
6. To come out, release the clasp. Uncross, lower, and straighten the legs.

Repeat on the second side.

safety

- Engage the thighs and feet to create stability in the knees.
- Extend out through the inner edge of the top foot.
- Relax the shoulders and throat even as the upper body engages to draw the legs in toward the chest.
- Lift the pelvic floor and tone the low belly.
- Allow the low back to round.
- To reduce the intensity of the stretch, interlace the fingers around the thigh instead of the calf and keep the arms straight.

refinement

Sucirandhrasana can be a deep hip opener if you bring your shin to your chest and keep it parallel to the floor and the top of your mat. To help bring your left knee and ankle equidistant to the floor, lean onto your right hip, and slide your left elbow up your leg toward your knee and push your elbow into your left thigh. For a more intense variation of *sucirandhrasana*, release your hands and bring your right shin vertical–heel over knee. Clasp your foot with your hands, and bend your knee until your heel is directly above your knee. Bend your elbows out to the sides and pull your shin to your chest. This variation of *sucirandhrasana* is a good preparatory pose for *eka pada galavasana*. *Sucirandhrasana* is also an appropriate alternate pose if *agnistambasana* is too intense for your hips or knees.

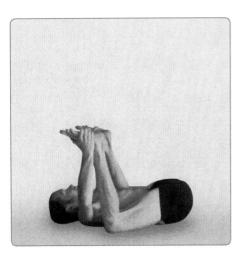

sukha balasana
happy baby pose

shape
(from *supta tadasana*)

1. Bend the knees, lift the feet, and with the arms to the insides of the legs, hold the outsides of the feet. Stack the heels directly above the knees.
2. Inhale fully. Exhale, bend the elbows and pull the knees toward/to the floor just outside of the torso.
3. Allow the low back to round. Look up. Hold the pose and breathe.
4. To come out, release the hands. Lower and straighten the legs.

safety

- Flex the feet and flare the toes.
- Push the feet into the hands and pull the feet with the hands.
- Isometrically kick the heels toward the sit bones to engage the hamstrings.
- Relax the shoulders, throat, and jaw.

refinement

To deepen the pose, reach your tailbone down toward the floor. Use your upper body strength to draw your knees to the floor, but keep your face soft and relaxed. *Sukha balasana* is a good preparatory pose for *kurmasana*, *dwi hasta bhujasana*, and *tittibhasana*.

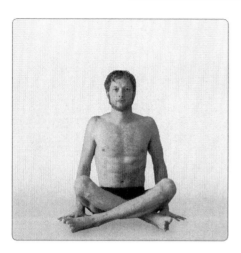

sukhasana
easy pose

shape
(from *dandasana*)

1. Place the hands or fingertips on the floor slightly wider than the shoulders.
2. Bend the knees and cross the legs by bringing the right foot on the floor about 12 inches in front of the left hip and the left foot just forward of the right knee in line with the right hip. Press the middle of the shins together.
3. Lower the knees to the sides—knees over feet.
4. Place the hands on the legs and look straight ahead. Hold the pose and breathe.
5. To come out, straighten the legs and place the hands next to the hips.

Repeat on the second side—change the cross of the legs.

safety

- Press the hands into the floor, lift the hips up, and move the sit bones back so the low back curves in. Lower the hips back down to the floor.
- If the low back does not curve in, sit up on one or more blankets—edge of blanket to mid-thigh, feet and ankles on floor.
- Press the outer edges of the feet down.
- Move the shoulder blades down the back.
- Stretch the spine up and lift the top of the sternum.
- Move the low belly in.
- Level the shoulders and center the crown of the head over the pelvic floor. Lift the chin slightly.
- Keep the shins parallel to the edge of the mat.

refinement

If placing your hands on your knees draws your shoulders forward, slide your hands back slightly to widen your collarbones and open across your chest. Keep your arms straight. *Sukhasana* is good preparation for *agnistambhasana*, which is a good preparation for *padmasana*. If you cannot perform *sukhasana*, do not attempt *padmasana*. While the name translates to "easy pose," *sukhasana* is not necessarily an easy pose. In fact, *sukhasana* is a difficult pose for many practitioners. Practice this one diligently until the difficult becomes doable. Heed these words from the *Tao De Ching*: "Confront the difficult while it is still easy."[1]

---

[1]   Stephen Mitchell, *Tao De Ching* (New York: Harper Perennial, 1988), passage 63.

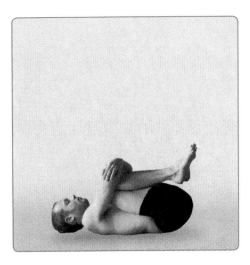

supta balasana
reclined baby pose

shape
(from *supta tadasana*)

1. Bend both knees, lift the feet off the floor, and bring the thighs toward/to the torso.
2. Wrap the arms around the shins. Hold the elbows with the hands.
3. Bring the inner edges of the feet together. Look up. Hold the pose and breathe.
4. To come out, release the arms and lower the legs.

safety

• Relax.

refinement

For safety I could have included things like: engage the feet, press the shins and elbows into each other, tone the pelvic floor and low belly, and so on and so forth. In this pose, such alignment cues would block the benefits, which are primarily relaxation and reflection. In hatha yoga we must learn to both fully engage and relax. Relaxation is a precious and often limited resource. Make hatha yoga your refuge of relaxation! *Supta balasana* is a great pose to practice just prior to *savasana*.

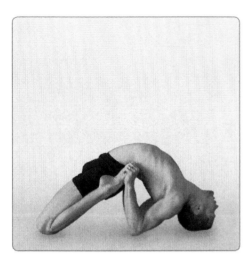

supta bhekasana
reclined frog pose

shape
(from *supta virasana*)

1. Lift the torso to lean onto the forearms with the upper arms vertical. Keep the chin tucked into the chest.
2. Press the forearms down to momentarily lift the hips, round the low back, and then lower the hips back down to the floor.
3. Lean to the left. Lift the right hip and leg off the floor to slide the right hand underneath the right foot with the palm up.
4. Lower the right knee back down to the floor but keep the right hip slightly elevated. Repeat on the other side.
5. One at a time, little by little, walk the knees back and lift the hands, feet, and hips.
6. Once the body weight is no longer on the forearms and is completely on the elbows, turn the hands out to the sides and then toward the head to clasp the toes and tops of the feet.
7. Curl the head back and lower the top of the head to the floor.
8. Look at the tip of the nose. Hold the pose for five breaths.
9. To come out, one at a time slide the feet down the inner edges of the forearms to the floor (otherwise the legs and feet will slam into the floor). Lift the head and walk the elbows back and place the forearms on the floor. Lift the torso vertical.

safety

- Keep the inner edges of the feet against the outer edges of the hips from start to finish.
- Engage the feet, spread the toes, and press the tops of the feet into the hands.
- Lift the tailbone and tone the low belly.
- Engage the glutes.
- Press the head into the floor.
- If there is pain or discomfort on the elbows, place a folded blanket underneath the elbows for extra padding.

refinement

Advanced practitioners can come into this pose from *setu bandha sarvangasana* and/or *sarvangasana*.

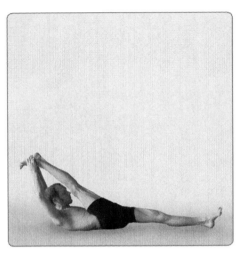
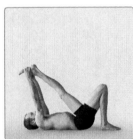

supta dwi hasta padasana
reclined two hand foot pose

forehead to shin

shape
(from *supta tadasana*)

1. Lift the right leg and interlace the fingers around the foot.
2. Straighten the arms and top leg.
3. Inhale fully. Exhale, pull the top leg toward the torso and lift the head off the floor to bring the forehead toward/to the shin. Look up. Hold the pose and breathe.
4. To come out, release the hands and lower the head and leg.

Repeat on the second side.

safety
- Engage the bottom leg and press the back of the leg into the floor. Point the kneecap directly up.
- Engage the glutes of the lifted leg.
- Lock the elbows and knees into a straight position.
- Press the hands and top foot into each other.
- Move the ribs and shoulders toward/to the floor.
- Lift the pelvic floor and tone the low belly.
- To reduce the intensity of the hamstring stretch of the top leg, keep the leg straight and use a strap to hold the foot. If it is still too intense, bend the knee of the bottom leg and place the foot on the floor.

refinement
This pose strengthens the abdomen and neck as much as it stretches the hamstrings of the top leg.

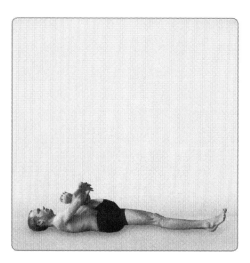

supta hindolasana
reclined baby cradle pose

shape
(from *supta tadasana*)

1. Bend both knees and bring the feet to the floor in front of the sit bones.
2. Lift the feet and bring the outer left ankle onto the right thigh just below the knee. Flex both feet.
3. Wrap the right elbow around the left foot and the left elbow around the left knee. Interlace the fingers around the shin.
4. Lower the right foot and lift the head.
5. Straighten the bottom leg and lift the foot up and in line with the head.
6. Keep the bottom leg straight and exhale, lower the head and heel to the floor.
7. Look up. Hold the pose and breathe.
8. To come out, release the clasp and lower the top leg to the floor.

Repeat on the second side.

safety

- If the arms cannot wrap around the top shin, hold the top foot with one hand and use the opposite hand to hold the outer shin.
- Engage the top thigh and foot to create stability in the knee.
- Press the inner edge of the top foot into the biceps.
- Squeeze the elbows in toward each other and pull the top shin toward the collarbones.
- Engage the bottom leg—point the kneecap and toes up, and press the back of the leg down.
- If the lower leg cannot straighten and lower to the floor, either keep the foot and head lifted with the leg straight, or bend the bottom knee and place the foot in front of the sit bone. Little by little, slide the foot away from the sit bone until the leg can eventually straighten with the head on the floor.

refinement

Bring your top shin parallel to the floor and the top of the mat. Continue to reach your top thigh away from your chest even as you draw the leg into the chest. Keep your bottom foot in line with your outer hip. *Supta hindolasana* is an excellent preparatory pose for *eka pada galavasana*. It is also a good alternate pose for *bhairavasana*.

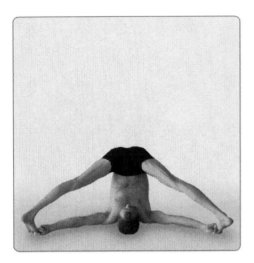

supta konasana
reclined angle pose

shape
(from *halasana*)

1. Separate the feet to capacity without bending the knees.
2. Hold the big toes with the first two fingers and thumbs.
3. Elevate the hips above the shoulders until the spine is vertical.
4. Straighten the arms and legs. Look up past the tip of the nose. Hold the pose and breathe.
5. To come out, release the hands and bring the feet together.

safety
- Keep the seventh cervical (the bony protrusion at the base of the neck) off the floor. If your seventh cervical touches the floor in *halasana*, place folded blankets below the torso and shoulders as described in *sarvangasana 1*.
- Press the shoulders down, in toward each other, and forward toward the head.
- Center the head and press the head down. Bring the chin vertical.
- Straighten and strengthen the legs.
- Extend the hips and spine up.
- Breathe evenly.

refinement
Props are a necessary option in many of the poses in the *sarvangasana* cycle. The downside of blankets in *halasana* and *supta konasana* is that the shoulders are higher than the feet, which makes for a more intense hamstring stretch. The paradox of props is that it can make a pose both less and more difficult. As Douglas Brooks, founder of Rajanaka Yoga, says, "Yoga is a paradox to be embraced."[1] Embrace the paradox, use props for *sarvangasana* and cycle! (You can even use props for *parsva sarvangasana* if you have shoulderstand pads available—they offer a solid enough foundation.)

[1]   Personal Douglas Brooks lecture notes.

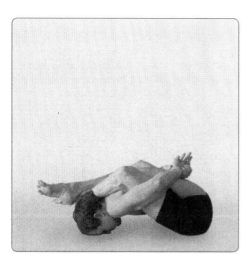

supta kurmasana
sleeping tortoise pose

shape
(from *dandasana*)

1. Separate the legs so the feet are slightly wider than the mat.
2. Inhale fully. Exhale, fold the torso forward between the legs. Keep the heels on the floor and bend the knees slightly.
3. One at a time, lower the shoulders beneath the knees. Bring the forehead to the floor and reach the arms out to the sides. Pause and breathe.
4. Bend the elbows and use the hands to draw the feet toward each other. Hook the right foot over the left foot or vice versa.
5. Lift the chest slightly and reach the arms back behind the hips—palms facing up. Wrap the arms behind the back and clasp the hands.
6. Walk the feet toward the head and place the head underneath the feet at the ankles.
7. Look toward the tip of the nose. Hold the pose and breathe.
8. To come out, inhale, lift the head. Release the hands and feet, and the shoulders from underneath the torso. Lift the torso vertical.

safety

- If the hands cannot clasp behind the back, use a strap or stretch the arms straight back or out to the sides.
- If the legs cannot hook in front of the head, draw the feet in as close together as possible and stretch the legs straight.
- Engage and flex the feet. Flare the outer two toes of each foot.
- Isometrically bend the knees to engage the hamstrings.
- Allow the spine to stretch deeply.
- Lift the pelvic floor and tone the low belly.

refinement

Switch the feet throughout the pose, especially if you are holding the pose for an extended period of time. Also, when practicing this pose repeatedly, it is easy to favor one side over the other. Instead of always bringing the same leg behind the head first, break the habit and use the less dominant side first. Another entry point for this pose is to lower the body from *dwi pada sirsasana,* which is the most efficient way to come into the pose, if you can do *dwi pada sirsasana.* For some, sitting upright is an easier position to bring the feet behind the head than folded over on the floor. For the rest, the above instructions beginning in *dandasana* offer various stages in which you can come into modified and less intense variations of the pose. It is possible to pause and hold the pose at any point leading up to the final instruction. *Supta kurmasana* puts definite pressure on the head, and this pressure is deeply calming.

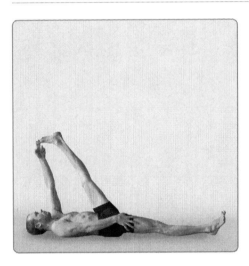

supta padangusthasana 1
reclined big toe pose 1

shape
(from *supta tadasana*)

1. Lift the right foot and hold the big toe with the first two fingers and thumb of the right hand.
2. Place the left hand on the left quads.
3. Straighten the arms and legs.
4. Pull the right shoulder toward/to the floor. Look up. Hold the pose and breathe.
5. To come out, release the arms and lower the leg.

Repeat on the second side.

safety
- Draw the kneecaps up to engage the legs.
- Lock the elbows and knees into a straight position.
- Press the bottom heel down and in.
- Turn the inner thigh of the lower leg down toward the floor.
- Turn the thigh of the lifted leg out to center the kneecap.
- Extend out through the inner edges and the toe mounds of both feet.
- Push the foot into the top hand and pull the foot with the hand.
- To reduce the intensity of the hamstring stretch, extend the right shoulder away from the floor or use a strap to hold the foot.
- Keep the chin slightly lifted. Pressing the chin toward the throat is often a sign of tension and/ or overworking.

refinement

Yoga can alleviate or exasperate weaknesses in the body. In order to turn weakness into strength, proper alignment is essential. Even proper alignment cannot protect you if you operate with force or past your capacity. Pay attention to what your body is telling you as you practice. Not enough is not enough and too much is too much.

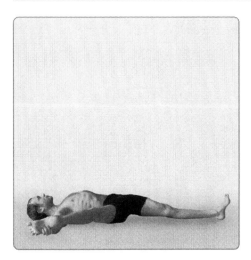

supta padangusthasana 2
reclined big toe pose 2

shape
(from *supta tadasana*)

1. Lift the right leg vertical. Clasp the outer edge of the foot with the right hand.
2. Extend the left arm out to the side—wrist in line with shoulder, palm facing up.
3. Straighten the arm and legs.
4. Inhale fully. Exhale, lower the right foot and arm out to the right side. Look up. Hold the pose and breathe.
5. To come out, inhale, lift the leg and arm vertical. Exhale, release the leg and arms.

Repeat on the second side.

safety

- If the hand cannot clasp the foot with straight legs, use a strap. Hold the strap as close to the foot as possible to straighten the arm.
- If the thigh of the bottom leg lifts away from the floor, raise the lifted leg until the back of the sacrum rests evenly on the floor.
- Engage the arms, legs, and left glutes.
- Lock the elbows and knees into a straight position.
- Press the hand and foot into each other.
- Isometrically squeeze the heels toward each other.
- Reach the inner edge of the bottom leg down. Point the toes directly up.
- Push the hip of the lifted leg down away from the ribcage. Roll the thigh out and point the kneecap and toes down slightly.
- Keep the chin vertical.

- To reduce the intensity of the hamstring stretch and/or the demands of the arm, place the foot at an appropriate height against a wall, or prop the outer leg up on a chair or block.

refinement

To strengthen your hands and arms, hold your big toe with your first two fingers and thumb instead of your outer foot. To stay in the pose for an extended period of time, place a block of appropriate height underneath your outer thigh to prop up your leg, and rest. Keep your feet and legs engaged. *Supta padangusthasana 2* is a good preparatory pose for *utthita hasta padangusthasana 2, vasisthasana,* and *eka pada koundinyasana 2.*

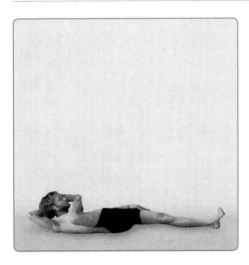

supta padangusthasana 3
reclined big toe pose 3

shape
(from *supta hindolasana*)

1. Hold the outer left foot with the right hand.
2. Lift the head and bring the left elbow behind the head. Clasp the left big toe with the first two fingers and thumb of the left hand. Press the head into the forearm.
3. Place the right hand on the right thigh. Look up. Hold the pose and breathe.
4. To come out, hold the top foot with the right hand. Lift the head and release the top arm. Straighten and lower the leg.

Repeat on the second side.

safety

- Flex the top foot and flare the outer two toes to stabilize the knee.
- Create a bending action in the top knee.
- Pull the big toe with the fingers and thumb.
- Straighten and strengthen the extended leg. Engage the glutes.
- Move the shoulder of the lifted arm back and down toward the floor.
- Rotate the abdomen away from the lifted thigh.
- Lift the pelvic floor and tone the low belly.
- To reduce the intensity of the pose, hold the top foot with the right elbow, bend the bottom knee, and place the foot on the floor.

- If the hand does not have enough strength to clasp the big toe or if there is pain in the toe, hold the heel with the opposite hand for additional support.

refinement

Point the toes of your extended leg up. Articulate the arches of your feet and rest your head on your upper elbow. *Supta padangusthasana 3* is a good preparatory pose for *akarna dhanurasana 1, viranchyasana 1 & 2,* and *buddhasana.* Advanced practitioners can move into this pose directly from *supta padangusthasana 1.*

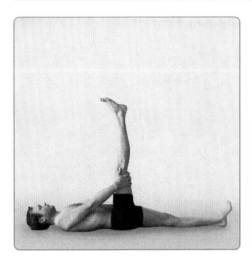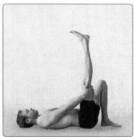

supta padangusthasana prep
reclined big toe pose

shape
(from *supta tadasana*)

1. Keep the right leg straight and lift the leg vertical—heel directly above hip.
2. Interlace the fingers around the back of the leg just below the knee.
3. Engage the feet—bring the feet halfway between a flexed and pointed position, and spread the toes.
4. Move the shoulders toward/to the floor. Look up. Hold the pose and breathe.
5. To come out, release the arms and lower the leg.

Repeat on the second side.

safety

- If the hands cannot clasp the thigh, bend the lower knee or use a strap around the top foot and straighten the arms and legs.
- Lock the elbows and knees into a straight position.
- Press the lower heel down and in.
- Turn the inner thigh of the lower leg down toward the floor.
- Turn the thigh of the lifted leg out to center the kneecap.
- Keep the chin slightly lifted. Pressing the chin toward the throat is often a sign of tension and/or overworking.

refinement

Point the toes of your bottom foot up. To use *supta padangusthasana prep* as a counter-pose to release the low back after backbends, press your thigh into your hands. *Supta padangusthasana prep* teaches the necessary alignment required in *virabhadrasana 3*, *dwi hasta padasana*, and *eka pada sirsasana* (headstand variation). These three poses together can then pave the way to *hanumanasana*.

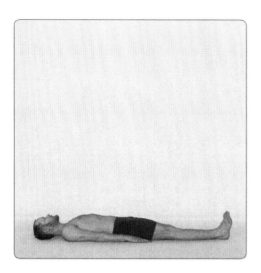

supta tadasana
reclined mountain pose

shape

1. Lie down on the back.
2. Straighten the legs and bring the inner ankles, heels, and feet together.
3. Straighten the arms alongside the torso and press the palms into the floor.
4. Bring the base of the chin vertical and look straight up.
5. Hold the pose and breathe.

safety

- Point the kneecaps and toes straight up.
- Press the inner legs and feet together.
- Extend out through the inner feet. Spread the toes.
- Tighten the kneecaps and elbows.
- Press the tailbone down toward the feet and tone the low belly.
- Lower the shoulder blades onto the back away from the ears.
- Extend down through the feet and up through the head.
- Center the head. Avoid turning the head to the left or right.

refinement

Supta tadasana is a great pose to understand the alignment of *tadasana*. It is a valuable pose in its own right when practiced with earnest and effort. *Supta tadasana* and *savasana* look similar yet feel like polar opposites. *Supta tadasana* is active and more extroverted. *Savasana* is more introverted and passive.

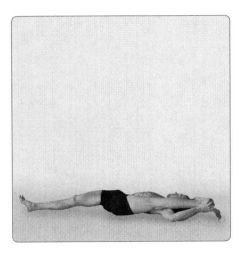

supta trivikramasana
reclined Vishnu's pose

shape
(from *supta tadasana*)

1. Keeping the legs straight, lift the right leg and hold the heel with the hands.
2. Keep the left heel on the floor and lift the head off the floor as high as possible.
3. Bend the arms slightly and pull the inner edge of the right calf to the ear.
4. Inhale, keep the left leg straight and lift the left foot as high as the right foot.
5. Exhale, lower the left heel, head, and right toes to the floor. Look up. Hold the pose and breathe.
6. To come out, lift the top leg, release the hands and lower the leg.

Repeat on the second side.

safety

- Move slowly and with sensitivity.
- Tone the thighs. Tighten the knees and lock the knees into a straight position.
- Point the front of the bottom leg up and the front of the top leg down.
- To reduce the intensity of the pose, bend the bottom knee and place the foot on the floor as close to the sit bone as necessary.
- To lower the top leg to the floor, use the hands to press the outer hip away from the shoulder and move the leg out slightly.

refinement

Keep your legs straight from start to finish. This pose shares a similar geometry to *hanumanasana*. While the shape of the legs is the same, in *hanumanasana* gravity helps bring the hips down. In *supta trivikramasana* however, you must use the strength of your legs and arms to bring your heel and toes to the floor. In addition, because there is very little weight on the feet, it is easy to distort and disengage the legs. The relationship of the torso to the legs is different as well. In *hanumanasana* the torso is upright between the legs. If *supta trivikramasana* were rotated in space with the front body to the floor, it would be obvious that the torso comes into a deep forward fold over the front leg. This reduces the stretch on the back hip flexors and psoas.

Learn to look for similarities and differences between sibling poses and discover how one's relationship to gravity can bring challenge or ease to different aspects of the pose.

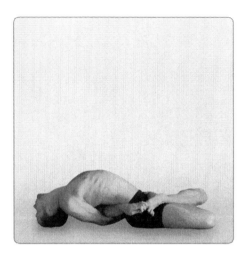

supta vajrasana
reclined thunderbolt pose

shape
(from *padmasana*)

1. With the right shin on top in *padmasana*, swing the right arm behind the back and hold the right big toe with the first two fingers and thumb.
2. Momentarily lean the torso forward. Swing the left arm behind the back, and hold the left big toe with the first two fingers and thumb.
3. Squeeze the knees toward each other until the thighs are nearly parallel to each other.
4. Lift the chest and slide the arms as low down the back as possible.
5. Inhale, lift the thighs. Exhale, roll back onto the elbows.
6. Keeping the clasp of the big toes with the first two fingers and thumbs, bring the top of the head to the floor to lower the legs.
7. Look at the tip of the nose. Hold the pose for five breaths.
8. To come out, release the clasp and lie down on the floor. Lift onto the elbows and lift the torso vertical.

Repeat on the second side—switch the cross of the legs.

safety
- If the hands cannot reach the toes behind the back, use two straps and wrap a strap around the top of each foot.
- To avoid over stretching the knees or shoulders, place a folded blanket below the knees and thighs and a folded blanket below the top of the head before coming into the pose.
- Engage the feet and flare the toes.
- Press the outer edges/tops of the feet down and clamp the knees closed.

refinement
To keep the clasp of the big toes with the fingers and to make this difficult pose quite doable, squeeze the knees and elbows toward each other.

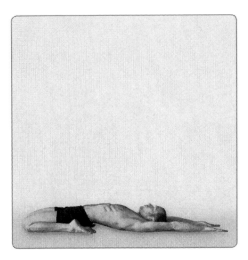

supta virasana
reclined hero pose

shape

1. Come onto the hands and knees with the arms and thighs vertical—shoulders directly over the wrists, hips directly over the knees.
2. Bring the knees together and feet outer hip-width apart.
3. Point the toes straight back and squeeze the ankles in.
4. Lower the hips to the floor between the feet.
5. With the hands, pull the skin underneath the knees forward and the skin underneath the feet out.
6. Inhale fully. Exhale, lean back and lower onto the forearms with the upper arms vertical—elbows below shoulders.
7. Lift the hips, round the low back, and lower the hips back down to the floor. Lift the chest. Pause and breathe.
8. Inhale fully. Exhale, lower the torso and head to the floor.
9. Straighten and stretch the arms overhead—wrists shoulder-width apart. Look up. Hold the pose and breathe.
10. To come out, place the hands on the floor near the hips, lift the head and come onto the forearms. Press the hands and forearms down to lift the torso.

safety

- Spread the toes and press the tops of the feet down.
- Squeeze the outer ankles in.
- Reach the tailbone forward toward the knees. Tone the low belly and relax the low back.
- If the sit bones cannot lower to the floor in *virasana*, place one or more folded blankets below the hips. Before lowering onto the forearms and down in *supta virasana*, remove half of the height of the props below the hips, and place a bolster or several folded blankets below the torso. Do not lower onto the back if the hips hover in mid-air or without first reducing any necessary props below the hips. These actions protect the low back.
- If there is any discomfort in the knees or low back, lie back onto a bolster or several folded blankets to elevate the torso. Separate the arms 30 degrees away the torso—palms facing up.
- If the hands or arms become numb with the arms overhead, bring the arms 30 degrees away from the torso—palms facing up.

refinement

Before lowering the hips to the floor, you may find it beneficial to lift the inner calves back and out with the hands so there is an equal amount of muscle on both sides of the shins. In *supta virasana* relax your body as much as possible without losing the alignment. Hold this pose for 1 to 15 minutes if possible. This pose is deeply calming and promotes both digestion and sleep.

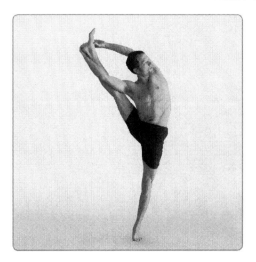

surya yantrasana
sundial pose

standing

shape
(from *tadasana*)

1. Balancing on the left foot, lift the right foot off the floor.
2. Hold the right outer heel with the right hand—arm to inside of leg.
3. Bend the standing leg slightly. Lift the right foot in line with the head.
4. Hold the outside of the right foot with the left hand.
5. Lift the left elbow above the head.
6. Move the head forward and press the back of the head into the upper arm.
7. Straighten the top leg, then straighten the standing leg.
8. Twist the abdomen away from the lifted leg. Turn the head to the left and look past the arm. Hold the pose and breathe.
9. To come out, exhale, look forward. Bend the standing leg slightly and release the head. Release the hands and lower the leg. Bring the arms to the sides.

Repeat on the second side.

safety

- To reduce the intensity of the hamstring stretch, bend the top knee.
- Before straightening the top leg, pull the foot with the hands and push the foot into the hands.
- Engage the standing leg—tone the thighs and lift the kneecap.
- Move the top elbow and shoulder back.
- Press the tailbone down and draw the low belly in.

refinement

It is the shadow on a sundial that tells the time. Similarly, it is our shadows, or darknesses, that can reveal the next step that we must undertake on our spiritual path. In this way, the discomfort we may experience in this pose is similar to the discomfort of facing our shadows. A yogin must navigate and not negate the dark side of practicing the dharma. One of the benefits of advanced asana is that we are required to make skillful choices in the midst of muck and mire.

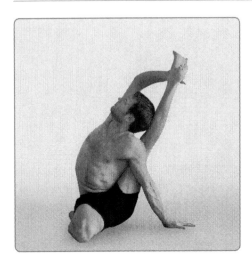

surya yantrasana
sundial pose

shape
(from *dandasana*)

1. Bend the right knee and place the inner ankle against the right outer hip. Lower the leg to the floor and point the foot back.
2. Lean to the left and pull the right glutes back with the right hand. Repeat on the other side.
3. Bend the left knee and hold the left heel with the right hand.
4. Hold the left calf with the left hand—arm to the inside of the leg.
5. Lift the foot and bring the left shoulder under the back of the knee.
6. Keeping the shoulder back, place the left palm on the floor behind and to the left of the hips. Straighten the left arm.
7. Hold the outside of the left foot with the right hand—palm to the top of the foot.
8. Press the lower hand down.
9. Straighten the left leg and reach the head forward between the arm and leg.
10. Inhale fully. Exhale, rotate the chest away from the extended leg and turn the chin toward the armpit. Look up. Hold the pose and breathe.
11. To come out, bend the top knee, lower the foot and look forward. Release the top hand and straighten the legs. Place the hands next to the hips.

Repeat on the second side.

safety

- If there is pain in the lower knee, practice *surya yantrasana* with the lower leg in *baddha konasana*. Pull the heel as close to the perineum as possible.

- To reduce the intensity of the hamstring stretch, straighten the leg slowly and do not force the leg straight. Instead, use a strap around the top foot before straightening the leg.
- Allow the sit bone to lift as needed.
- Pull the top foot back with the hand and press the top foot forward into the hand.
- Pull the outer edge of the top foot with the fingers. Extend the inner edge of the top foot up with the thumb.

refinement

As your top leg straightens, rotate your leg in and move your left sit bone back. Lower your hip. Lift your top elbow away from your head to move your head through your arm and leg.

Surya yantrasana requires both strength and flexibility in the thighs, hips, hamstrings, and shoulders. If you cannot even begin to approach the form of some of these poses, then they will not offer their benefits. If you have tight thighs, hamstrings, and shoulders, attempting this pose will likely cause more problems than benefits. I've said it before and I'll say it again: All that hatha yoga has to offer can be found in the basic poses. The more advanced poses are not more valuable. Another way of saying it: As the poses get more difficult, the risks increase while the rewards essentially remain the same.

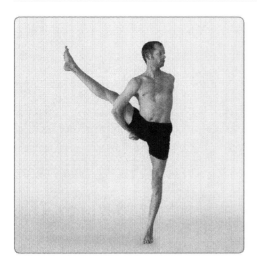

svarga dvijasana
bird of paradise pose

shape
(from *lunge pose*)

1. Pivot the back heel down and turn the foot in 30 degrees.
2. Place both hands on the floor inside of the front foot and fold the torso inside the front thigh.
3. Hold the back of the right calf with the right hand.
4. Bring the right shoulder underneath the right knee—top of shoulder to back of calf.
5. Place the back of the right hand on the outer right hip.
6. Swing the left arm behind the torso. Hold the left wrist with the right hand.
7. Look down and step the left foot forward next to the right foot—feet outer hip-width apart.
8. Bend both knees.

9. Balancing on the left foot, lift the right foot off the floor and stand upright.
10. Straighten the standing leg.
11. Lift the right shin parallel to the floor. Pause and breathe, then straighten the lifted leg completely.
12. Turn the head to the left and gaze past the left shoulder. Hold the pose and breathe.

To come out, exhale, look forward. Bend the standing knee and lower the top foot next to the standing foot—feet parallel, hip-width apart. Hop the left foot back to a long stance. Release the hands and place them on either side of the front foot. Lift the back heel.Repeat on the second side.

safety

- Strengthen the standing leg—lift the kneecap.
- Before straightening the lifted leg, engage the arms. Shrug the right shoulder up and back.
- Press the elbow into the knee, knee into the elbow.
- If the hamstrings are tight or if there is pain or discomfort in the shoulder when clasping the leg, keep the lifted leg bent.
- If it is difficult to balance, keep the gaze straight ahead.

refinement

Turn your navel away from your top leg. Flex your lifted foot, and flare your outer two toes to empower the leg. If there is ample flexibility in your opposite shoulder, slide your arm up the leg to stand even more upright. Learn to move into and out of poses with care and grace. Use your breath to facilitate each movement. Lifting the foot off the floor in *svarga dvijasana* takes incredible strength in the quadriceps of the standing leg, as well as in the low back. Meet the demand for strength with slow, executed movements rather than jerky or bouncy actions, which will throw off the balance in this pose. Similarly, place as much value on the exit of the pose as the entrance (and the pose itself). Learning to move with precision and grace will build strength in the body and develop focus in the mind. This is a good preparatory pose for *parsvaika pada sirsasana, marichyasana 1, malasana 1,* and *surya yantrasana.*

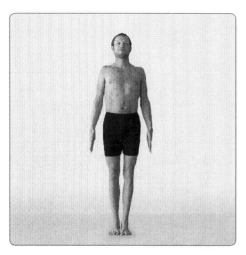
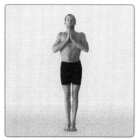

tadasana
mountain pose

shape

1. Bring the inner edges of the feet together.
2. Bring the arms by the sides.
3. Straighten the arms and legs.
4. Lift the chin slightly. Look straight ahead. Hold the pose and breathe.

safety

- Distribute the weight evenly on the feet. In other words, do not lean forward, back, or to one side or the other.
- Press the big toes down, flare the outer two toes—create space between the toes.
- Engage the thighs, lift the kneecaps.
- Squeeze the feet and legs together.
- Engage the glutes.
- Move the tailbone down and the low belly in.
- Move the base of the sternum back and lift the chest.
- Lock the knees and elbows into a straight position.

refinement

A primary purpose of this pose is to get poised for practice. Stretch your entire spine. Extend your head away from your hips. Soften your eyes and jaw. Consciously deepen your breath. One effective way to deepen your breath is by practicing *ujjayi pranayama* (which translates to "victoriously uprising"). To do *ujjayi*, create an aspirant sound with your breath, just as you do when you whisper. Hearing the sound of your breath can help you enhance and refine your practice. Dearth of sound means you are holding your breath—a likely sign of too much effort. At the same time, a loud, exaggerated breath can also mean overexertion; trying too hard is one of the easiest things to do in this practice. In general, breathe deeply and evenly in each pose. Some of the more challenging poses will require a labored breath to meet their demands. Awareness of your breath serves as a barometer of both the quantity and quality of your effort. If doing *ujjayi pranayama* creates tension in your face, throat, or jaw, simply breathe normally.

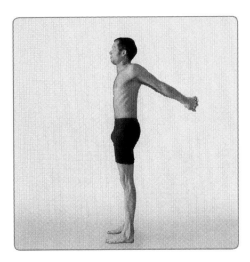

tadasana
mountain pose

hands bound

shape
(from *tadasana*)

1. Interlace the fingers behind the hips.
2. Bend the elbows, rest the hands on the sacrum.
3. Lift the shoulders and squeeze the shoulder blades together on the back.
4. Straighten the arms.
5. Look down, lift the arms up and back.
6. Lift the chin, look straight ahead. Hold the pose and breathe.
7. To come out, exhale, release the hands.

Repeat with the alternate clasp.

safety
- Engage the thighs—lift the kneecaps.
- Engage the glutes.
- Move the tailbone down and the low belly in.
- When looking down, engage the abdominal muscles and move the base of the sternum back. Keeping the base of the sternum back, lift the chest and chin, and look straight ahead.
- If the shoulder blades move apart, if the shoulders round, or if there is any pain in the shoulders, bend the elbows.

refinement
Extend your wrists, elbows, and shoulders back. This pose is a good preparation for *setu bandha sarvangasana, uttana mayurasana prep,* and *sarvangasana 2.*

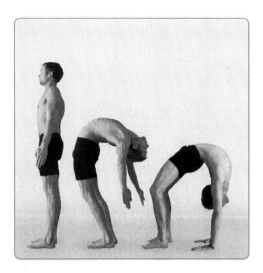

tadasana to urdhva dhanurasana
from mountain to upward-facing bow pose (dropback)

shape
(from *tadasana*)

1. Separate the feet outer hip-width apart. Point the palms forward. Inhale, squeeze the shoulder blades together toward the spine and lift the chest. Exhale, curl the head and torso back until the floor behind the feet becomes visible.
2. Widen the arms out to the sides to bring the arms back overhead and softly lower the hands to the floor—forearms vertical.
3. Hold this pose for five or more breaths.
4. Rock the chest and hips back and forth several times.
5. As the hips rock forward, inhale, transfer the weight of the body onto the feet and bring the arms alongside the hips. Keep the chest lifted and lift the torso. Once the torso is upright, lift the head.

safety

- Do not attempt this pose unless it is possible to practice *urdhva dhanurasana 1* with straight arms.
- Keep the legs straight for as long as possible and lock the elbows into a straight position from start to finish (if the elbows bend as the hands touch the floor, the head could hit the floor).
- Press the inner edges of the feet down. Move the inner and tops of the thighs back.
- Engage the glutes. Extend the tailbone down and push the hips forward.
- Lift the pelvic floor and tone the low belly.
- Stretch the spine and lift the chest.
- Keep the neck muscles engaged—do not relax the neck.
- If standing back up is too difficult, bend the elbows and tuck the chin into the chest to lower onto the floor after performing the dropback.

refinement

Just before lowering your hands to the floor, it may be helpful to temporarily lift your heels off the floor. This will transfer all of the weight into your feet, which will make lowering your hands to the floor safer, softer, and less scary. It is also possible to learn to drop-back and return to standing by walking the hands up and down a wall.

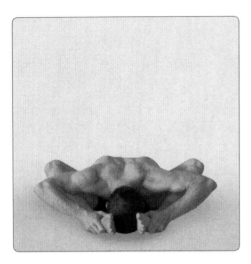

tarasana
omega/star pose

shape
(from *baddha konasana*)

1. Slide the feet approximately 12 inches forward.
2. Hold the feet with the hands and separate them six inches apart.
3. Inhale fully. Exhale, fold the torso forward and round the back.
4. Place the forehead on the floor between the feet. Hold the pose and breathe.
5. To come out, lift the head and torso vertical. Bring the feet together and draw the heels toward the hips.

safety
- Press the outer edges of the feet down.
- Isometrically pull the feet up with the hands and squeeze the feet toward the hips.
- Tilt the pelvis forward.
- Move the inner thighs down.
- Lift the pelvic floor and tone the low belly.

refinement
This pose can also be done with the feet together. The action of joining the head to the feet is significant in many ways. Whether the feet and head meet in a backbend such as *eka pada rajakapotasana 1*, or in a forward fold such as *tarasana*, the body creates an unbroken circuit of energy, called a *mudra*. Most *mudras* are hand gestures that place the hands and fingers in specific shapes to achieve a particular energetic outcome.

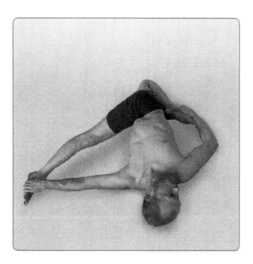

tibetan weaponry pose

shape
(from *supta tadasana*)

1. Bring the right arm out to the side—wrist in line with shoulder, palm facing up.
2. Lift the right leg vertical and hold the inside of the foot with the left hand.
3. Push the left heel down and shift the hips a few inches to the right.
4. Inhale fully. Exhale, roll onto the outer left hip and lower the right foot and left hand to the left and to the floor.
5. Bring the outer left hip, leg, and foot in line with the head.
6. Straighten the arms and legs.
7. Bend the left knee, hold the foot with the right hand, and press the left heel into the left glutes. Keep the left thigh parallel to the long edge of the mat.
8. Lower the right shoulder to the floor. Turn the head to look past the right shoulder. Hold the pose and breathe.
9. To come out, release the left foot and straighten the leg. Inhale, lift the right leg and arm vertical. Return the hips to center. Exhale, lower the leg and arm.

Repeat on the second side.

safety
- If the top foot does not reach the floor, place it on a wall at an appropriate height or rest the leg on a block or bolster. Keep both shoulders on the floor.
- Contract the quads and tighten the hamstrings of the extended leg.
- Push the foot into the hand and push the hand into the foot.
- Extend out through the inner edge of the extended foot. Flare the outer two toes.
- To reduce the intensity of the quad stretch, move the left foot away from the hip.
- To reduce the intensity of the hamstring stretch of the extended leg, use a strap and/or lower the top foot toward the bottom knee. Keep the leg straight.

refinement

This is among the most effective poses for reducing stress for me. That is because I store most of my stress in my legs. One of the benefits of this practice is that it increases body awareness. After even just a few months of practice, most practitioners know exactly where they tend to store stress and what poses help to reduce it. That knowledge is itself a form of weaponry.

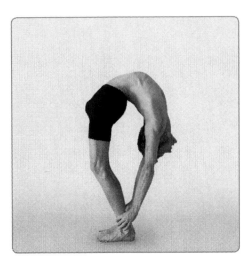

tiriang mukhottanasana
oblique backbend pose

shape
(from *tadasana*)

1. Separate the feet outer hip-width apart.
2. Bend backward and, one at a time, clasp the ankles with the hands.
3. Straighten the arms and legs as much as possible.
4. Curl the head back. Look down toward the floor. Hold the pose and breathe.
5. To come out, keep the chest full and inhale, lift the torso vertical. Once the torso is upright, lift the head.

safety

- Engage the feet and press the inner edges of the feet down. Flare the outer two toes.
- Tone the legs. Move the inner thighs back.
- Contract the glutes and press the tailbone forward.
- Lift the pelvic floor and tone the low belly.
- Move the base of the sternum back and lengthen the spine.
- Tighten the elbows and move the upper arms back.

refinement

When I first started practicing this pose, I thought it would be easier to drop-back from *tadasana* to *urdhva dhanurasana 1*, and then walk the hands back to the ankles. What I found was the balance was difficult and, for me, it was easier to drop-back and grab the ankles directly. *Padangustha dhanurasana* is a good preparatory pose for *tiriang mukhottanasana*.

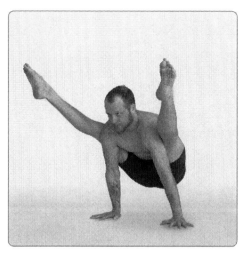

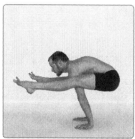

tittibhasana
firefly pose

shape
(from *tadasana*)

1. Separate the outer edges of the feet as wide as the mat.
2. Inhale fully. Exhale, fold the torso over the legs.
3. Widen and bend the knees to bring the shoulders below the knees. Hold the backs of the calves with the hands.
4. Place the thumbs on the centers of the calves and fingers to the outer shins. Press the calves forward and in with the thumbs.
5. One at a time, bring the shoulders behind the knees.
6. Bend the knees and lower the hips. Place the hands on the floor, shoulder-width apart, behind the feet. Separate the fingers and point the index fingers straight ahead.
7. Bring the weight of the body to the hands and lift the feet off the floor.
8. Straighten the arms. Lift and straighten the legs.
9. Look between the eyebrows. Hold the pose and breathe.
10. To come out, exhale, bend the knees and place the feet on the floor. Release the hands and lift to stand.

safety

- Press the fingertips and the perimeter of the palms into the floor with equal pressure.
- Flex the feet and flare the toes.
- Move the shoulders back.
- Spin the inner thighs down and move the heels out as the legs straighten.
- Straighten and strengthen the legs—engage the quads.
- Lift the pelvic floor and tone the low belly.

refinement

To prepare for *tittibhasana*, start with *baddha tittibhasana, eka pada sirsasana, dwi pada sirsasana*, and *yoganidrasana*. Getting the shoulders as far behind the knees and legs as possible is what is required to lift the legs vertical in *tittibhasana*.

Another variation of *tittibhasana* is to reach your torso and head forward to lift your hips up and back. This will lift your legs parallel to the floor. Use your hands to push away from the floor. Actively round your back by engaging your core and reaching your front body toward your back body. Extend out through your legs and feet. One key difference between the two variations of *tittibhasana* with legs vertical and legs horizontal, is that the legs horizontal position requires an immense amount of core strength to lift the hips as high as the feet.

Advanced practitioners can press up into *adho mukha vrksasana* for 15 to 30 seconds. Exhale, slowly lower into *uttanasana*. Inhale, lift the torso to return to *tadasana*.

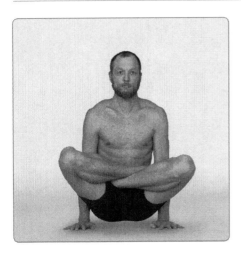

tolasana
scale pose

shape
(from *padmasana*)

1. Place the hands on the floor directly below the shoulders on the outside of the hips.
2. Lean back and point the knees up.
3. Inhale fully. Exhale, lean forward and lift the hips and thighs away from the floor. Press the hands and shoulders down.
4. Look straight ahead. Hold the pose and breathe.
5. To come out, exhale, bend the elbows to lower the hips to the floor.

Repeat on the second side—switch the cross of the legs.

safety

- Press the fingertips and the perimeter of the palms into the floor with firm and equal pressure.
- Press the outer edges/tops of the feet into the upper thighs. Squeeze the heels toward the hips.
- Flare the toes.
- Lift the pelvic floor and engage the abdomen.
- To decrease the difficulty of the pose, place the hands on blocks.

refinement

There are more than fifty asanas that require *ardha padmasana* or *padmasana*. Once you can perform those poses, you enter into a new realm of asana possibility.

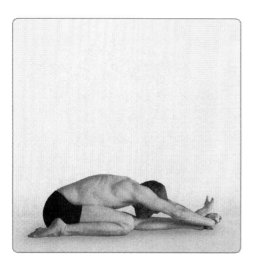

triang mukhaikapada paschimottanasana
three limbs face to one leg back stretched out pose

shape
(from *dandasana*)

1. Bend the right knee and place the inner ankle against the right outer hip. Lower the leg to the floor and point the foot back.
2. Lean to the left and pull the right glutes back with the right hand. Repeat on the other side.
3. Bring the knees together and thighs parallel.
4. Inhale, lift the arms. Exhale, fold the torso forward and hold the left foot with both hands. If possible, hold the right wrist with the left hand and extend the elbows out to the sides.
5. Inhale fully. Exhale, fold the torso over the legs. Place the forehead toward/to the knee. Pause here for a few breaths, then bring the chin toward/to the shin. Look down. Hold the pose and breathe.
6. To come out, release the hands and place the hands on the floor underneath the shoulders. Inhale, lift the head and torso upright. Straighten both legs and place the hands by the hips.

Repeat on the second side.

safety

- Before folding forward, the low back must curve in. If the low back rounds, sit up on one or more folded blankets—foot off the blanket.
- Use the hands to spin the inner left thigh down and the hamstrings muscles out before folding forward.
- Press the right heel into the outer hip.
- Tone the left quads and press the back of the knee.
- Pull the front foot with the hands and push the foot into the hands. Press both sit bones evenly into the floor.
- Lift the pelvic floor and tone the low belly.

refinement

Triang mukhaikapada paschimottanasana combines *virasana* with *paschimottanasana*. Learn the alignment and mechanics of each of these poses to inform and qualify *triang mukhaikapada paschimottanasana*.

No pose can be learned in isolation, one pose informs another. Each pose exists individually and is also intricately related to the full gamut of asana. Each breath has two primary aspects: the inhale and exhale. Those two things together make up one breath. The same can be said for poses like *utthita trikonasana* and *parivrtta trikonasana*, or *sirsasana 1* and *sarvangasana 1*. Together they, in a sense, make one complete pose. This, of course, is my opinion, not a fact. And even if it were a fact, that wouldn't make it true because as Douglas Brooks says, "Most facts eventually get replaced by better facts."[1]

---

[1]   Personal Douglas Brooks lecture notes.

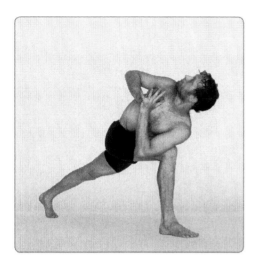

twisted lunge pose

shape
(from *lunge pose*)

1. Hold the upper right thigh with the right hand—thumb on top of thigh, fingers on outer thigh.
2. Inhale, lift the torso and left arm vertical.
3. Exhale, twist the torso to the right and place the outer left shoulder against the outer right knee.
4. Press the palms together—point the right elbow up.
5. Rotate the right shoulder over the left shoulder.
6. Tone the low belly and turn the abdomen and ribs to the right.
7. Shrug the right shoulder up and back. Look up. Hold the pose and breathe.
8. To come out, exhale, look down. Inhale, release the hands to the floor.

Repeat on the second side.

safety

- Squeeze the feet toward each other.
- Engage the back leg and glutes.
- Isometrically turn the front foot clockwise, tilt the right knee out, and move the right hip back and down.
- Without moving the front knee, move the back heel forward until it is vertical.
- Move the tailbone down and low belly in.
- Move the base of the sternum back, stretch up through the chest.
- To stabilize the spine and deepen the twist, press the hands together and press the elbow into the knee and the knee into the elbow.

refinement

Press your front heel down and back foot down and in. Move your hips to the left until your front thigh is parallel to the long edge of the mat. Keep your head and hips centered. The head tends to swing to the right while the hips swing to the left. Extend your head away from your hips to lengthen your spine. Allow your breath to breathe itself. In most twists it will be difficult to breathe evenly. Breathe as deeply and evenly as possible.

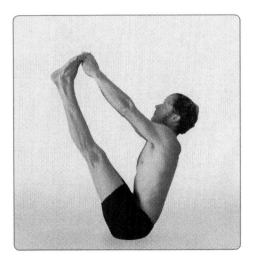

ubhaya padangusthasana
both big toes pose

shape
(from *dandasana*)

1. Bend the knees and bring the arms to the insides of the legs.
2. Hold the big toes with the first two fingers and thumbs of both hands.
3. Lean back and lift the feet off the floor. Bring the shins parallel to the floor and flex the feet.
4. Balancing on the backs of the sit bones, straighten the legs and arms. Lift the low back and chest, and look up. Hold the pose and breathe.
5. To come out, exhale, bend the knees. Release the hands and lower the arms and legs. Stretch the legs straight and bring the inner feet together. Place the hands next to the hips.

safety
- To reduce the intensity of the hamstring stretch, separate the feet outer hip-width apart, or, if needed, as wide as the mat.
- With the shins still parallel to the floor, press the big toes and fingers together.
- Lift the shoulders up and back.
- Before straightening the legs, the low back must be curved in. If the low back is rounding, do not proceed further into this pose.
- Straighten and strengthen the legs and arms.
- Tighten the knees and tone the thighs.
- Lift the pelvic floor and tone the low belly.

refinement
From *ubhaya padangusthasana*, inhale, roll back into *halasana* with your first two fingers and thumbs holding the big toes. Exhale, roll back into *ubhaya padangusthasana*, pause and balance. Do this five times in a row. At first your knees will likely bend as you move from *halasana* into *ubhaya padangusthasana*. Eventually keep the legs straight from start to finish. Rolling across the low back in this way invigorates the spine and energizes the mind.

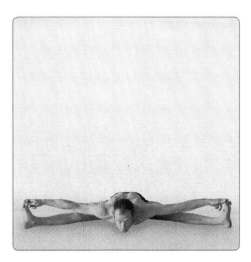

upavishta konasana
seated angle pose

shape
(from *dandasana,* facing long edge of mat)

1. Widen the legs to a 90-degree angle or beyond.
2. Press the hands down and lift the hips off the floor slightly.
3. Move the top of the pelvis forward and the sit bones back. Lower the hips.
4. Keep the hips down and flex and point the feet in rapid succession to widen the legs. Press the calves into the floor and lift the heels as the feet flex. Press the heels into the floor as the feet point. This action will drag the hips, glutes, and hamstrings back. (See *ardha baddha padma paschimottanasana.*)
5. Inhale fully. Exhale, fold the torso forward and place the chin on the floor.
6. Hold the big toes with the first two fingers and thumbs.
7. Look forward. Hold the pose and breathe.
8. To come out, place the hands below the shoulders. Inhale, use the arms to lift the torso upright. Use the hands to draw the legs together and place the hands next to the hips. Straighten the legs.

safety
- If the low back rounds while seated upright with the legs apart or while reaching the hands to the feet, sit on one or more blankets and bring the legs slightly closer together.
- Engage the legs—press the backs of the knees down.
- Press the big toes and fingers into each other.
- Lift the shoulders up.
- The kneecaps tend to fall in rather than point directly up. Engage the quads and isometrically spin the thighs out to externally rotate the legs. Keep the feet pointing up.
- Press the tailbone down and forward; lift the low belly.
- If the chin does not reach the floor, rest the chin on one or more blocks.

refinement
Engage your feet. Push your big toe mounds forward and spread your toes. Stretch your spine to lengthen the front of your torso. Spin your biceps up. To animate the pose, hoist your legs and torso into an upright position so that you are balancing on your hips. Lift your chest and balance

here for five breaths. Then in one movement, return into *upavishta konasana* by landing on your calves without allowing your heels to touch the floor. Depending on what is optimal, practitioners can use this pose to build strength and heat, or to rest, relax, and restore.

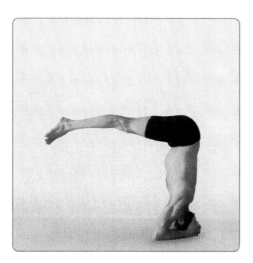

urdhva dandasana in sirsasana
upward staff in headstand pose

shape
(from *sirsasana 1*)

1. Inhale fully. Exhale, lower the legs parallel to the floor.
2. Keep the hips directly above the head. Look forward. Hold the pose and breathe.
3. To come out, lift the legs vertical.

safety

- Do not allow the upper back to round, which can compress the neck.
- Press the forearms and wrists down. Lift the shoulders up.
- Extend down through the head.
- Straighten and strengthen the legs.
- Press the inner feet, ankles, and knees together.
- Engage the abdomen and move the base of the sternum back.
- Extend up through the spine and out through the feet.
- Breathe evenly. Relax the eyes and jaw.
- If the balance is difficult, practice against or near a wall.

refinement

Keeping your hips above your head in this pose can be a good way to prepare for *eka pada sirsasana*. Even so, it is also fine if your hips move back beyond the head, which is easier and no less beneficial. Sometimes the path of least resistance is indeed the best path. Trying too hard to attain a certain form can limit what the pose has to offer. Yoga is considered both a science and an art. When it comes to asana, do not let the science diminish the art. Each one should inform and empower the other. Even the alignment itself is not an indisputable science. Be experiential and experimental in your practice. Notice what works and what does not work for you. Your practice is, after all, your practice! Take ownership of it. One of my guiding mottos in life is what I call "from own to offer." You cannot offer something you do not own. But if you own something you can give that away. Take ownership of your practice and offer it to yourself and others.

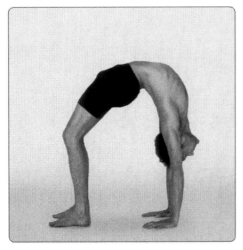
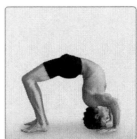

urdhva dhanurasana 1
upward-facing bow pose 1

shape
(from *supta tadasana*)

1. Bend the knees and place the feet on the floor just in front of the hips. Point the toes straight ahead.
2. Place the hands flat on the floor beside the head—thumbs facing in.
3. Bring the elbows to a vertical position and separate the hands slightly wider than the shoulders. Point the index fingers straight back.
4. Without moving the hands or feet, lift the hips and place the top of the head on the floor. Walk the hands in toward the feet.
5. Move the hips up and forward—toward the head—to capacity.
6. Press the hands down and forward, and simultaneously move the shoulders down and back.
7. Extend the chest forward and roll toward the forehead slightly.
8. Inhale fully. Exhale, straighten the arms and lift the heels.
9. Walk the feet in slightly until the forearms are vertical.
10. Lower the heels to the floor.
11. Curl the head back and look between the eyebrows. Hold the pose and breathe.
12. To come out, walk the feet out slightly and lift the chin toward the chest. Exhale, bend the elbows and lower the torso to the floor.

safety

- If the arms cannot straighten, pause with the crown of the head on the floor between the hands to develop strength and flexibility in the shoulders and arms.
- Press the fingertips and the perimeter of the palms into the floor with equal pressure.
- Push the thumbs and the mounds of the index fingers into the floor.
- Strengthen the arms and lock the elbows into a straight position.
- Isometrically squeeze the heels toward the hands.
- Flare the outer two toes and squeeze the shins in.
- Keep the knees outer hip-width apart, and extend the inner thighs and the inner edges of the feet down.
- Engage the glutes and abdomen and lift the tailbone.
- Move the base of the sternum back and stretch the entire spine. Move the hips and chest away from each another.

refinement

If you are interested in getting into the fullest expression of this pose, bring your shins and forearms vertical and extend the chest forward beyond the wrists. I would recommend that most students only practice the basic belly-down backbends and *urdhva dhanurasana 1* for the first several years of their practice. In my opinion, progressing into the more advanced backbends without first refining these basic poses is unwise. To never progress beyond them might be the healthiest choice for many practitioners.

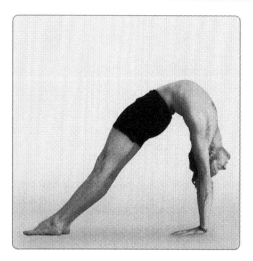

urdhva dhanurasana 2
upward-facing bow pose 2

shape
(from *urdhva dhanurasana 1*)

1. One at a time, slide the feet forward and straighten the legs.
2. Curl the head back and look between the eyebrows. Hold the pose and breathe.
3. To come out, walk the feet back directly below the knees.

safety

- Press the fingertips and the perimeter of the palms down with equal pressure.
- Push the thumbs and mounds of the index fingers into the floor.
- Strengthen the arms and legs and lock the elbows and knees into a straight position.
- Simultaneously extend the shoulders back and the chest forward.
- Isometrically squeeze the shins in and flare the outer two toes.
- Extend the inner thighs and the inner edges of the feet down.
- Engage the glutes and abdomen and lift the tailbone.
- Move the base of the sternum back and stretch the entire spine.

refinement

This is an excellent preparatory pose for *dwi pada viparita dandasana*.

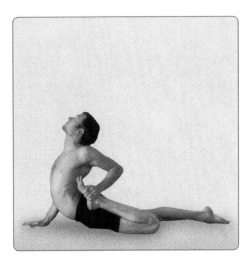

urdhva eka pada bhekasana
upward one leg frog pose

shape

1. Lower the front body to the floor—legs straight, feet outer hip-width apart.
2. Place the right forearm on the floor parallel to the top of the mat —elbow directly below shoulder.
3. Bend the left knee and hold the foot with the left hand. Bring the heel to the top of the left glutes. Pause and breathe.
4. Bring the hand to the inner edge of the foot and place the thumb around the arch of the foot, fingers around the outer edge of the foot. Point the elbow up.
5. Inhale fully. Exhale, lower the inner edge of the left heel to the outer left hip.
6. Look straight ahead. Hold the pose and breathe.
7. To come out, release the hand and straighten the bent leg.

Repeat on the second side.

safety

- Lock the extended leg into a strong and straight position.
- Tone and lift the inner thighs.
- Press the tailbone down, lift the low belly, and contract the glutes.
- Press the extended foot and front forearm down. Pull the front forearm toward the hips to lift the chest up and forward.
- Extend the bent knee and chest away from the hips.
- Square the torso and shoulders to the top of the mat. Move both shoulders up and back.
- If there is pain or discomfort in the bent knee, widen the knee slightly. If there is still pain, discontinue the pose.
- If there is pain or discomfort in the low back, walk the front forearm forward so the elbow is in front of the shoulder and the torso and chest lowers.

refinement

Advanced practitioners can wrap the fingers around the top of the toes and press the heel into the floor. Thus far I have not recognized any benefit from practicing *urdhva eka pada bhekasana*. Why practice it at all then? I practice it because I know there is a good chance that one day something will click and I will suddenly experience the value of the pose. I make it a point to practice poses that I don't seem to resonate with. For example, I basically regarded *bharadvajasana 1* as a waste of time for yoga years. Now, it is among my favorite poses to both practice and teach. So, it just goes to show, you never know.

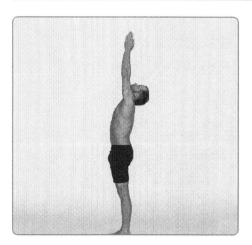

urdhva hastasana
raised hands pose

shape
(from *tadasana*)

1. Inhale, extend the arms overhead until the elbows are directly above the shoulders.
2. Separate the fingers or keep the fingers closed.
3. Squeeze the elbows straight. Look up past the hands. Hold the pose and breathe.
4. To come out, exhale, look forward and lower the arms.

safety

- Press the big toes down and flare the outer two toes.
- Squeeze the feet and legs together.
- Engage the thighs, lift the kneecaps.
- Engage the glutes.
- Move the tailbone down and the low belly in.
- Move the base of sternum back and lift the chest. When the arms are overhead, there is a tendency to push the base of the sternum and front ribs forward.
- Lock the knees and elbows into a straight position.
- Extend the arms up and back.
- If looking up is too intense for the neck, look straight ahead.

refinement

To gain more strength and stretch in your shoulders, interlace your fingers and release your thumbs and index fingers. *Urdhva hastasana* offers a significant shoulder stretch that can prepare practitioners for poses like *adho mukha vrksasana*, *pincha mayurasana*, and *urdhva dhanurasana*. The shoulder stretch comes from three things: 1) squeezing the arms straight, 2) extending the arms up and back, and 3) lifting the elbows directly above the shoulders. The next time you do *urdhva hastasana*, look up at your elbows, and chances are they will be in front of your shoulders. If your front ribs jut forward when you bring your elbows directly above your shoulders, bring the base of your sternum back and allow the wrists to come forward. Keep your arms straight and lift your chest. While this pose looks simple, it may require regular, consistent practice to open the shoulders and get the elbows directly above the shoulders.

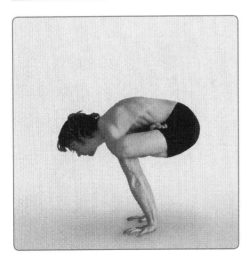

urdhva kukkutasana
raised rooster pose

shape
(from *sirsasana 2*)

1. Extend the inner edge of the right leg back and move the tailbone in.
2. With momentum, swing the left leg into *ardha padmasana*.
3. Move the left knee back slightly.
4. With momentum, swing the right leg into *padmasana*. Pause and breathe.
5. Inhale fully. Exhale, lower the knees toward the arms. Place the knees/upper shins as close to the armpits as possible.
6. Lift the head slightly and lower the hips until the legs are on the arms and the thighs are parallel to the floor. Pause and breathe.
7. Transfer the weight onto the hands and slowly lift the head off the floor.
8. Isometrically squeeze the forearms in toward each other to straighten the arms. Round the back to capacity. Look forward. Hold the pose and breathe.
9. To come out, bend the elbows and lower the head to the floor. Lift the hips and bring the spine and legs vertical. Uncross the legs.

Repeat on the second side.

safety
- Press the fingertips and the perimeter of the palms into the floor with firm and equal pressure.
- Press the outer edges/tops of the feet into the thighs. Flare the toes.
- Squeeze the heels toward the hips to clamp the knees closed.
- Engage the abdomen. Move the tailbone down and forward.
- Lift the pelvic floor.

refinement
If you cannot yet come into *padmasana* from *sirsasana 2*, enter into *sirsasana 2* from *galavasana*

and proceed from there. Be prepared to fall onto your hips as you lift your head off the floor. If you cannot fall softly, put a folded blanket under your hips for padding. An alternative entry point is from *padmasana*. Place your hands in front of your legs directly in front of the upper shins. Lean forward and walk your knees up the arms little by little. This entry point is more difficult and it is unlikely you will be able to get your knees as high up your arms than if you came into the pose from *sirsasana* 2. But if you can't come into *sirsasana* 2, this is worth a shot.

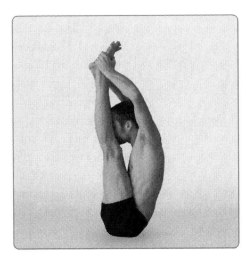

urdhva mukha paschimottanasana 1
upward-facing back stretched out pose 1

shape
(from *dandasana*)

1. Bend the knees and bring the arms to the insides the legs. Hold the outer edges of the feet with the hands.
2. Lean back and lift the feet off the floor. Bring the shins parallel to the floor and flex the feet.
3. Straighten the legs and arms. Inhale, lift the low back and chest. Pause and breathe.
4. Exhale, bend the elbows out to the sides and draw the legs in to bring the face toward/to the shins.
5. Look at the floor through the shins to enhance your balance. Hold the pose and breathe.
6. To come out, straighten the arms, release the hands, and lower the legs to the floor. Place the hands next to the hips.

safety

- To reduce the intensity of the stretch, separate the feet outer hip-width apart or more.
- While the shins are still parallel to the floor, pull the feet with the hands and push the feet into the hands.
- Curve the low back in and up. Before straightening the legs, the low back must be curved in. If the low back is rounding, do not proceed further into the pose.
- Lift the shoulders up and back.
- Straighten and strengthen the legs—tighten the knees and tone the thighs.
- Lift the pelvic floor and tone the low belly.

refinement

This pose is a difficult balance. Just as falling apart is part of the path, falling over is a part of this pose. From *urdhva mukha paschimottanasana 1*, inhale, roll back into *halasana* holding the outer edges of the feet. Inhale. Exhale, push off the floor with the head and toes, and roll back into *urdhva mukha paschimottanasana 1*. Do this five times in a row. This is much more difficult than going from *halasana* into *ubhaya padangusthasana*.

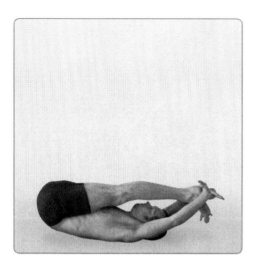

urdhva mukha paschimottanasana 2
upward-facing back stretched out pose 2

shape
(from *dandasana*)

1. Bend the knees and bring the arms to the insides of the legs.
2. Hold the outer edges of the feet.
3. Lean back and lift the feet off the floor. Bring the shins parallel to the floor and flex the feet.
4. Balancing on the backs of the sit bones, straighten the legs and arms. Lift the low back and chest. Pause and breathe.
5. Roll onto the upper back and rest the back and the head on the floor.
6. Bring the legs parallel to the floor and move the hips down and forward as much as possible.
7. Hold the right wrist with the left hand or vice versa. Look straight up. Hold the pose and breathe.
8. To come out, release the clasp and grab the outer edges of the feet. Roll up and balance on the backs of the sit bones.
9. Release the hands, lower the legs to the floor, and place the hands next to the hips.

safety

- To reduce the intensity of the stretch, separate the feet outer hip-width apart or wider. Bend the knees and keep the feet and hips equidistant to the floor.
- Tone the legs—tighten the knees.
- Press the hands and feet into each other.
- Bend and extend the elbows out to the sides to lengthen the spine.

refinement

For a more intense variation, lift your head and pull it between your shins. This will strengthen the front of the torso from the pubic bone to the collarbones, as well as the front of the neck. There are very few poses that require the neck to actively engage in this way.

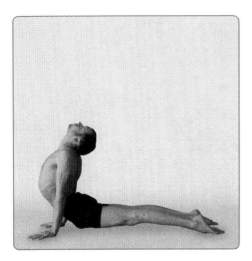

urdhva mukha svanasana
upward-facing dog pose

shape

1. Bring the front body to the floor.
2. Straighten the legs, bring the feet outer hip-width apart, and point the toes straight back.
3. Place the hands on the floor outer shoulder-width apart with the wrists directly below the elbows—forearms vertical.
4. Separate the fingers and point the index fingers straight ahead.
5. Inhale, look forward and lift the chest to bring the shoulders as high as the elbows. Squeeze the shoulder blades toward the spine.
6. On the following inhale, reach the chest forward and straighten the arms to lift the hips and thighs off the floor. Exhale, curl the head back.
7. Look back. Hold the pose and breathe.
8. To come out, exhale, lower the hips and torso to the floor.

safety

- Press the fingertips and the perimeter of the palms into the floor with even pressure.
- Point the toes straight back and isometrically squeeze the ankles in.
- Press the feet down and toward each other.
- Lock the arms and legs into a straight position.
- Point the kneecaps straight down.
- Press the tailbone down and lift the low belly up.
- Contract the glutes.
- Press the hands, especially the mounds of the index fingers, and the tops of the feet down.
- Lift the shoulders up and back. Point the biceps forward.
- Stretch the spine and lift the chest.
- If there is any pain or discomfort in the neck, look straight ahead.
- To reduce the intensity of the pose, place the hands on blocks.

refinement

For a deeper backbend, walk your hands back toward your waistline. *Bhujangasana 1* is a much deeper backbend than *urdhva mukha svanasana*. *Bhujangasana 1* requires more bending in the back, whereas *urdhva mukha svanasana* is more about strengthening the back.

The following is a sequence inspired by *urdhva mukha svanasana* that I often perform toward the end of practice: *bharadvajasana 1, lolasana, mayurasana, gomukhasana, urdhva mukha svanasana, paschimottanasana, purvottanasana, purvotanasana* prep, *setu bandha sarvangasana, urdhva mukha paschimottanasana 2, visvavajrasana, supta balasana, savasana.*

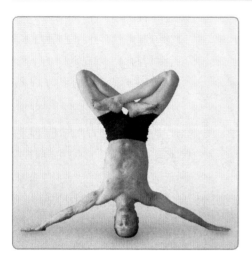

urdhva padmasana in prasarita hasta sirsasana
raised lotus in spread hands headstand

shape
(from *prasarita hasta sirsasana*)

1. Move the right leg back slightly.
2. In one movement, bring the left leg into *ardha padmasana.*
3. Move the left knee back slightly. In one movement, bring the right leg into *padmasana.*
4. Look forward. Hold the pose and breathe.
5. Recross the legs and hold the pose and breathe.
6. To come out, straighten the legs and lower the legs to the floor. Rest with the hips and forehead down in *balasana.*

safety

*   Press the hands down and lift the shoulders up.
*   Extend down through the head, and stretch up through the legs and knees.
*   Press the outer edges/tops of the feet into the thighs and squeeze the heels toward each other.
*   Engage the glutes and abdomen.
*   Move the base of the sternum back and the tailbone forward.
*   Keep the breath even and the eyes steady.
*   If the balance is difficult, practice against or near a wall.

refinement

The key to balancing in *urdhva padmasana* in *prasarita hasta sirsasana* is through the hands. If you start to fall back, press the thumbs into the floor. If you start to fall forward, press your pinkies into the floor. Although this pose looks like a difficult balance, it is relatively easy compared to *sirsasana 3, baddha hasta sirsasana,* and *mukta hasta sirsasana.*

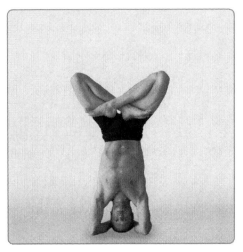
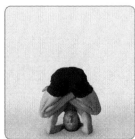

urdhva padmasana in sirsasana
raised lotus in headstand pose

shape
(from *sirsasana 1*)

1. Move the right leg back slightly.
2. With momentum, swing the left foot into *ardha padmasana*.
3. Move the left knee back slightly.
4. With momentum, swing the right leg into *padmasana*. Look forward. Hold the pose and breathe.
5. To come out, release and straighten the legs to vertical.

Repeat on the second side—switch the cross of the legs.

safety
- Press the wrists and forearms down. Lift the shoulders up.
- Extend down through the head and up through the hips and knees.
- Move the base of the sternum back and tone the abdomen. Press the tailbone forward.
- Squeeze the knees in toward each other to tighten the legs.
- Press the outer edges/tops of the feet into the thighs and squeeze the heels toward each other.
- If the balance is difficult, practice against or near a wall.

refinement
In seated *padmasana*, the thighs and torso are at a 90-degree angle. In *urdhva padmasana in sirsasana* the thighs and torso are both vertical to the floor, which opens the front of the quads more than the seated variation of *padmasana*. This pose is similar to resting lion pose.

To lower from *urdhva padmasana in sirsasana* into *pindasana in sirsasana* press the wrists into the floor and tone the abs as you lower the shins slowly to the arms. Be prepared for your weight to shift from the head toward the elbows and for the possibility of your hips falling suddenly to the floor. *Pindasana in sirsasana* is a good preparatory pose for *karandavasana* and *urdhva kukkutasana*. I often lower my hips all the way to the floor as a safe way of coming out of the *pindasana* variation.

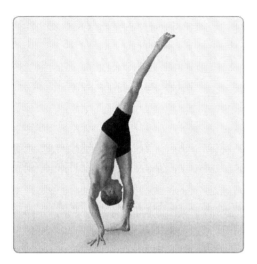

urdhva prasarita ekapadasana
standing split pose

shape
(from *tadasana*)

1. Inhale fully. Exhale, fold the torso over the legs.
2. Bring the fingertips to the floor directly below the shoulders.
3. Lift the left leg to capacity. Point the foot.
4. Hold the back of the calf with the right hand.
5. Inhale fully. Exhale, draw the forehead toward/to the shin and point the left elbow out to the side. Hold the pose and breathe.
6. To come out, place the right hand on the floor below the shoulder. Release the left leg to the floor. Inhale, lift the torso to stand.

Repeat on the second side.

safety

*   Engage the legs—lift the kneecaps.
*   Turn the thigh of the standing leg out so the kneecap faces forward.
*   To reduce the intensity of the hamstring stretch, lower the top leg.
*   Avoid hyperextension in the standing leg.

refinement

To deepen the forward fold, engage your abdomen and round your back. Press your lower hand into your calf and push your calf into the hand. For a greater challenge, hold your lower calf or ankle with both hands. To deepen the hamstring stretch, bring the hip of the lifted leg down and square the hips.

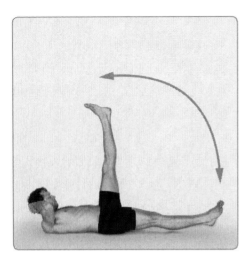

urdhva prasarita padasana
upward extended legs pose

shape
(from *dandasana*)

1. Roll onto the back and bring the feet above the head.
2. Lift the head off the floor. Interlace the fingers behind the head and point the elbows up.
3. Inhale, lower the feet just above the floor.
4. Exhale, lift the feet above the head. As the feet lift above the head, lift the hips up off the floor momentarily. Repeat several times and breathe.
5. To come out, roll up to sit. Straighten the legs and arms, and place the hands next to the hips.

safety
- Bend the knees if needed.
- For extra back support, straighten the arms and place the palms flat on the floor under the glutes. As the feet lower, press the hands and wrists into the glutes.
- Engage the legs fully.
- Squeeze the legs together. Press the inner edges of the feet together including the heels.
- Tone the low belly as the legs lower. Draw the navel toward the spine.

refinement
The most effective way to develop strength in this pose is to lower and lift your legs slowly. Use strength rather than momentum. Use your abdomen rather than your face and jaw. Strengthening the abdomen is an important part of this practice. In backbends, the abdomen gets stretched to capacity. It is important that the abdomen also gets strengthened to capacity. Stretch without strength leads to strain. A strong abdomen promotes a strong and supple spine.

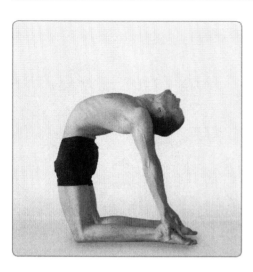

ustrasana
camel pose

shape

1. Come into an upright kneeling position—knees outer hip-width apart and shins parallel.
2. Bring the tops of the feet onto the floor and point the toes straight back.
3. Inhale, lift the chest. Exhale, curl the torso and head and hold the feet with the hands.
4. Look between the eyebrows. Hold the pose and breathe.
5. To come out, inhale, lift the torso. Once the torso is upright, lift the head.

safety

- Isometrically squeeze the shins and heels in, and flare the outer two toes.
- Move the inner thighs back, engage the glutes, and move the hips forward.
- Press the tops of the feet down and lift the chest up.
- Engage the pelvic floor and low belly.
- Keep the neck muscles engaged.
- If the hands cannot reach the feet, curl the toes under and hold the heels.
- If curling the head back is too intense for the neck, look straight up or straight ahead.

refinement

For a slightly more difficult variation, press the palms into the soles of your feet. Another way to come into and out of *ustrasana* is from *virasana* (my personal preference). Hold your feet from start to finish.

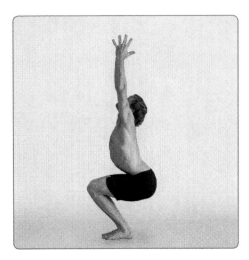

utkatasana
powerful pose

shape
(from *tadasana*)

1. Inhale, lift the arms overhead—elbows directly above the shoulders.
2. Press the palms together. Squeeze the elbows straight.
3. Exhale, bend the knees and lower the hips until the thighs are parallel to the floor.
4. Press the feet, ankles, and knees together.
5. Move the base of the sternum back and lift the chest.
6. Look straight ahead or up past the hands. Hold the pose and breathe.
7. To come out, inhale, straighten the legs. Exhale, release the arms by the sides.

safety

- If there is pain or discomfort in the knees or difficulty with balance, separate the feet hip-width apart. Keep the feet parallel.
- Move the tailbone down and draw the low belly in.
- Reach the sit bones down instead of up and back.
- If the shoulders are tight, separate the hands shoulder-width apart. If there is still discomfort in the shoulders, keep the arms straight, but lower the wrists slightly.

refinement

To gain more strength and stretch in your shoulders, interlace your fingers and release your thumbs and index fingers or simply overlap your thumbs. Stretch your spine. Lift your shoulders. Extend your hands up. It is common for practitioners to hold the breath when facing the difficulty of this pose. Focus on breathing deeply and evenly.

When I was growing up, my dad was fond of saying, "Hard work ain't easy." Well, the same goes here: Hatha work ain't easy! And yet, it can look easy when looking at these photographs. What you cannot see in these photographs is the effort it took to get into them.

When I look at photos of B. K. S. Iyengar in *Light On Yoga*, I contemplate his effort. His expression of each pose did not come easily or for free. For example, in the above pose, if I did not put all of my effort into moving the tailbone down and drawing the low belly in, the base of my sternum would rest on the top of my thighs. Resisting an extreme backbend in this pose required all of my effort. At the same time, this action moves the arms forward. So, to simultaneously do these seemingly opposing actions—moving the tailbone down while lifting your arms up and back—will feel like you are working against yourself. In fact, you are working for alignment. You will know you are in the full form of this pose when it becomes a precarious balancing pose.

During the photoshoot for *utkatasana,* I fell over 15 to 20 times before I was able to hold the form and balance. Once in awhile, practice a pose like *utkatasana* as if it is game day: Do it again and again and go for the full expression of the pose.

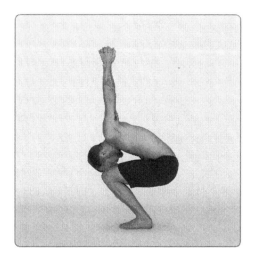

utkatasana
powerful pose

hands bound

shape
(from *tadasana*)

1. Interlace the fingers behind the hips. Pull the wrists apart, or for a deeper shoulder stretch, press the palms together.
2. Bend the elbows, rest the hands on the sacrum.
3. Lift the shoulders and squeeze the shoulder blades together on the back.
4. Engage and straighten the arms.
5. Look straight down and round the back.
6. Lift the arms up and back.
7. Lift the chest into the chin and lock the chin into the chest.
8. Inhale fully. Exhale, bend the knees, lower the thighs parallel to the floor.
9. Place the forehead on the knees.
10. Round the back—move the ribs away from the thighs.
11. Lift the arms vertical to the floor. Hold the pose and breathe.
12. To come out, inhale, lift the forehead off the knees and look forward. Exhale, stand and release the hands.

Repeat with the alternate clasp.

safety

- Press the big toes down.
- Squeeze the feet, ankles, and knees together.
- Move the shoulders up and back away from the head.
- Move the tailbone down and low belly in.

refinement

Extend your hands up. This is one of the most effective warm-up poses since many poses require that the legs, spine, and shoulders be warm. Try this pose for five complete breaths and you will find that the body is quickly heated.

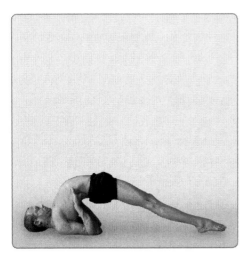 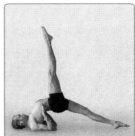

uttana mayurasana
stretched out peacock pose

shape
(from *sarvangasana 1*)

1. Inhale fully. Exhale, bend the knees, lift the chest, and slowly drop the feet to the floor behind the back.
2. Bring the heels directly below the knees. Pause and breathe.
3. Walk the feet out until the legs are nearly straight. Point the feet.
4. Hold the pose and breathe for 15 to 30 seconds.
5. To come out, bend both knees and walk the feet in toward the hands until the shins are vertical. Inhale, lift both legs vertical.

safety

- Keep the seventh cervical (the bony protrusion at the base of the neck) off the floor. If your seventh cervical touches the floor, place folded blankets below the torso and shoulders as described in *sarvangasana 1*.
- Press the shoulders down, in toward each other, and forward toward the head.
- Center the head and press the head down. Bring the chin vertical.
- Lift the chest toward the chin until the base of the chin and chest touch. Do not press the chin into the chest.
- If there is pressure or discomfort in the wrists, place the index fingers and thumbs at the

edges of the ribs while still in *sarvangasana 1*. Actively lift the torso with the hands instead of passively taking the weight of the torso into the hands.

- Press the outer edges of the hands forward and up to strengthen the wrists and deepen the backbend.
- Engage the glutes and legs.
- Extend the hips and spine up.
- Squeeze the inner knees, ankles, and feet together.
- Press the feet down and forward; lift the hips up and back.
- Breathe evenly.
- If it is too difficult to exit the pose by kicking the feet up at the same time, kick the feet up one at a time to return to *sarvangasana 1*.

refinement

Advanced practitioners can lift one leg vertical, then the other.

Uttana mayurasana is unique in that the neck is in a forward fold position while the rest of the spine is in a backbend. The position of the hands is also unique, and often puts intense pressure on the wrists. One way to remove some of the pressure on the wrists is to bend deeply in your upper back. Bending more deeply in your upper back, however, will put more pressure on your neck. The remedy? Intensify all the actions of alignment. The amount of effort to put forth is the amount of effort required to attain alignment. In yoga, the quantity of effort must always be balanced with quality of effort.

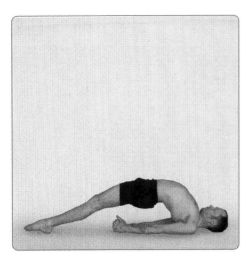

uttana mayurasana prep
stretched out peacock pose

hands bound

shape

1. Lie down on the back, bend the knees, and bring the heels directly below the knees—shins vertical.
2. Inhale, lift the hips. Interlace the fingers below the sacrum.
3. One at a time, walk the shoulders up toward the head and in toward the spine. zDo this several times until the chest is fully lifted.
4. Inhale, lift the hips and chest up and back toward the head.
5. Keep the hips lifted and, one at a time, walk the feet forward to straighten the legs. Bring the feet together and point the toes.
6. Look up. Hold the pose and breathe.
7. To come out, bend the knees and walk the feet back until the shins are vertical. Release the hands and exhale, lower the hips.

safety

- Tighten and tone the legs. Point the kneecaps up and spin the inner thighs down.
- Bring the shoulders toward the head to avoid overstretching the neck.
- Press the head, shoulders, wrists, and heels down.
- Lift the chin, chest, and hips up and back.
- Engage the glutes.
- Center the head and avoid turning the head from side to side.
- Keep the base of the chin vertical.
- If the shoulders are tight, hold the outer edges of the mat with the hands instead of interlacing the fingers. Separating the hands will help bring the shoulder blades together, which will prevent overstretching the neck.

refinement

Just as peanut butter goes with chocolate, this pose goes well with *purvottanasana* and *urdhva mukha svanasana*. It also serves as a good modification for the full form of *uttana mayurasana*.

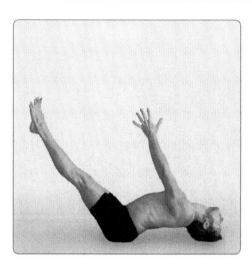

uttana padasana
stretched out legs pose

shape
(from *supta tadasana*)

1. With the arms alongside the torso, press the elbows into the floor, lift the chest, and bring the top of the head to the floor.
2. Inhale, lift the legs and arms 60 degrees away from the floor.
3. Bring the palms together and separate the fingers.
4. Look between the eyebrows. Hold the pose and breathe.
5. To come out, exhale, lower the arms, legs, and torso to the floor.

safety

- Straighten and strengthen the arms and legs—lock the knees and elbows into a straight position.
- Press the inner legs and feet together.
- Bring the feet halfway between a flexed and pointed position. Spread the toes.
- Press the head down, and lift the legs, chest, and arms.
- Extend out through the inner feet and the fingers.
- Center the head. Do not turn the head once it is bearing weight.
- Lift the pelvic floor and tone the low belly.
- If there is any pain or discomfort in the neck or jaw, keep the forearms on the floor to minimize the weight placed on the head.

refinement

After a workshop in which I taught *uttana padasana,* a student called out, "That was weird." What makes one pose seem strange and another one seem normal? Back in the 1970s, mainstream America regarded all yoga as weird. Now, yoga is considered not only normal but even hip or cool. If you practice what seems like a peripheral pose enough times it can quickly become standard to your sequence. At YogaOasis, the studio I direct in Tucson, we teach *mayurasana* on a regular basis. At first students thought it was weird. Now when we teach it, 75 percent of the students go right into it without giving it another thought. Pose preference can create practice patterns that limit possibility and creativity.

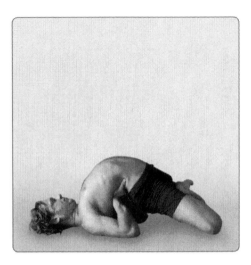

uttana padma mayurasana
stretched out lotus peacock pose

shape
(from *sarvangasana 1*)

1. Move the right leg back slightly.
2. In one movement, bring the left leg into *ardha padmasana*.
3. Move the left knee back slightly and in one movement, bring the right leg into *padmasana*.
4. Lean the torso back into the hands so the weight of the body moves onto the elbows.
5. Keep the legs vertical but lower the hips until the sacrum is parallel to the floor. Point the knees up.
6. Inhale, expand the chest toward the chin.
7. Exhale, lower the knees to the floor. Look past the tip of the nose. Hold the pose and breathe.
8. To come out, inhale lift the legs and torso vertical. Exhale, release and straighten the legs.

Repeat on the second side—switch the cross of the legs.

safety

- Press the shoulders down, in toward each other, and forward toward the head.
- Center the head and press the head down. Bring the chin vertical.
- Before lowering the torso, bring the hands as low on the back as possible. If the fingers and thumbs are higher than the top of the ribcage, do not proceed.
- Engage the biceps and press the hands into the torso. Press the outer edges of the hands forward and up.
- Press the outer edges/tops of the feet into the thighs. Squeeze the heels toward the hips.
- Do not hold the breath.
- Soften the eyes and jaw as much as possible.

refinement

Uttana padma mayurasana is difficult even for the very flexible. In addition to a deep backbend, this pose requires immense strength in the core in order to lower into and come out of the pose with control. One technique to work toward this pose is to curl your head back as you lower your knees to the floor. Prop yourself up on your elbows and the top of your head. Inhale fully. Exhale, lower the shoulders and back of the head to the floor if possible. Also, if you widen your elbows it will take some pressure off the wrists. In *Matrika* magazine, Douglas Brooks writes,

"For Hanuman the impossible is yet another possibility."[1] This pose is impossible. Be a hatha hanuman and make it a possibility. Though, I for one, wouldn't necessarily recommend it.

[1]   Douglas Brooks, "Hanuman: Yoga in the Forest of Mythic Consciousness," *Matrika*, Spring 2006 Volume 2.

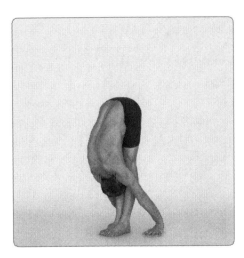

uttanasana
forward fold pose

shape
(from *tadasana*)

1. Inhale fully. Exhale, fold the torso forward.
2. Place the fingertips on the floor next to, or even behind, the feet.
3. Bend the elbows out to the sides, or if possible, straighten the arms.
4. Bring the face toward/to the shins.
5. Bring the weight forward until the hips are directly over the heels.
6. Straighten the legs completely. Hold the pose and breathe.
7. To come out, inhale, lift the torso to stand.

safety

- Squeeze the feet and legs together.
- Engage the legs, especially the thighs.
- Lift the kneecaps up.
- Lock the legs into a straight position.
- Press the tops of the feet down to engage the calves.
- Move the tailbone down and the low belly in.
- There are several variations for practitioners with tight hamstrings. Separate the feet outer hip-width apart before folding forward. Widen the knees slightly wider than the ankles. If the hands dangle above the floor, bend the knees as much as necessary. Alternatively, place the hands on blocks, first below the shoulders and later to the outsides of the feet. If the low back still rounds with the hands elevated on blocks, place the hands on a wall and fold to a 90-degree angle, keeping the knees as bent as necessary to maintain a long, straight spine.
- Over time, begin to straighten the legs little by little. Little by little does not mean in a matter of seconds. Gaining flexibility in the hamstrings, can take weeks, months, even years of regular practice. Patience is paramount to practice. Being too focused on flexibility can turn stretches into strains. Yoga requires that you go from a competitive to contemplative mindset.

refinement

Press your fingertips down and forward. Allow a deep stretch to occur in the backs of your legs and spine. This pose reveals stored tension in our bodies so we can consciously release it. Even a few breaths in this pose can clear your mind and leave you feeling relaxed and rejuvenated.

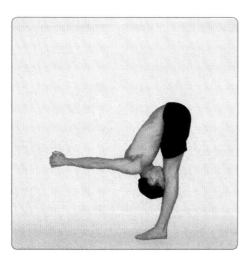

uttanasana
forward fold pose

hands bound

shape
(from *tadasana*)

1. Interlace the hands behind the hips; press the palms together or stretch the wrists apart.
2. Bend the elbows, rest the hands on the sacrum.
3. Lift the shoulders, and squeeze the shoulder blades together on the back.
4. Inhale, straighten the arms.
5. Exhale, fold the torso forward.
6. Engage the abdominals to pull the torso toward/to the legs—place the face between the shins.
7. Bring the weight forward until the hips are directly over the heels.
8. Lift the shoulder blades up; extend the shoulders and hands toward floor. Hold the pose and breathe.
9. To come out, inhale, lift the torso to stand. Exhale, release the hands.

Repeat with the alternate clasp.

safety

- Squeeze the feet and legs together.
- Engage the thighs—lift the kneecaps.
- Press the tailbone down and lift the low belly.
- To reduce the intensity of the stretch, bend the knees to a 45-degree angle and rest the torso on the thighs.

refinement

Stretch your shoulders to capacity by extending your shoulders toward the floor as you lift your shoulder blades up.

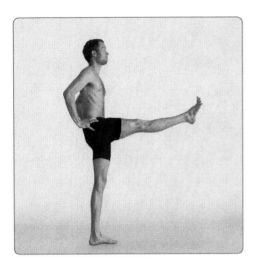

utthita eka padasana

extended one foot pose

shape

(from *tadasana*)

1. Place the hands on the hips.
2. Keeping the right leg straight, lift the right foot as high as the hips.
3. Bring the foot halfway between a flexed and pointed position. Spread the toes.
4. Look straight ahead. Hold the pose and breathe.
5. To come out, exhale, release the leg and bring the arms by the sides.

Repeat on the second side.

safety

- As much as possible, use the strength of the abdomen to lift the leg, which will support the hip flexors.
- If the hip flexors are tight or tweaked, lift the foot only part way or bend the lifted leg to a 90-degree angle.
- Do not lean back.
- Push the hands down and lift the chest.

refinement

Tight and tweaked hip flexors, which may be aggravated by this pose, are common among athletes and those who spend an excessive amount of time driving or sitting at a desk. A more accessible variation of this pose is the supine version, *supta padangushtasana prep*.

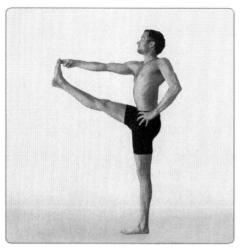
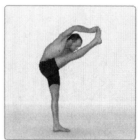

utthita hasta padangusthasana 1
extended hand to big toe pose 1

shape
(from *tadasana*)

1. Place the left hand on the left hip.
2. Balancing on the left foot, lift the right foot, and hold the big toe with the first two fingers and thumb of the right hand.
3. Stand upright.
4. Lift the right shin parallel to the floor.
5. Straighten the top leg.
6. Look straight ahead. Hold the pose and breathe.
7. To come out, exhale, release the leg. Bring the arms by the sides.

Repeat on the second side.

safety

- Engage the standing leg—lift the kneecap.
- Use the fingers to pull the toe, and at the same time, push the toe into the fingers.
- Reach the inner edge of the lifted foot forward, the outer edge back.
- Move the top of the standing thigh back until the leg is perfectly vertical—outer knee directly above outer ankle and outer hip directly above outer knee.
- Drop the outer hip of the lifted leg down.
- To avoid pain in the right shoulder, pull the right shoulder blade onto the back and lift the chest. The shoulder will still be forward of the body, but the integration of the shoulder, back, and chest will help protect the front of the shoulder.
- Lift the left shoulder up and back.
- Engage the abdominal muscles, move the base of the sternum back, and lift the chest.
- To reduce the intensity of the hamstring stretch, use a strap around the lifted foot and hold the strap as close to the foot as possible. Keep the arm straight and do not allow the torso to lean back.

refinement

This is one of the most intense hamstring stretches found in all of the standing poses. It is a great preparatory pose for *eka pada sirsasana, krounchasana, akarna dhanurasana 2, hanumanasana,* and *supta trivikramasana*. It is also a good culmination pose after *supta padangusthasana* and cycle. For a more advanced variation, fold the torso and place the forehead on the lifted shin.

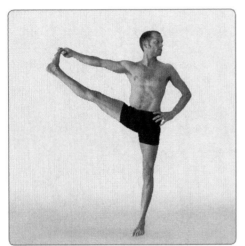
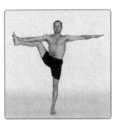
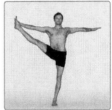
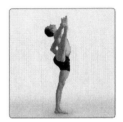

utthita hasta padangusthasana 2
extended hand to big toe pose 2

shape
(from *tadasana*)

1. Place the left hand on the left hip.
2. Balancing on the left foot, lift the right foot and hold the big toe with the first two fingers and thumb of the right hand.
3. Stand upright and move the right leg out to the side.
4. Lift the right shin parallel to the floor.
5. Flex the foot and straighten the lifted leg.
6. Move the top of the standing thigh back and press the tailbone down.
7. Turn the head to the left and look past the shoulder. Hold the pose and breathe.
8. To come out, inhale, look forward. Exhale, release the foot and bring the arms by the sides.

Repeat on the second side.

safety
- Engage the standing leg—lift the kneecap.
- Pull the right foot with the right hand and push the foot into the hand to engage the lifted leg.
- Isometrically extend the right heel down to strengthen the hamstrings.
- Tilt the right foot out slightly.
- To reduce the intensity of the hamstring stretch, keep the top knee bent and hold the outer edge of the foot instead of the big toe.

refinement
Drop the sit bone of your lifted leg down and level your hips. The tendency is to distort the hips in order to lift the top leg even higher. For a more advanced variation, curl your head and upper torso back. Look back.

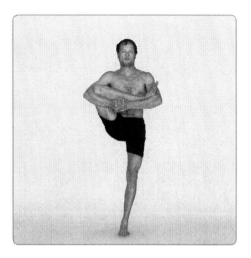

utthita hindolasana
extended baby cradle pose

shape
(from *tadasana*)

1. Lift the right knee and hold the ankle with the right hand—arm to the inside of the leg.
2. Bend the standing knee and place the right foot into the crease of the left elbow. Bend the elbow to cradle the foot.
3. Wrap the right arm around the right knee—inner elbow to knee.
4. Interlace the fingers around the shin.
5. Straighten the standing leg and stand upright.
6. Lift the shin toward the chest.
7. Look forward. Hold the pose and breathe.
8. To come out, exhale, release the hands and arms, and lower the leg. Bring the arms by the sides.

Repeat on the second side.

safety

- Press the outer edge of the top foot into the crease of the left elbow and the inner edge of the foot into the left bicep.
- Flex the top foot, especially the outer two toes, to protect the knee.
- Squeeze the elbows in.
- Move the hip of the lifted leg down and forward.
- Lift the shoulders up and back.
- To reduce the intensity in the hips, hold the right foot with the left hand. Slide the left hand under the calf and hold the outer right shin—fingers pointing up.
- To lift the torso more upright, bend the knee of the standing leg.

refinement

Bring your shin parallel to your chest by lifting your foot with your elbow. To increase the stretch in your hip, lift your top heel higher than your top knee. I used to always instruct students to lift the torso as upright as possible until I realized that what is possible is not necessarily optimal. To quote Professor Douglas Brooks, "Just because you can, doesn't mean you should."[1]

---

[1] Personal communication with Douglas Brooks, Tucson, Arizona, April 2011.

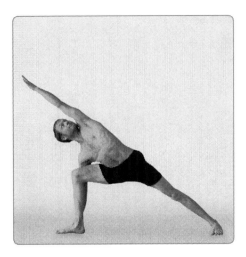

utthita parsvakonasana
extended side angle pose

shape
(from *tadasana*, facing long edge of mat)

1. Inhale, bend the knees.
2. Exhale, take a wide stance. Lift the arms parallel to the floor.
3. Turn the left foot in 30 degrees, right foot out 90 degrees.
4. Make a straight line from the front heel to the arch of the back foot.
5. Inhale, look past the right fingertips.
6. Exhale, bend the right knee to 90 degrees—knee over heel.
7. Place the right hand on the floor to the outside of the front foot.
8. Extend the left arm up and forward, over the face.
9. Straighten the arms. Point the top palm down and the bottom biceps forward toward the top of the mat.
10. Inhale, look up; turn the chin to the armpit. Hold the pose and breathe.
11. To come out, look down. Lift the top arm vertical. Without moving the arms, inhale and lift the torso. Exhale, straighten the front leg and parallel the feet. Inhale, bend the knees. Exhale, bring the feet together and lower the arms.

Repeat on the second side.

safety
- Do not allow the front knee to move beyond the heel.
- Press the back foot and front heel down; squeeze the feet toward each other.
- If the right hip is higher than the right knee, lengthen the stance via the back foot until the front thigh is parallel to the floor.
- Tone the back leg—tighten the back knee without hyperextending.
- It is important to keep both sides of the torso long. The tendency is for the lower waist to shorten and collapse, and for the left ribs to round and overstretch. To avoid this, place the right hand or fingertips on a block. This additional height will create more space in the waist and torso, especially on the lower side.
- Move the tailbone down and low belly in.
- Move the base of the sternum back, stretch up through the chest.
- Move the top shoulder back until the armpit is hollow.

- If looking up is too intense for the neck or jaw, look down.

refinement

Bring your awareness to your back foot and top hand and stretch them in opposite directions. Tighten your back knee and top elbow, and extend them away from your hips.

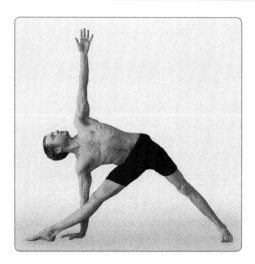

utthita trikonasana
extended triangle pose

shape
(from *tadasana*, facing long edge of mat)

1. Inhale, bend the knees.
2. Exhale, take a wide stance. Lift the arms parallel to the floor.
3. Turn the left foot in 30 degrees, the right foot out 90 degrees.
4. Make a straight line from the front heel to the arch of the back foot.
5. Inhale, look past the right fingertips.
6. Exhale, hinge the torso sideways at the hips. Place the right palm flat on the floor.
7. Rotate the left shoulder over the right shoulder—arms vertical.
8. Rotate the abdomen and ribs up.
9. Look up past the top thumb.
10. Make a straight line from the hips to the head so the torso is parallel to the long edge of the mat.
11. Point both biceps toward the top of the mat. Hold the pose and breathe.
12. To come out, look down at the floor. Inhale, lift the torso to vertical. Exhale, parallel the feet. Inhale, bend the knees. Exhale, bring the feet together and lower the arms.

Repeat on the second side.

safety

- Contract the quads, tighten the kneecaps and hamstrings.
- Lift the right kneecap and keep it lifted. In other words: no droopy kneecaps! To stretch without strain requires steady strength.
- The center of the front kneecap should face directly forward. For most people, the kneecap tends to fall in and down. To avoid this, press the inner edge of the front foot down, and turn

the front thigh out until the kneecap faces forward.

- Press the back foot down—make it almost as heavy as the front foot.
- Engage the abdominal muscles, and move the base of the sternum back.
- If placing the palm flat on the floor is too intense on the front hamstrings, bring the fingertips to the floor, or place the hand on a block or even a chair. Choose an appropriate hand position that allows the front leg to completely straighten while maintaining length in the spine.
- If looking up is too intense for the neck or jaw, look down.

refinement

Keep your knees and elbows locked into a straight position. Press your feet down and apart. Extend your right palm or fingertips into the floor, reach your left hand up. Extend your head away from your hips and lengthen your entire spine. What requires more often has more to offer.

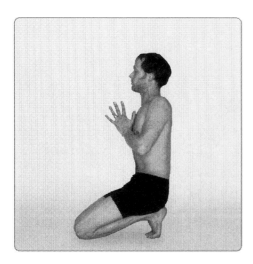

vajrasana
thunderbolt pose

elevated

shape
(from *bharmanasana*)

1. Bring the knees and feet together and curl the toes under—heels vertical.
2. Inhale fully. Exhale, lower the hips onto the heels.
3. Lift the torso upright.
4. Place the hands on the knees, press the palms together in front of the chest, or straighten the arms and place the palms together overhead. Look forward. Hold the pose and breathe.
5. To come out, release the hands to the floor in front of the knees. Walk the hands forward until the hips are directly above the knees and the shoulders are above the wrists. Separate the knees and feet hip-width apart. Bring the tops of the feet to the floor.

safety

- If this pose puts too much pressure on the toes, place a tightly rolled-up blanket underneath the toe mounds.
  Squeeze the legs and feet together.
- Press the tailbone down and move the low belly in.
- Move the base of the sternum back and lift the chest.
- Relax the shoulder blades down the back, away from the ears.

refinement
Broaden your collarbones. Lift your chin slightly and center your head directly over your torso and pelvic floor. This pose is excellent medicine for the toes and is one of the few ways to safely stretch the bottoms of your feet and toes. Stay in the pose longer than you think. If your toes and feet are strong, practice lifting your knees off the floor to balance. When it is time to come out, lower your knees slowly to develop precision in your practice. This simple action will quickly develop strength as well as stretch in the feet.

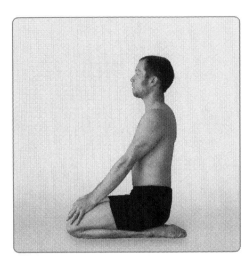

vajrasana
thunderbolt pose

shape
(from *bharmanasana*)

1. Bring the inner knees, ankles, and big toes together.
2. Lower the hips to the heels.
3. Place the hands on the knees and straighten the arms. Look forward. Hold the pose and breathe.
4. To come out, release the hands to the floor in front of the legs—hands shoulder-width apart. Separate the knees and ankles hip-width apart—shoulders over wrists, hips over knees.

safety

- To reduce the intensity on the knees, separate the knees and feet outer hip-width apart and/ or sit on one or more folded blankets.
- If the tops of the feet are tight and do not fully touch the floor, place a rolled-up blanket of appropriate height beneath the lower shins/ankles.
- If there is discomfort in the legs, place a folded blanket under the shins for padding.

refinement

Engage your hamstrings and squeeze your thighs toward each other. Keep your heels vertical and do not allow your feet to sickle. This small action of engaging the feet keeps the body and mind alert. I was once in a yoga class where the teacher said, "If you can't do *vajrasana* comfortably, do it every day until you can. It will prevent future problems in your feet and knees." Anytime I perform or teach this pose, I remember that moment. It's interesting how something a yoga instructor says in a class becomes a gem that we carry with us as a guide. *Vajrasana* requires the same flexibility and strength in the tops of the feet as some of the more advanced poses such as *virasana, bhujangasana, hanumanasana,* and the *eka pada rajakapotasana prep* series, in which the heels are vertical and the outer and inner ankles are balanced. The alignment of the feet directly affects the alignment in the legs and pelvis. Being able to safely bear the weight of the body on the tops of the feet can also prepare students for poses like *purvottanasana, uttana mayurasana* prep, and *dwi pada viparita dandasana,* which require extreme flexibility in the tops of the feet.

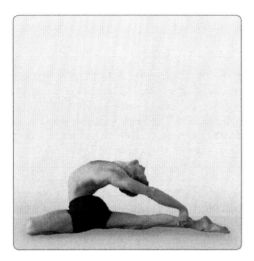

valakhilyasana
celestial spirit pose

shape
(from *adho mukha svanasana*)

1. Inhale fully. Exhale, bring the left knee to the floor to the left of and just behind the left hand—knee slightly wider than the left hip.
2. Lower the left sit bone and leg to the floor.
3. Point the left foot and press the left heel to the front of the right hip.
4. Lower the front of the right thigh to the floor—leg parallel to the long edge of the mat. Point the foot straight back.
5. Inhale, lift the torso to a vertical position. Bend the back knee to lift the shin vertical.
6. Place the palms together behind the head, point the fingers straight back, and separate the elbows shoulder-width apart.
7. Inhale fully. Exhale, curl the head and torso back and clasp the foot with the hands. If possible, flex the foot and slide the hands down to the ankle.
8. Press the forehead into the heel. Pause and breathe.
9. In one smooth movement, keep holding the back foot and exhale, straighten the back leg and arms. Lower the back leg and the top of the foot to the floor.
10. Look back. Hold the pose and breathe.
11. To come out, keep the chest full and inhale, bend the back leg to lift the torso. Exhale, lower the arms and back foot to the floor.
12. Place the hands on the floor in front of the top shin. Separate the hands shoulder-width apart, curl the back toes under, and push the hands down and forward to push the hips up and back.

Repeat on the second side.

safety
- To reduce the intensity of this pose, allow the hips to lift away from the floor.
- Move the right hip forward and the left hip back to square the hips.
- Press the outer edge/top of the front foot down and clamp the front knee closed.
- Isometrically squeeze the knees toward each other.
- Press the tailbone down, engage the glutes, and lift the low belly.
- Move the base of the sternum back and stretch the spine and chest up while simultaneously

moving the shoulders back.
- For a more accessible entry, wrap a strap around the back foot and inhale, lift the arms vertical. Lower the back foot to the floor and walk the hands down the strap toward the foot.

refinement

For what it's worth, creating sacred space can turn the impossible into a possibility. For example, during one of the last photo shoots for the *From Tadasana to Savasana* poster, I was attempting *valakhilyasana*—which I like to call *Kali-kill-u-asana*. I was able to get my back toes on the floor. I wasn't, however, able to get my shin and the top of my foot to the floor. After many attempts I concluded without a shadow of a doubt that THAT asana was impossible for me. My friends in the room assured me I could do it. But how the hatha-hell would they know? I knew there was no way, no chance. In a state of defeat I gazed at a photo of Bhagawan Nityananda, a great yogi saint. I had put that photo of Bhagawan Nityananda on the *puja* (altar) that morning to inspire me. As I gazed at Bhagawan Nityananda, I felt my awareness soften. I started to feel a powerful energy that took me into a realm of my heart I had never been—what felt like a wellspring of possibility. Then, like moving from the depths of water back to the surface, my awareness rose back into the room. In that short period of time I went through a deep inner shift. I turned to Milo with a smile and said, "I can do it." As I went into the pose all the previous obstacles were still there. Only now, instead of a stop sign, it was a yield sign. Instead of a red light, it was a yellow light. The deep recognition that I could do it kept me guru-going all the way into the final form.

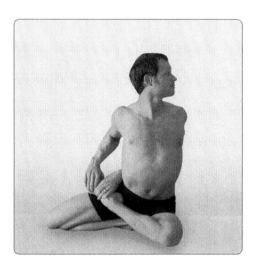

vamadevasana 1
Sage Vamadeva's pose 1

shape
(from *ardha mulabandhasana*, upright)

1. With the right foot in *ardha mulabandhasana*, place the right hand on the floor behind the hips and the left hand in front of the hips.
2. Lift the hips. Push the right heel and the hips forward.
3. Lift the hips even more and, keeping the mound of the big toe in place, tilt the right heel toward the floor to lower the inner edge of the right foot and ankle to the floor below the pelvis. Lower the hips to sit on the outer right ankle.
4. Bend the left knee and bring the foot in front of the pubic bone.
5. Keeping the left knee on the floor, bring the left foot into *ardha padmasana* position.
6. Inhale fully. Exhale, swing the left arm around the back and hold the left foot with the hand. Hold the left foot with the right hand as well.
7. Inhale, lift the spine. Exhale, twist the torso to the left. Look past the shoulder. Hold the pose and breathe.
8. To come out, inhale, look forward. Exhale, release the hands and lower the top foot to the floor in front of the pubic bone. Lean to the side and release the foot and leg. Straighten the legs.

Repeat on the second side.

safety
- If the foot does not flex into a vertical, do not attempt this pose.
- Continue bearing weight in the hands until the front foot is bent in toward the pelvis.
- Before attempting this pose, perform a full forward-fold, twist, and hip-opening sequence to warm up.
- Attain the flexed foot position via the hip and not the knee.

refinement
This pose is so counterintuitive to the body and mind that it will take several attempts just to get a feel for it. Once you do, it is strangely not as difficult as it might seem. Still, exercise caution and move slowly as you lower your hips.

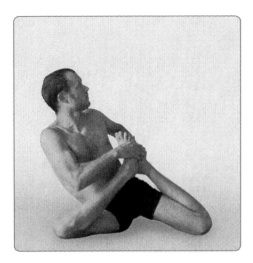

vamadevasana 2
Sage Vamadeva's pose 2

shape
(from *dandasana*)

1. Widen the legs and lean onto the right hip.
2. Bend the left knee and use the left hand to bring the inner heel to the outer left hip. Spin the hand so the fingers point in the same direction as the toes—palm to top of foot.
3. Place the right hand to the floor outside the right hip. Bend the right knee and bring the heel to the pubic bone. Hold the top of the foot with the hand.
4. Move the left thigh to the left in line with the front knee—thigh parallel to the long edges of the mat.
5. Lean the torso forward and to the right so that most of the body weight is on the right hip.
6. Lift the feet up and press the soles of the feet together.
7. Inhale fully. Exhale, twist the torso to the left. Look past the left shoulder. Hold the pose and breathe.
8. To come out, inhale, look forward. Exhale, release the hands and separate the feet. Straighten the legs.

Repeat on the second side.

safety

- Keep the knees on the floor from start to finish.
- Bring the back inner heel and outer hip as close together as possible.
- To lift the front foot, roll the thigh out to protect the knee.
- Activate the feet and clamp the knees closed.
- Lift the pelvic floor and tone the low belly.

refinement

Your breath will likely become quick and shallow. Attempt to breathe normally and evenly. If you detect stress or strain, emphasize the exhalations to help you become calm in the midst of discomfort, a skill that is certainly valuable off the mat. Again and again these poses put us into stressful situations that require us to become calm and focused if we choose to survive and thrive in this practice. I know of a man who told his wife that he was thinking of giving up his yoga practice. His wife, who did not practice hatha yoga, urged him to continue practicing.

He asked her why, considering his classes were in the evening and meant giving up family time. She said that his yoga practice afforded him less quantity but more quality family time. I often say that *sadhana* (spiritual practice) is *seva* (service for the benefit of others). If practiced properly, the work we do on ourselves in this practice becomes an immediate offering to all those around us.

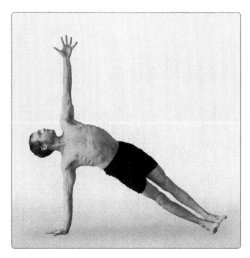
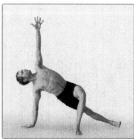

vasisthasana
Sage Vasistha's pose

legs together

shape
(from *plank pose*)

1. Bring the feet together.
2. Keeping the feet together, roll onto the outer edge of the right foot and place the left hand on the left hip—left foot on top of right foot. Balance on the right hand and the outer edge of the right foot.
3. Squeeze the inner edges of the feet together.
4. Lift the left arm vertical.
5. Look up past the top hand.
6. To come out, lower the left foot and left hand to the floor.

Repeat on the second side.

safety

- To reduce the pressure on the lower wrist, move the hand a few inches forward—toward the top of the mat—so that the wrist is in front of the shoulder.
- Separate the fingers of the bottom hand. Point the biceps and the index finger straight ahead.
- Press the fingertips and the perimeter of the lower palm evenly into the floor—press the mound of the index finger down and lift the outer wrist.
- Press the lower hand down and forward—toward the top of the mat—and lift the hips up.
- Press the tailbone forward and lift the low belly.
- Move the base of the sternum back and lengthen the spine.
- If looking up is too intense for the neck or jaw, look down.
- If it is too difficult to stack the legs and keep the top foot flexed, bend the top knee and place the foot on the floor—heel below knee.

refinement

Poses that put pressure on the wrist have the potential to resolve and prevent wrist problems— when practiced with good alignment. However, these poses can also cause the very symptoms they resolve. That is the paradox of hatha yoga. Good alignment is therefore paramount. Patience, self-acceptance, and sensitivity must become part and parcel of your practice.

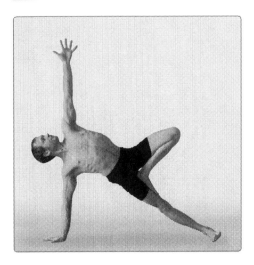

vasisthasana
Sage Vasistha's pose

top leg in tree

shape
(from *vasisthasana*, legs together)

1. Bend the left knee completely and hold the ankle with the left hand. Place the sole of the foot on the upper inner right thigh. Point the left knee up.
2. Lift the left arm vertical.
3. Straighten the arms and bottom leg.
4. Look up past the top hand. Hold the pose and breathe.
5. To come out, straighten and lower the left leg, and squeeze the legs together.

Repeat on the second side.

safety

- To reduce the pressure on the lower wrist, move the hand a few inches forward—toward the top of the mat—so that the wrist is in front of the shoulder.
- Separate the fingers of the bottom hand. Point the index finger and biceps straight ahead.
- Press the fingertips and the perimeter of the lower palm evenly into the floor—press the mound of the index finger down and lift the outer wrist.
- Press the lower hand down. Lift the hips up and back to bring more weight into the bottom foot.
- Press the foot and inner thigh into each other.
- Engage the abdomen and move the base of the sternum back.
- If looking up is too intense for the neck or jaw, look down.

refinement

To lift your hips to capacity, place the sole of the bottom foot flat on the floor. Practice arm balances like you do standing poses. In other words, do one side of the pose, come back to center, and then move to the other side. Practitioners have a tendency to sit down and take breaks between arm balances. Imagine how that would affect your practice if you sat down to rest between the right and left sides of *trikonasana*? It would break your flow and focus. One of the key benefits to doing several arm balances in a row is the stamina and will power it develops. That won't happen if you rest between each arm balance. My friend Ross Evans, the inventor of the Xtracycle, filmed the initial shoot for the photographs of these poses. Because he was filming, he wanted me to move from one pose to the next without stopping. I therefore had to do most of the arm balances in a row. About half way through, my arms were on fire and I felt exhausted. But I kept pushing and pushing until I hit a wellspring of momentum. By the time I finished, I felt vibrant and focused. The challenge of hatha yoga often offers the very change we seek. The price is practice, practice, and more practice.

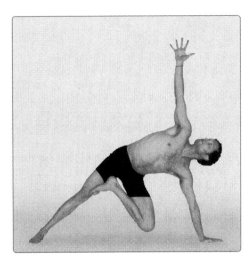

vasisthasana
Sage Vasistha's pose

bottom leg in tree

shape
(from *vasisthasana*, top leg in tree)

1. Lower the left hand to the floor and roll onto the toe mounds of the right foot—heel lifted. This will bring you into plank pose with one leg in tree.
2. Roll onto the inner edge of the right foot and place the sole of the foot on the floor. Point the bent knee straight down.
3. Lift the right arm vertical. Look up past the hand. Hold the pose and breathe.
4. To come out, lower the top hand to the floor and roll onto the toe mounds of the back foot. Balancing on the lower hand, roll onto the outer edge of the foot and extend the left arm up.

Repeat on the second side.

safety
- To reduce the pressure on the lower wrist, move the hand a few inches forward—toward the top of the mat—so that the wrist is in front of the shoulder.
- Separate the fingers of the bottom hand. Point the index finger and biceps straight ahead.
- Press the fingertips and the perimeter of the palm evenly into the floor—press the mound of the index finger down and lift the outer wrist.
- Press the bottom hand and foot down. Lift the hips up and back.
- Push the foot and inner thigh into each other.
- Move the tailbone forward and tone the low belly. Move the base of the sternum back.
- If looking up is too intense for the neck or jaw, look down.

refinement
This pose is surprisingly challenging for the core and obliques, especially if you actively lift your bottom knee away from the floor. While lowering the knee to the floor may seem like a nice rest and reduces the arm and core strength required, balancing becomes more difficult. Shorten the distance between your bottom hand and foot to reduce the difficulty of the pose. Lengthen the distance to increase the difficulty.

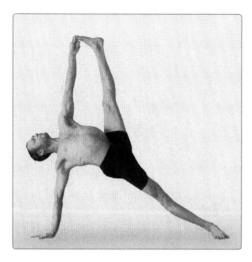
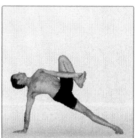

vasisthasana
Sage Vasistha's pose

shape
(from *vasisthasana*, legs together)

1. Bend the left knee. Bring the left arm to the inside of the leg and hold the big toe with the first two fingers and thumb.
2. Push the lower hand down and bend the bottom knee to place the sole of the bottom foot flat on the floor. Keep the foot on the floor and straighten the leg.
3. Point the top knee up. Pause and breathe.
4. Inhale, straighten the top leg.
5. Stretch out through the inner edge of the top foot. Look up. Hold the pose and breathe.
6. To come out, release the hand and lower the leg. Squeeze the legs together.

Repeat on the second side.

safety
- To reduce the pressure on the lower wrist, move the hand a few inches forward—toward the top of the mat—so that the wrist is in front of the shoulder.
- Separate the fingers of the bottom hand. Point the index finger and biceps straight ahead.
- Press the fingertips and the perimeter of the palm evenly into the floor—press the mound of the index finger down and lift the outer wrist.
- Push the lower hand down and lift the hips up and back.
- Press the left big toe and fingers into each other to engage the top leg.
- Move the tailbone forward and tone the low belly. Press the base of the sternum back.
- If the hamstrings are tight, do not attempt to straighten the top leg completely. Keeping the knee bent, use the hand to pull the foot in toward the hip, while pushing the foot into the hand to create a stretch.
- If looking up is too intense for the neck or jaw, look down.

refinement
Learn to come into and out of each pose with precision and control, especially arm balances or difficult balancing poses like *vasisthasana*. It is common to fall out of these types of poses due to the demands of the pose, but coming out of a pose step by step just as you do when entering a pose can offer you a great deal in terms of strength and alignment. *Vasisthasana* is an excellent

preparatory pose for *camatkarasana* and *urdhva dhanurasana*. It also works well in sequence with *utthita hasta padangustasana 2* and *anantasana*.

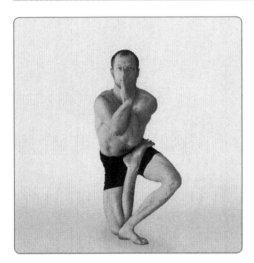

vatayanasana
mythical horse pose

shape
(from *dandasana*)

1. Bring the right palm to the inner right knee.
2. Pull the knee as far right and back as possible so that the legs come into an obtuse angle—outer leg and knee to floor.
3. With the hands, lift the right foot and place the outer right foot on the upper inner left thigh at the crease of the groin. Point the right knee forward and lower the leg.
4. Keep the right knee on the floor and place the left heel just in front of the left sit bone—knee pointing up. Turn the left foot out 60 degrees.
5. Place both hands next to the hips. Push the hands down and lift the hips up and back.
6. Place the right knee on the floor next to the left heel.
7. Bring the left hand to the left knee. Lift the torso upright and balance.
8. Bring the arms into *garudasana* arms: Swing the right elbow under the left elbow, cross and wrap the left wrist around the right wrist, and press the palms together—thumbs toward the face. Look forward. Hold the pose and breathe.
9. To come out, release the arms to the floor, lower the hips and straighten the legs.

Repeat on the second side—switch the cross of the arms and legs.

safety
- If the leg does not fold into *ardha padmasana* or if the knee hovers above the floor in *ardha padmasana*, do not attempt this pose.
- To reduce the intensity of the pose and the difficulty of the balance, move the standing foot out 12 inches away from the lower knee.
- If there is pain or discomfort in the top ankle or to reduce the difficulty of the balance, lower the top knee to the floor and point the foot back.
- If necessary, bring one or both hands to a wall for balance.
- Clamp both knees.

- Flex the top foot and spread the toes. Push the thigh into the top of the foot and the foot into the thigh.
- Press the tailbone down, tone the low belly, and lift the pelvic floor.
- If there is pain or discomfort in the shoulders or wrists, or if the hand position is not accessible, swing the elbow under the other elbow and press the backs of the hands and arms together.

refinement

Garudasana, ardha matsyendrasana 2, and paripurna matsyendrasana are good preparatory poses for *vatayanasana*. Practice *vatayanasana* with caution because the *ardha padmasana* leg bears weight in the knee. As you enter into the realm of advanced asana it is essential that you contemplate your aim. When looking at some of the more advanced poses, ask yourself, "Why do I want to do this?" Contemplate the potential risk and reward. A key teaching in this practice is that you must make a profit. In other words, you must get more than you give. When that happens, you will have more to give, so don't worry, it is a selfless not selfish teaching. In my experience this practice is very powerful; it is both generous and generative.

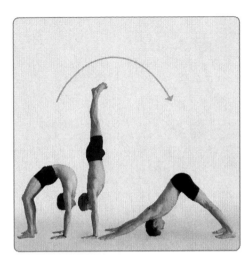

viparita chakrasana from urdhva dhanurasana
reverse wheel pose from upward-facing bow pose (tick tock)

shape
(from *urdhva dhanurasana 1*)

1. Rock the chest and hips back and forth.
2. Transfer the full weight of the body onto the hands. Exhale, kick the legs up and over.
3. As the feet touch the floor, immediately bend the knees and transfer the weight of the body onto the feet.
4. Bend the knees and jump up and over into *urdhva dhanurasana 1*. Land as softly on the feet as possible.

safety

*   Press the fingertips and the perimeter of the palms down with equal pressure.
*   Just before the feet leave the floor, press the fingertips down, extend the shoulders back toward the legs, and squeeze the elbows in.
*   Strengthen the legs.
*   Lift the pelvic floor and tone the low belly.
*   Keep the head back as the hips move up and over into *adho mukha svanasana*.

refinement

They say that *timing is everything*, and in the case of *viparita chakrasana*, that is definitely the case. The window of opportunity to jump from *urdhva dhanurasana 1* into *adho mukha svanasana* is a split second. More often than not, practitioners attempt to jump too soon. Do not jump until your arms and chest are vertical to the floor. Once you can practice this pose with ease, do 5 to 15 sets in a row. Advanced practitioners can jump up and over from *urdhva dhanurasana* into *eka pada koundinyasana 2* in one fluid movement.

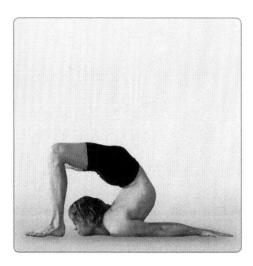

viparita salabhasana
inverted locust pose

shape
(from *viparita salabhasana prep*, legs vertical)

1. Inhale fully. Exhale, bend the knees and lower the feet to the floor in front of the head—feet outer hip-width apart.
2. Look past the feet. Hold the pose and breathe.
3. To come out, inhale, lift the heels and kick the legs up to vertical position. Lower the legs and release the hands.

safety

- Press the fingertips and the perimeter of the palms into the floor with equal pressure.
- Press the shoulders down and forward.
- Extend the inner thighs and the inner edges of the feet down.
- Engage the glutes and lift the tailbone. Draw the low belly in.
- Stretch the knees away from the hips.
- Flare the outer two toes.
- Move the base of the sternum back. Do not overly stretch or strain any part of the spine.

refinement

It is possible to practice this pose against a wall and walk the feet and knees down the wall until the feet can eventually lower to the floor. In order to get your feet to the floor, it is necessary to lift the front of the ribs into nearly a vertical position. If your ribs remain on the floor your low back will be forced to over-bend.

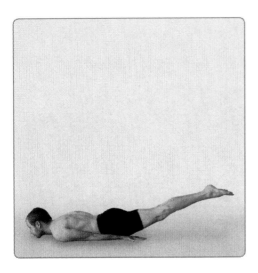

viparita salabhasana prep
inverted locust pose

shape

1. Bring the front body and chin to the floor.
2. Extend the arms alongside the body with the palms facing down.
3. Move the knees forward slightly, lift the hips, and bring the outer edges of the hands together underneath the legs.
4. Slide the elbows underneath the torso.
5. Lower the hips onto the arms, straighten the legs, and bring the inner edges of the feet together.
6. Inhale, lift the legs to capacity. Look forward. Hold the pose and breathe.
7. To come out, exhale, lower the legs. Lift the hips to release the hands.

safety

- Press the fingertips and the perimeter of the palms into the floor with equal pressure.
- Press the inner edges of the feet and heels together.
- Press the tailbone and hips down. Engage the glutes.
- To reduce pressure on the elbows, point the palms up instead of down.
- If there is pain or discomfort in the neck, place the forehead on the floor and look down.
- If there is pain or discomfort at the front of the shoulders, widen the hands.

refinement

Press your hands down and forward—toward your head—to lift your feet. Extend out through your inner feet and initiate lifting the legs from the inner thighs. *Viparita salabhasana prep* is a good preparatory pose for *mayurasana* and *hamsasana*.

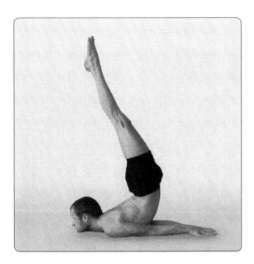

viparita salabhasana prep
inverted locust pose

legs vertical

shape

1. Bring the front body and chin onto the floor.
2. Extend the arms alongside the body—palms facing down.
3. Lift the hips and one at a time, bring the outer edges of the hands together underneath the legs. Move the elbows as close together as possible.
4. Lower the hips, straighten the legs, and bring the inner edges of the feet together.
5. Press the arms and hands down and inhale, lift the legs up. Bring the heels directly over the head.
6. Look forward. Hold the pose and breathe.
7. To come out, exhale, lower the legs and release the hands.

safety

- Press the fingertips and the perimeter of the palms into the floor with equal pressure.
- Press the inner edges of the feet together. Move the inner thighs back.
- Engage the glutes and move the tailbone in.
- Strengthen the legs and stretch them up to capacity.
- Press the shoulders down and forward.
- Breathe as evenly as possible.

refinement

To make this pose more accessible, place a shoulderstand pad or folded blankets under the arms, shoulders, and chest. Be sure the neck and chin are in front of (and off) the props. Like in shoulderstand, these props will take a great deal of pressure off the neck.

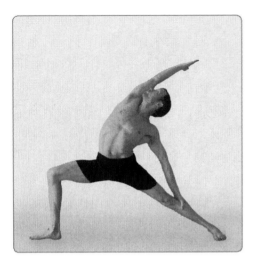

viparita virabhadrasana
reverse warrior pose

shape
(from *virabhadrasana 2*)

1. Place the left hand on the outer left leg above or below the knee.
2. Inhale, lift the right arm vertical, palm facing back. Exhale, lean the torso and right arm back.
3. Straighten both arms, point the right bicep back.
4. Lift the chin and look up. Hold the pose and breathe.
5. To come out, inhale, lift the torso vertical, arms parallel.

Repeat on the second side.

safety

- Bring the front knee directly over the front heel.
- Tilt the front shin out so the shin is perfectly vertical.
- Press the back foot down, lock the back leg into straight position, and engage the back glutes.
- Move the tailbone down and draw the low belly in.
- Bring the left shoulder blade down the back away from the ear.
- Move the base of the sternum back.
- Avoid overstretching or compressing either side of the torso.

refinement

The tendency in the pose is to distort the hips. Square your hips to the long edge of the mat. Reach your front sit bone toward your front knee. Extend your left hand down and your top hand up. Extend your head away from your hips. Stretch your entire spine.

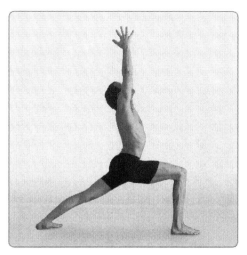 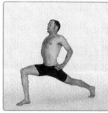 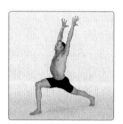

virabhadrasana 1
warrior pose 1

shape
(from *tadasana,* facing long edge of mat)

1. Lift the arms vertical—elbows directly above shoulders.
2. Press the palms together.
3. Inhale, bend the knees.
4. Exhale, take a wide stance shorter than *trikonasana.*
5. Turn the left foot in 60 degrees, right foot out 90 degrees. Pivot the hips to face the same direction as the front foot—right hip back, left hip forward.
6. Inhale fully.
7. Exhale, bend the right knee directly above the heel—right thigh parallel to floor.
8. Look up past the thumbs. Hold the pose and breathe.
9. To come out, inhale, straighten the front leg. Exhale, parallel the feet. Bring the feet together and lower the arms.

Repeat on the second side.

safety
- If the front knee moves beyond the front heel, lengthen the stance via the back foot until the front shin is perfectly vertical.
- Press the back foot down and engage the left glutes.
- Lock the back knee into a straight position.
- Press the tailbone down and draw low belly in.
- Move the base of the sternum back and lift the chest.
- If the hips open out to the side and do not square to the front of the mat, lift the back heel vertical.
- If the shoulders are tight, separate the hands shoulder-width apart.
- If looking up is too intense for the neck, look straight ahead.

refinement
To gain more power, interlace your fingers and release your thumbs and index fingers. Or, simply interlock your thumbs with your hands in *anjali mudra.* Tighten your back knee and elbows, then stretch them away from your hips. Stretch your entire spine. *Virabhadrasana 1* is often taught

from lunge pose. In my experience, the alignment of the pose is more accessible when entered from *tadasana*. It puts less strain on the front hip flexors and evenly stretches the back hip flexors. It is also easier to establish and keep strength in the torso as you approach the backbending aspect of this pose.

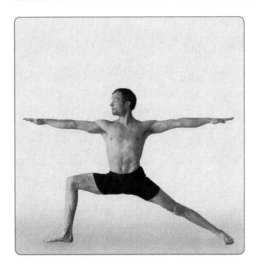

virabhadrasana 2
warrior pose 2

shape
(from *tadasana*, facing long edge of mat)

1. Inhale, bend the knees.
2. Exhale, take a wide stance.
3. Lift the arms parallel to the floor.
4. Point the palms and biceps up. Keeping the biceps pointing up, point the palms down.
5. Turn the back foot in 30 degrees, the front foot out 90 degrees.
6. Inhale, look past the right hand.
7. Exhale, bend the front knee above the heel—shin vertical, thigh parallel to the floor and the outer edge of mat. Hold the pose and breathe.
8. To come out, inhale, straighten the front leg. Exhale, parallel the feet. Bring the feet together and lower the arms.

Repeat on the second side.

safety
- The front knee must be above front heel—knee beyond heel is not a stable position.
- If the right hip is higher than the right knee, lengthen the stance via the back foot until the thigh is parallel to the floor.
- The front shin must be straight up and down—the knee tends to tilt in.
- Press the back foot down, lock the back leg into a straight position, and engage the back glutes.
- Move the tailbone down and draw the low belly in.
- Move the base of the sternum back and lift the chest.

refinement

Center your torso over your hips—the torso tends to lean forward over the bent leg. Square your hips to the long edge of the mat. Push the outer edge of your back foot down and move your right hip back. Reach your right sit bone toward your front knee. Extend your hands out.

In this pose, the back arm can represent the past, the front arm the future, and the torso the present moment. Yoga offers perspectives that can turn the past—no matter how difficult—into potential, the future into fortunate, and the present moment into momentum. Such perspective is a precious resource.

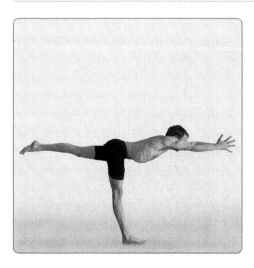

virabhadrasana 3
warrior pose 3

shape
(from *tadasana*)

1. Inhale, lift the arms overhead—elbows directly above the shoulders.
2. Press the palms together. Squeeze the elbows straight.
3. Exhale, lean forward. Step the left foot back and point the foot. Rest the tips of the toes on the floor behind you.
4. Square the hips—left hip forward, right hip back.
5. Inhale fully. Exhale, bring the arms, torso, and back leg parallel to the floor. Lift the back foot and hands slightly higher than the shoulders and hips.
6. Look straight ahead. Hold the pose and breathe.
7. To come out, exhale, lift the torso to stand. Release the arms by the sides.

Repeat on the second side.

safety

- Engage the legs and lock them into a straight position.
- Lift the kneecap of the standing leg.
- Engage the glutes of the lifted leg.
- If it is too taxing to square the hips and point the back knee down, allow the kneecap of the top leg to face out slightly.

- Rotate the thigh of the standing leg out until the kneecap faces forward and pull the right hip back (the standing leg tends to turn in).
- Move the tailbone down and draw the low belly in.
- To reduce the intensity in the hamstrings of the standing leg, bend the knee slightly.
- To reduce the stretch in the shoulders, separate the hands shoulder-width apart. Point the palms in.
- To reduce the intensity in the lower back, bring the arms back along the sides of the torso. Point the palms in.

refinement

To gain more strength and stretch in your shoulders, interlace your fingers and release your thumbs and index fingers, or overlap your thumbs. Extend your hands and feet away from your hips. Be soft, yet determined in your eyes. This pithy posture leaves no room for kind of/sort of. In a well-known yoga text called *Bhagavad Gita*, it says, "On this path no effort is wasted, no gain is ever reversed; even a little of this practice will shelter you from great sorrow."[1] What is wasted, however, is the effort you did not make. And what cannot be given to you is that which you have not gained.

---

[1]   Stephen Mitchell, *Bhagavad Gita: A New Translation* (New York: Three Rivers Press, 2002), 2.40.

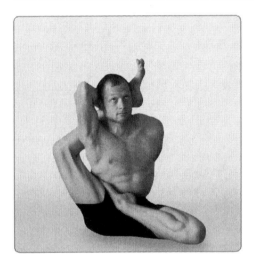

viranchyasana 1
Sage Viranchi's pose 1

shape
(from *dandasana*)

1. Bring the left leg into *ardha padmasana*.
2. Bend the right knee and place the right foot just in front of the left shin. Lift the foot and hold the foot with the left hand.
3. Lean back to bring both thighs vertical to the floor—point the knees up.
4. Bring the right arm to the inside of the right leg and hold the calf with the hand.
5. Round the back and bring the right shoulder under the right knee.
6. Place the right hand on the floor outside of the right hip.

7. Use the left hand to lift the right foot up and over the head. Use the right shoulder to move the right shin back.
8. Turn the head to the left and place the right shin on the back of the neck. Turn the head to look forward.
9. Slowly lower the *ardha padmasana* knee to the floor.
10. Swing the left arm behind the back and place the left hand high up on the back.
11. Lift the right arm vertical, bend the elbow, and reach for the left hand. Clasp the hands behind the back. Look between the eyebrows. Hold the pose and breathe.
12. To come out, exhale, release the hands next to the hips. Release the top leg from behind the head and straighten both legs.

Repeat on the second side.

safety

- Engage both feet, especially the top foot.
- Isometrically bend the top knee to engage the hamstrings.
- Flare the outer two toes of the top foot.
- Press the shoulder and neck into the top ankle.
- For the leg in *ardha padmasana*, press the top of the foot into the thigh and the outer edge of the foot down.
- Squeeze the bottom knee.
- If the leg in *ardha padmasana* does not lower to the floor, place a blanket underneath the knee.
- Lift the pelvic floor and tone the low belly.

refinement

It is a daunting task just to attempt to get into and out of these asanas. It is amazing that there was a time when these forms did not yet exist. They were just pure potential, pure possibility. Potential and possibility only have power when realized. You may have the potential to do a certain pose, but until you do it, that potential is of no use. Some say that many of these poses were the spontaneous results of yogins in deep meditation and that as the *kundalini* awakened, or to awaken the *kundalini*, yogins would spontaneously move into these forms. Others say these were simply exercises to prepare the body for meditation, or to make the body strong enough to withstand the awakening of *kundalini*. Although I cannot personally speak to the realm of *kundalini*, I can say that when I shape-shift, I definitely experience a positive state-shift. I've always had a particular adoration of *viranchyasana 1*.

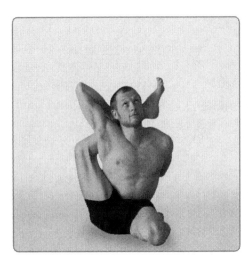

viranchyasana 2
Sage Viranchi's pose 2

shape
(from *dandasana*)

1. Bend the left knee and place the inner ankle against the outer hip. Lower the leg to the floor and point the foot back.
2. Lean to the right and pull the left glutes back with the right hand.
3. Bend the right knee out to the side.
4. Bring the right arm to the inside of the leg and hold the back of the calf with the hand.
5. Round the back and bring the right shoulder underneath the right knee.
6. Place the right hand on the floor outside of the right hip.
7. Use the left hand to lift the right foot up and over the head. Use the right shoulder to move the right shin back.
8. Turn the head to the left and slide the right shin over the head and onto the back of the neck. Turn the head and look straight ahead.
9. Swing the left arm behind the back and place the left hand as high up on the back as possible.
10. Inhale, lift the right arm vertical, bend the elbow, and reach for the left hand. Clasp the hands.
11. Look between the eyebrows. Hold the pose and breathe.
12. To come out, inhale, lift the right arm vertical. Exhale, make a fist with the left hand. Push the back of the hand into the back and slide the fist down the back and to the side. Release the fist. Release the top leg and straighten both legs.

Repeat on the second side.

safety
- Engage both feet, especially the top foot.
- Isometrically bend the top knee to engage the hamstrings.
- Flare the outer two toes of the top foot.
- Press the shoulder and neck into the top ankle.
- For the leg in *virasana*, point the toes straight back, press the inner heel against the outer hip, and point the knee straight ahead.
- If the hands cannot clasp behind the back, use a strap.
- Lift the pelvic floor and tone the low belly.

refinement

When I look at photos of myself performing these yoga poses, I can see where I lacked awareness. In *viranchyasana 1*, I would move my top elbow back directly above the shoulder instead of slightly forward. In *viranchyasana 2*, I would move my top elbow in so that my upper arm was vertical. I would also rotate my abdomen up and to the right slightly, so on and so forth. Despite these seemingly imperfections, this is actually what I love about the practice: There is no way to get it picture perfect. As Richard Freeman once said, "There are no ends to these postures. As soon as you think you've got it, you've lost it."[1]

1   Richard Freeman, "Yoga Primary Series," (Boulder, CO: Sounds True, 2004), DVD.

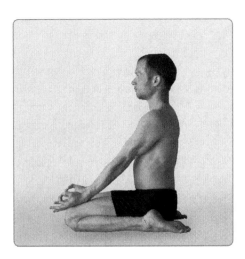

virasana
hero pose

shape
(from *bharmanasana*)

1. Bring the knees together and separate the inner edges of the feet outer hip-width apart. Press the tops of the feet into the floor.
2. Lower the hips halfway to the feet and bring the top of the head to the floor. Place the palms on the center of each calf directly behind the knee—fingers pointing forward.
3. Press the calf muscles down and back, as the hips lower to the floor between the feet.
4. Inhale, lift the torso to a vertical position.
5. Place the backs of the hands on the knees. Look forward. Hold the pose and breathe.
6. To come out, release the hands to the floor shoulder-width apart. Walk the hands forward to come onto the hands and knees—shoulders over wrists, hips over knees. Separate the knees and feet hip-width apart.

safety
- If there is pain or discomfort in the knees, separate the knees and/or place a folded blanket under the sit bones, between the feet. Sit on the edge of the blanket with most of the blanket behind the back and keep the feet on the floor/mat.
- To reduce the intensity in the ankles, place a rolled-up blanket underneath the tops of the feet/lower shins. Over time, work toward removing the blankets.
- Clamp the knees closed to engage the hamstrings.
- Keep the thighs parallel and point the toes straight back.
- Squeeze the heels in until they are vertical.
- Lift the pelvic floor and tone the low belly.

refinement
Pull the skin under your knees forward and up. Pull the skin underneath your feet out and up. Pull the flesh under your sit bones back. All of these actions will create space in the body to bring the sit bones comfortably to the floor or blankets. If the pose is uncomfortable in your knees, use props to protect your knees from injury. The point of props is to meet you where you are to take you further into a given pose. Props can offer temporary support, like training wheels on a bicycle, and at the same time, do not indicate inferiority or handicap. *Virasana* can teach us that being a hero does not mean withstanding pain for no gain.

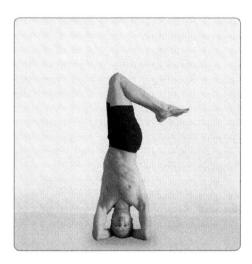

virasana in parsva sirsasana
hero in turned headstand pose

shape
(from *sirsasana 1*)

1. Inhale fully. Exhale, bend the knees and bring the heels toward/to the sit bones. Turn the hips to the left. Hold for 30 to 60 seconds.
2. Inhale, return to center.
3. Exhale, turn the hips to the right. Hold for 30 to 60 seconds.
4. Inhale, return to center. Straighten the legs.

safety
- Press the forearms and wrists down. Lift the shoulders up.
- Extend down through the head.
- One shoulder tends to push forward and the other back in order to achieve the twist. Keep the shoulders squared and facing forward.
- Press the inner feet, ankles, and knees together.
- Extend the thighs up and back.
- Engage the abdomen, and move the base of the sternum back and tailbone forward.
- Keep the hips and knees directly above the head.
- Breathe evenly. Relax the eyes and jaw.
- If the balance is difficult, practice against or near a wall.

refinement
Virasana in *parsva sirsasana* is a good preparatory pose for headstand drop over and *vrischikasana 1*. Bending the knees in *virasana* while inverted often causes the spine and torso to collapse. The above safety instructions ensure that you resist the tendency to backbend, which becomes all the more difficult when twisting. Such resistance is essential when performing poses such as headstand drop over and *vrischikasana 1*.

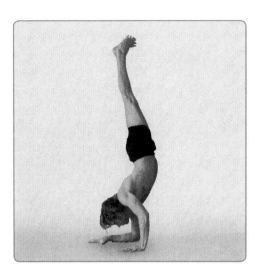

visama pincha mayurasana
uneven peacock feather pose

shape
(from *pincha mayurasana*)

1. Transfer most of the body weight onto the right forearm.
2. In one quick movement, lift the left forearm and place the hand shoulder-width apart from the right elbow. Look forward. Hold the pose and breathe.
3. To come out, lower the legs and release the hands.

Repeat on the second side.

safety

- Engage the feet—flare the toes.
- Press the inner edges of the feet and the legs together.
- Engage the glutes and abdomen.
- Press the tailbone in.

refinement

It is easier to first place the hands and then kick up into this pose. One of my favorite quotes from F. Scott Fitzgerald's novel *Tender is the Night* is, "[She] was the product of much ingenuity and toil."[1] To make a pose like *visama pincha mayurasana* easier takes away what it both requires and offers: ingenuity and toil. It may be helpful to keep this yoga motto in mind: falling apart is part of the pose!

---

[1]   F. Scott Fitzgerald, *Tender is the Night* (New York: Charles Scribner's Sons, 1996).

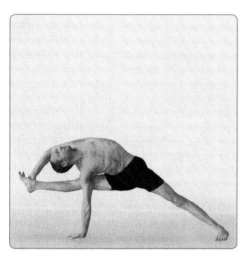
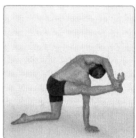

visvamitrasana
Sage Visvamitra's pose

shape
(from *lunge pose*)

1. With the right foot forward, pivot the back heel down. Point the toes straight out.
2. Place the right arm to the inside of the right leg and lower the torso to the same height as the right thigh.
3. Press the right thumb into the center of the right calf.
4. Move the calf to the left and bring the right shoulder underneath the right knee.
5. Place the right hand on the floor outside of the front foot. Place the left hand on the floor inside the front foot.
6. Straighten the arms and lean the weight of the body onto the right hand and foot.
7. Lift the right foot off the floor. Hold the outer edge of the right foot with the left hand.
8. Press the right shoulder and knee together and straighten the right leg parallel to the floor.
9. Tone the abdomen and twist the torso up.
10. Look up. Hold the pose and breathe.
11. To come out, look down. Bend the right knee, lower the top hand and foot to the floor. Release the right arm and place the hand on the floor outside of the right leg. Lift the back heel.

Repeat on the second side.

safety

- If the hamstrings are tight, do not attempt to straighten the top leg completely. Keeping the knee bent, use the hand to pull the foot in toward the hip, while pushing the foot into the hand to create a stretch.
- Separate the fingers of the bottom hand. Point the index finger and biceps straight ahead.
- Press the fingertips and the perimeter of the right hand evenly into the floor—press the mound of the index finger down and lift the outer wrist up.
- Before straightening the top leg, press the knee and shoulder into each other. Engage the hamstrings.
- Pull the foot with the hand and push the foot into the hand.
- Press the back foot down. Lift the back thigh up.

refinement

This is among my favorite poses to practice. Even so, I only teach it during advanced intensives because there are so many potential risks involved. To reduce the risk of injury to the shoulder and hamstrings, bring your left knee to the floor with your left thigh vertical. Bend the knee to a 90-degree angle. Press your right foot into a wall. Place your right hand on a block if necessary. Extend your left arm forward, across your face like in *parsvakonasana*.

Consider viewing hatha yoga as a sport instead of as a remedy for injury and health issues. In that context, when injury occurs in your practice it simply goes with the territory. The aim of hatha yoga is certainly not to injure you. Nor is that the aim of any sport. However, in both sports and yoga, injury does occur. In my view that is not necessarily a problem. As Lee Lozowick says, "Don't make a problem out of what is not a problem." In most, if not all sports, there is an opponent. In yoga, the opponent might be misalignment, weakness, injury, imbalance, etc. Some days the yoga wins. Some days the misalignment wins. If you practice poses as difficult as *visvamitrasana* and beyond, you must be aware of the possibility of injury.

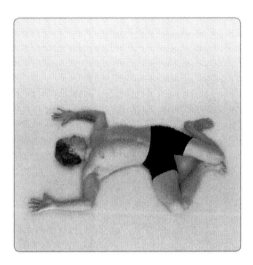

visvavajrasana
double diamond pose

shape
(from *supta tadasana*)

1. Bend the elbows to a 90-degree angle—fingers and palms pointing up.
2. Bend the knees and place the feet on the floor in front of the sit bones.
3. Separate the feet outer hip-width apart.
4. Move the hips 4 to 6 inches to the left.
5. Without moving the feet, exhale, lower the knees to the right—left knee to arch of right foot.
6. Turn the head to the left and look past the shoulder. Hold the pose and breathe.
7. To come out, inhale, look forward and lift the knees vertical. Exhale, straighten the arms and legs.

Repeat on the second side.

safety

· If necessary, engage the feet and isometrically squeeze the feet toward the hips.
  If there is no discomfort in the knees, simply relax.

refinement

To deepen the stretch, place your right foot on top of your left knee and press your knee down. From your outer hip, extend out through your top knee. This pose is inherently calming. It is like dimming bright lights for the nervous system. Become heavy and soft, and soak up the relaxation—a precious, and all too often scarce, resource in our lives. Due to the relaxing nature of *visvavajrasana*, it is useful to perform it toward the end of practice.

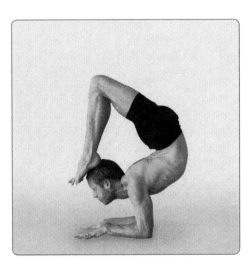

vrischikasana 1
scorpion pose 1

shape
(from *pincha mayurasana*)

1. Bend the knees and separate the knees outer hip-width apart. Bring the inner edges of the feet together.
2. Move the chest down and forward, lift the chin, and curl the head back.
3. Inhale fully. Exhale, lower the soles of the feet to the top of the head.
4. Look straight ahead. Hold the pose and breathe.
5. To come out, inhale, lift the legs vertical.

safety
- Keep the forearms parallel and the upper arms vertical.
- Press the inner wrists into the floor.
- Press the inner edges of the feet together and flare the outer two toes.
- Extend the inner thighs down. Press the inner edges of the feet down.
- Press the tailbone down, engage the glutes, and lift the low belly. Tone the pelvic floor.
- Move the base of the sternum back and stretch the spine and chest up.
- Extend the knees away from the hips.
- Breathe as evenly as possible.
- If the feet cannot reach the head, practice against a wall and walk the feet, and eventually the knees, down the wall.

refinement
Students often widen their knees in order to touch their head with their feet. Do just the opposite. Bring your knees outer hip-width apart or even slightly narrower than your hips. Although this may cause your feet to move further from your head, it will benefit your spine and sacrum. Make the goal of getting your feet to your head in *vrischikasana 1* a guide without destination.

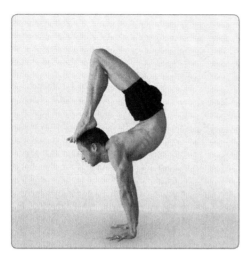
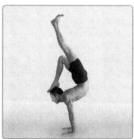

vrischikasana 2
scorpion pose 2

shape
(from *adho mukha vrksasana*)

1. Bend the knees and separate the knees outer hip-width apart. Bring the inner edges of the feet together.
2. Move the chest down and forward until the sternum is level to the floor.
3. Inhale, lift the chin and curl the head back. Exhale, lower the soles of the feet to the head.
4. Look straight ahead. Hold the pose and breathe.
5. To come out, inhale, lift the legs vertical.

safety

- Press the tips of the fingers and perimeter of the palms down with equal pressure.
- Lock the elbows into a straight position.
- Press the inner edges of the feet together and flare the outer two toes.
- Extend the inner thighs down. Press the inner edges of the feet down.
- Press the tailbone down, engage the glutes, and lift the low belly. Tone the pelvic floor.
- Move the chest down and forward. Extend the head and knees up.
- Move the base of the sternum back and stretch the spine and chest up.
- Bend deeply and evenly in the entire spine.

refinement

I recommend that you not even attempt this pose until you can balance in *adho mukha vrksasana* in the middle of the room for 60 seconds.

Advanced practitioners can bend the elbows and lower the chest to hover just above the floor. After a few breaths, come into *chaturanga dandasana*. Another variation of this pose is *eka pada vrischikasana 2*. From *vrischikasana 2*, lift your left foot up and straighten your leg. Hold for a few breaths and then switch legs. Advanced practitioners can bend the knee and cross the ankle just above the knee of the opposite leg.

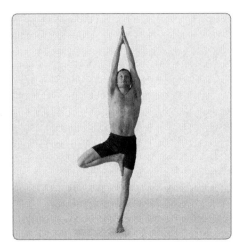
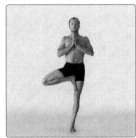

vrksasana
tree pose

shape
(from *tadasana*)

1. Place the left hand on the left hip.
2. Lift the right knee and hold the ankle with the right hand—arm to the inside of the leg.
3. Point the knee out to the side and lift the knee higher than the hips.
4. Place the sole of the right foot against the left inner thigh—toes pointing down.
5. Bring the palms together at the middle of the sternum. Inhale, lift the arms overhead—elbows directly above shoulders.
6. Press the palms together and squeeze the elbows straight.
7. Lift the chin slightly and look straight ahead. Hold the pose and breathe.
8. To come out, exhale, release the hands and lower the leg.

Repeat on the second side.

safety
- Avoid placing the foot against the knee.
- Engage the thigh of the standing leg—lift the kneecap.
- Press the foot into the thigh—make the thigh, like the trunk of a tree, circumferentially strong.
- Engage the glutes of the standing leg.
- Move the hip of the standing leg down and forward.
- Move the base of the sternum back and lift the chest.
- Move the tailbone down and draw the low belly in.
- If it is difficult to balance, lower the hands to the middle of the sternum in *anjali mudra*, or place one hand on a wall.

refinement
To gain more strength and stretch in your shoulders, interlace your fingers and release your thumbs and index fingers. Or overlap your thumbs. Stretch your hands up to fully strengthen, stretch, and remove stress from your shoulders. To enhance your balance, focus your gaze on a single point on the floor. Your body may sway and waiver, but if you keep your focus steady, you may be able to balance from beginning to end. To challenge your balance, close your eyes. Symbolically think of your body as the tree and your focus as the roots that hold the tree steady, even as it sways. *Vrksasana* is one of the safest and most effective poses for developing balance and poise.

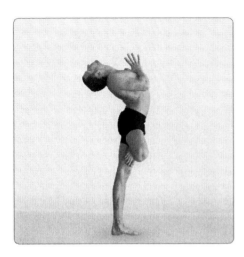

vrksasana
tree pose

hands in anjali mudra, backbend

shape
(from *vrksasana*)

1. Bring the palms together at the middle of the sternum.
2. Inhale fully. Exhale, lift the chest and curl back. Repeat as necessary to backbend in the upper back.
3. Look up or even back. Hold the pose and breathe.
4. To come out, inhale, lift the head and chest. Exhale, release the leg and bring the arms by the sides.

Repeat on the second side.

safety

- Strengthen the standing leg—lift the kneecap.
- Move the tailbone down and draw the low belly in.
- Shrug the shoulders up and back.
- Slide the sides of the throat back and lift the chin to bring the head back.

refinement

Lift your chest into your hands and fully stretch your spine. Move your hips forward to come into a deeper backbend. This variation of *vrksasana* will challenge and enhance your balance.

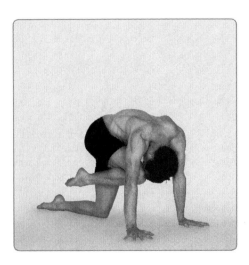

vyaghrasana
tiger pose

forehead to knee

shape
(from *bharmanasana*)

1. Inhale fully. Exhale, round the back, and bring the chin to the chest and right knee to the forehead.
2. Lift the back heel—right shin parallel to the floor.
3. Look toward the base of the sternum. Hold the pose and breathe.
4. To come out, inhale, look forward. Exhale, release the right knee to the floor in line with the left knee. Bring the spine to a neutral position.

Repeat on the second side.

safety
*   Press the fingertips and the roots of the index fingers down.
*   Move the tailbone down and forward. Lift the low belly and pelvic floor.
*   Lift the base of the sternum up.
*   Point the lifted foot and clamp the knee closed to stabilize the knee and engage the hamstrings. Engaging the hamstrings will empower the abdomen and make this movement less intense on the hip flexors.
*   If there is discomfort in the knees, place a blanket underneath the knees for additional padding.

refinement
Ideally *vyaghrasana* will strengthen your hip flexors and abdomen. If, however, your hip flexors are strained, this pose may not be a good choice for you. Keep your shoulders over your wrists and touch your knee to your forehead. The tendency for many practitioners is to bring the knee close to the forehead, but not exert the effort required to complete the movement by bringing the knee and forehead together. Practice coming into and out of *vyaghrasana* with your breath. Inhale, lift your leg parallel to the floor. Exhale, round your back into *vyaghrasana*. Continue like this for several breaths and repeat on the second side.

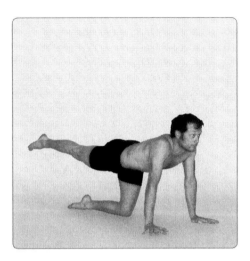

vyaghrasana
tiger pose

shape

1. Come onto the hands and knees with the arms and thighs vertical—shoulders directly over the wrists, hips directly over the knees.
2. Separate the hands slightly wider than shoulder-distance apart. Straighten the arms.
3. Separate the knees and feet outer hip-width apart.
4. Bring the tops of the feet onto the floor. Point the toes straight back and squeeze the ankles in until the heels are vertical.
5. Inhale, lift the chin and the right leg parallel to the floor. Point the foot and look straight ahead. Hold the pose and breathe.
6. To come out, exhale, lower the lifted leg and place the knee directly below the hips.

Repeat on the second side.

safety

- Separate the fingers and point the index fingers forward. Press the entire perimeter of the palms down, especially the mounds of the index fingers.
- Lock the elbows and lifted knee into a straight position.
- Press the lower knee, shin, and the top of the foot down.
- Engage the glutes of the lifted leg.
- Point the lifted kneecap down.
- Press the tailbone down and lift the low belly.
- Move the base of the sternum up and extend the chest forward. Stretch the entire spine.

refinement

Isometrically press your hands down and back to stretch your chest up and forward. The hip of the lifted leg tends to drop lower than the hip of the bent knee. Lower your lifted leg slightly until it is truly parallel to the floor, level your hips, and engage your core to stabilize your pelvis. From the pelvis, extend back through your lifted leg and foot. Spread your toes. *Vyaghrasana* is a great way to warm up the arms, low back, and hamstrings. It works well in a *surya namaskar* sequence.

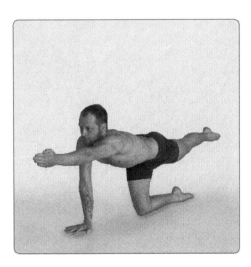

vyaghrasana
tiger pose

same leg and arm

shape

1. Come onto the hands and knees with the arms and thighs vertical—shoulders directly over the wrists, hips directly over the knees.
2. Separate the hands slightly wider than shoulder-distance apart. Straighten the arms.
3. Separate the knees and feet outer hip-width apart.
4. Bring the tops of the feet onto the floor. Point the toes straight back and squeeze the ankles in until the heels are vertical.
5. Inhale, lift the chin and the left leg parallel to the floor. Point the foot and look straight ahead.
6. Transfer the weight onto the right hand and knee.
7. Inhale, lift the left arm forward—arm parallel to the floor. Point the palm in. Hold the pose and breathe.
8. To come out, exhale, lower the lifted arm and leg.

Repeat on the second side.

safety

- Separate the fingers of the bottom hand and point the index finger forward. Press the entire perimeter of the palm down, especially the mound of the index finger.
- Lock the elbows and lifted knee into a straight position.
- Press the lower knee, shin, and the top of the foot down.
- Engage the glutes of the lifted leg.
- Point the lifted kneecap down.
- Press the tailbone down and lift the low belly.
- Move the base of the sternum up and extend the chest forward. Stretch the entire spine.
- Extend the back foot and front hand away from the hips.

refinement

I was a wrestler in high school and noticed that unlike many of their opponents, the top wrestlers were comfortable with being slightly off balance. They chose to navigate instead of negate potentially precarious situations, which is often why they won match after match. They ventured outside the box of the normal moves and techniques. They often even invented moves on the spot, which caught their opponents off guard. To explore the endless possibilities of our potential, we must become comfortable with being a little off center.

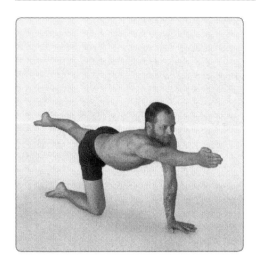

vyaghrasana
tiger pose

opposite leg and arm

shape

1. Come onto the hands and knees with the arms and thighs vertical—shoulders directly over the wrists, hips directly over the knees.
2. Separate the hands slightly wider than shoulder-distance apart. Straighten the arms.
3. Separate the knees and feet outer hip-width apart.
4. Bring the tops of the feet onto the floor. Point the toes straight back and squeeze the ankles in until the heels are vertical.
5. Inhale, lift the chin and the left leg parallel to the floor. Point the toes straight down.
6. Transfer the weight onto the left hand and lift the right arm forward, parallel to the floor. Point the palm in.
7. Look forward. Hold the pose and breathe.
8. To come out, exhale, lower the lifted arm and leg.

Repeat on the second side.

safety

- Separate the fingers of the bottom hand and point the index finger forward. Press the entire perimeter of the palm down, especially the mound of the index finger.
- Lock the elbows and lifted knee into a straight position.
- Press the lower knee, shin, and the top of the foot down.
- Engage the glutes of the lifted leg.

- Point the lifted kneecap down.
- Press the tailbone down and lift the low belly.
- Move the base of the sternum up and extend the chest forward. Stretch the entire spine.
- Lift the shoulder of the lower arm up toward the ear.
- Extend the back foot and front hand away from the hips.

refinement

Vyaghrasana warms up the arms, back, and hamstrings. Perform this pose before or during *surya namaskar*. If you disengage the core, the belly and organs of the abdomen will drop away from the spine, and the lifted arm and leg will likely lift to counterbalance a low center of gravity. Strengthen your core in this light backbend to discover the necessary actions to protect the low back as you progress into deeper backbends.

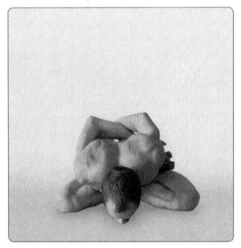 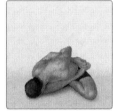 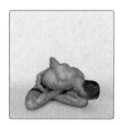

yoga mudrasana
yoga seal pose

shape
(from *padmasana*, right foot on top)

1. Inhale fully. Exhale, swing the right arm behind the back and hold the right big toe with the first two fingers and thumb of the right hand.
2. Lean forward slightly. Exhale, swing the left arm behind the back. Hold the left big toe with the first two fingers and thumb of the left hand.
3. Inhale, lift the torso upright.
4. Exhale, fold the torso forward and place the chin on the floor. Look past the tip of the nose. Hold the pose and breathe.
5. To come out, inhale, lift the head. Release the hands and lift the torso upright.

Repeat on the second side— change the cross of the legs and use the other hand to clasp the top foot first.

safety

- Press the outer edges/tops of the feet down and the heels into the groin.
- Pull the feet back with the hands. Squeeze the knees in.

- Lift the pelvic floor and tone the low belly.
- Lift the shoulders up. Squeeze the elbows in.
- If the hands do not reach the feet behind the back, bring both hands behind the back and use the left hand to pull the right hand to the right big toe. Swing the left arm behind the back. Lean forward over the right knee so the left sit bone lifts. Use the left forearm to slide the right wrist up the back. Rock back and forth to work the left hand to the big toe. Or, use two straps around the tops of the feet.

refinement

Try this: Before folding forward into the pose, exhale, lower your chin to your left knee. Inhale, lift your torso back to center. Exhale, lower your chin to your right knee. Do this five times to each side, then come back to center. Press your tailbone down and low belly in, lift your chest and curl the head back. Look up and hold this for five breaths. Exhale, fold the torso forward. (See variations.)

Need a reason to practice *yoga mudrasana*? In *Light On Yoga,* B. K. S. Iyengar says, "This asana is especially useful in awakening Kundalini."[1] There you go.

1   B. K. S. Iyengar, *Light on Yoga* (New York: Schocken Books, 1977) p. 144.

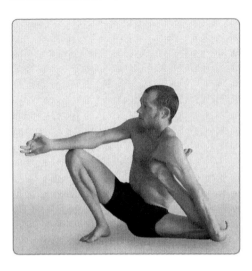

yogadandasana
yoga staff pose

shape
(from *dandasana*)

1. Bend the right knee and place the heel in front of and a couple inches to the right of the sit bone. Turn the foot out 60 degrees and point the knee up.
2. Place the left palm on the inside of the left knee. Pull the knee as far left and back as possible so the heel is near the pubic bone—outer leg and knee on floor.
3. Inhale, lean to the right. Exhale, bring the arch of the left foot to the left armpit. This may take several attempts.
4. With momentum, swing the left hand to the left knee. Lean to the left and lower the left thigh to the floor.
5. Place the right forearm on the right knee. Bring the right thumb and index finger together. Look past the right hand. Hold the pose and breathe.
6. To come out, release the hands and foot. Straighten the legs.

Repeat on the second side.

safety

*   When bringing the foot to the armpit, lift the foot by pushing the back of the upper arm into the foot. Hold the lifted foot with the right hand and reach the left arm forward to bring the armpit toward the foot.
*   Do not reach for the knee with the left hand until the left foot is in the armpit.
*   Engage and flex the lifted foot. Push the foot into the armpit and the armpit into the foot.
*   Isometrically pull the top heel down to engage the hamstrings.
*   Roll the thigh of the lower leg out and allow the right sit bone to lift.
*   Lift the pelvic floor and tone the low belly.

refinement

To burn up the tension in your hips, hold this pose for three minutes on each side. A quest question I used to ask myself often when I practiced: What do I need to do in order to get into this particular shape? And how will getting into this shape shift my physical, mental, emotional, and spiritual state?

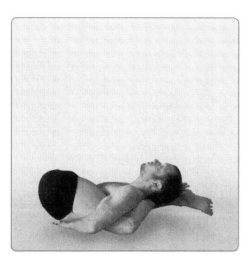

yoganidrasana
yoga sleep pose

shape

1. Lie down on the back.
2. Bend the right knee and place the foot several inches in front of the right sit bone—knee pointing up.
3. Lift the left leg off the floor and bend the knee. Hold the heel with the right hand.
4. Lift the head and torso and place the left knee underneath the left shoulder. Pull the leg as far behind the arm and back as possible.
5. Bring the chin into the chest and place the left ankle behind the head. Lift the head.
6. Lift the right leg off the floor and hold the heel with the left hand. Place the right knee underneath the right shoulder. Pull the leg as far behind the arm and back as possible. Hook the right ankle below the left ankle.
7. Wrap the arms beneath the low back and clasp the hands. Look up. Hold the pose and breathe.
8. To come out, release the hands and bring the chin to the chest. Release the top foot and then the bottom foot. Lower the legs.

Repeat on the second side—switch the cross of the legs.

safety

- If the second foot does not clasp the first foot, practice *eka pada sirsasana* on each side instead.
- Engage the feet. Flex the ankles to keep the feet hooked. Flare the outer two toes of each foot.
- Isometrically bend the knees to engage the hamstrings.
- If the hands cannot clasp beneath the back, use a strap.
- Allow the spine to stretch deeply.
- Lift the pelvic floor and tone the low belly.

refinement

If you are looking forward instead of up, it is likely that your neck is over compensating for tight hips. Make sure both shoulders are in front of your legs in order to create more space for your torso and head. Then press your head back into your legs until you are looking straight up. *Yoganidrasana* puts immense pressure on the diaphragm. Breathe deeply and evenly to evoke a sense of rest and relaxation.

A-Z index

arranged alphabetically by Sanskrit name

Sanskrit name
english translation
variant (if applicable)
visual index categories
page number

A-Z index

A

adho mukha svanasana
downward-facing dog pose
forward folds
36

adho mukha vrksasana
downward-facing tree pose / handstand pose
arm balances, inversions
37

agnistambhasana
firelog pose
forward folds, seated
38

akarna dhanurasana 1
archer's pose 1
forward folds, seated, core
40

akarna dhanurasana 2
archer's pose 2
forward folds, seated, core
41

anantasana
endless pose
core
42

anjaneyasana
monkey lunge pose
standing, backbends
44

ardha baddha padma paschimottanasana
half bound lotus back stretched out pose
forward folds, seated
45

ardha baddha padmottanasana
half bound lotus stretched out pose
standing, forward folds
47

ardha chandrachapasana
half moon bow pose
standing, backbends
48

ardha chandrasana
half moon pose
standing
49

ardha matsyendrasana 1
half Lord of the Fishes pose 1
twists, seated
51

ardha matsyendrasana 1
half Lord of the Fishes pose 1
hips on feet, clasping front foot
twists, seated
52

ardha matsyendrasana 1 prep
half Lord of the Fishes pose 1
twists, seated
54

ardha matsyendrasana 2
half Lord of the Fishes pose 2
forward folds, twists, seated
55

ardha matsyendrasana 3
half Lord of the Fishes pose 3
twists, seated
56

ardha mulabandhasana
half root lock pose
seated
58

ardha mulabandhasana
half root lock pose
forward fold
forward folds, seated
59

ardha navasana
half boat pose
forward folds, seated, core
60

ardha padmasana
half lotus pose
standing
standing
61

acknowledgements

Dagda, Creo and Bronwin for your patience; Lee Lozowick for the leverage of lineage; MiLo for your perseverance; Ellen, Gretel and Joanne for being meticulous; Beth and Lynette for being so surya supportive; Beth, Katie, Travis, Courtney, Xóchitl, and Jenai for putting the shape, safety, and refinement instructions to the test; B.K.S. Iyengar for your formidable form; mom and dad for your support; Rachel for being Laksmi; Margaret for keeping me sane; Christina for teaching with me; the yo community for manifesting so much for so many!

– Darren Rhodes

Mucho thanks to Juliana, Jenai, Xóchitl, Dee, Mom, Dad, Ellen, Adam, and Sandra for all your love, wisdom, patience and invaluable support.

– Milo

about Yo Productions

Yo Productions was founded by Darren Rhodes and Michael Longstaff (MiLo) as the publishing arm of YogaOasis studios in Tucson, AZ. We create products to inform, inspire, and uplift your yoga practice.

Since 2006, we have offered an array of yoga educational materials:
the *yogahour* app/audio classes (on CD/mp3/ iPhone app), the *Yoga Resource* Kindle/iBook, and the *Penchant for Practice* poster.
www.shopatyo.com

Facebook
Yo Productions
Darren Rhodes Yoga

Study with Darren Rhodes
Experience Darren's unique & informational teaching in workshops or teacher trainings:
www.yogaoasis.com

Contact MiLo
MiLo specializes in creative multimedia production, photography and design.
www.milostudios.org

Please send all inquiries, comments, complaints and praise to:
info@yo-productions.com

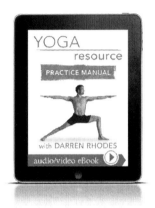
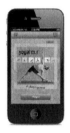
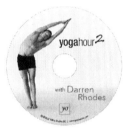
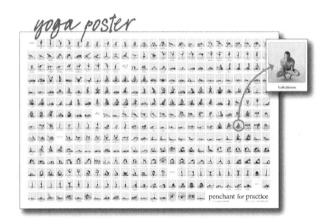
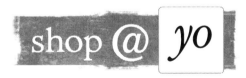

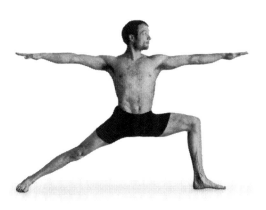

please practice

Made in the USA
Monee, IL
27 January 2020